Rotational Vestibular Assessment

Core Clinical Concepts in Audiology

Series Editor
Brad A. Stach, PhD

Basic Audiometry

Acoustic Immittance Measures
Lisa Hunter, PhD, FAAA, and Navid Shahnaz, PhD, Aud(C)

Speech Audiometry
Gary D. Lawson, PhD, and Mary E. Peterson, AuD

Basic Audiometry Learning Manual
Mark DeRuiter, MBA, PhD, and Virginia Ramachandran, AuD, PhD

Pure-Tone Audiometry and Masking
Maureen Valente, PhD

Electrodiagnostic Audiology

Otoacoustic Emissions: Principles, Procedures, and Protocols
Sumitrajit Dhar, PhD, and James W. Hall III, PhD

Objective Assessment of Hearing
James W. Hall III, PhD, and De Wet Swanepoel, PhD

Cochlear Implants

Programming Cochlear Implants, Second Edition
Jace Wolfe, PhD, and Erin C. Schafer, PhD

Cochlear Implant Patient Assessment: Evaluation of Candidacy, Performance, and Outcomes
René H. Gifford, PhD

Objective Measures in Cochlear Implants
Michelle L. Hughes, PhD, CCC-A

Balance and Vestibular Assessment

Electronystagmography/Videonystagmography (ENG/VNG)
Devin L. McCaslin, PhD

Vestibular Learning Manual
Bre Lynn Myers, AuD

Pediatric Audiology

Comprehensive Handbook of Pediatric Audiology
Anne Marie Tharpe, PhD, and Richard Seewald, PhD

Foundations of Pediatric Audiology
Fred H. Bess, PhD, and Judith S. Gravel, PhD

Rotational Vestibular Assessment

Christopher K. Zalewski, PhD

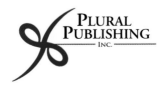

PLURAL PUBLISHING INC.

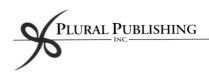

PLURAL PUBLISHING
INC.

5521 Ruffin Road
San Diego, CA 92123

e-mail: info@pluralpublishing.com
Website: http://www.pluralpublishing.com

Typeset in 11/13 Palatino by Flanagan's Publishing Services, Inc.
Printed in Korea through Four Colour Print Group, Louisville, Ky.

Cover image from: Darwin, Erasmus. *Zoonomia; Or, the Laws of Organic Life* (3rd ed.), Vol IV. London, UK. 1801.

Library of Congress Cataloging-in-Publication Data:

Names: Zalewksi, Christopher K., author.
Title: Rotational vestibular assessment / Christopher K. Zalewksi.
Description: San Diego, CA : Plural Publishing, [2018] | Includes
  bibliographical references and index.
Identifiers: LCCN 2017033239 | ISBN 9781597567978 (alk. paper) | ISBN
  1597567973 (alk. paper)
Subjects: | MESH: Vestibular Function Tests--methods | Vestibular
  Nerve--physiology | Vestibular Nuclei--physiology
Classification: LCC RF123 | NLM WV 255 | DDC 617.8--dc23
LC record available at https://lccn.loc.gov/2017033239

Contents

Preface

The last one and one-half decades have seen a significant advancement in the range of clinical assessment techniques for the identification of vestibular pathology. Such changes have demanded a concomitant expansion in our understanding of vestibular anatomy, physiology, and symptomatology. To meet this growing need, many academic doctoral programs have augmented their curriculum to include a comprehensive course (or courses) on the assessment and management of vestibular function. Concurrently, our construct of what constitutes a comprehensive vestibular assessment during routine clinical practice has also swelled over the past 10 to 15 years with the addition of cervical and ocular VEMP testing, vHIT testing, and more enhanced rotational test paradigms. Collectively, this evolution of vestibular knowledge and clinical assessment techniques have significantly increased the need for specialized academic and clinical resources. In fact, rotational vestibular assessment is a perfect example of this evolutionary resource need.

When asked if I would be willing to write a textbook on rotational testing, I thought back to my first rotational assessment 15 years earlier. There was little in the way of didactic writing on the subject. Aside from a few chapters in Shepard & Telian's text *Practical Management of the Balance Disordered Patient* and in Jacobson, Newman, and Kartush's text *Handbook of Balance Function Testing* (1st ed.), there was not a single text dedicated to the subject of rotational testing. Fifteen years later, and (unfortunately) the same can still be said. As such, I agreed to this project with one singular goal; to write a comprehensive text that would not only detail the various tests associated with rotational assessment, but also intertwine a comprehensive understanding of how the vestibular system's anatomy and physiology function with respect to each rotational test. In doing so, this text will hopefully provide the vestibular clinician with a greater understanding of vestibular function, and disease.

A tremendous amount of science has brought us to our current understanding of vestibular function (and dysfunction). This text explores the humble beginnings of vestibular science, and the brilliant scientists and physicians who advanced this understanding. The first chapter begins by highlighting the progression of human rotation from the eightieth century, to the discovery of the vestibular sixth sense. Ever since the acceptance of the vestibular sixth sense, rotational testing has continued to evolve throughout the twentieth and twenty-first centuries to better meet the challenges of diagnosing complex vestibular pathology.

Rotational testing continues to hold a unique position in the comprehensive vestibular assessment. Between its natural acceleration stimuli and its detailed outcomes measures, its analysis is unparalleled for the identification of peripheral and central vestibular disease. This textbook details the various tests conducted during rotational assessment, most notably sinusoidal acceleration testing and velocity step testing. It also explores more specialized rotational tests of visual-vestibular interaction, as well as tests of otolith function (e.g., unilateral centrifugation testing, as well as a brief overview of off-vertical axis rotational testing). It includes a detailed discusion on the anatomy and physiology of the peripheral and central vestibular systems, as well as a thorough review of the vestibular ocular reflex (VOR). It was written from the point of view of a vestibular clinician, for the vestibular clinician.

As with all things, as rotational testing continues to advance into the twenty-first century, it will be essential to stay current with our understanding of the various assessment techniques and outcomes measures associated with normal and abnormal vestibular function. It is my hope you will find this text to be a step toward that direction.

Some of the material found in this textbook is supplemented with a PluralPlus companion website that provides a selection of videos showing the various rotational tests, which illustrates the rotational stimuli and the VOR response generated during each test. When viewing each video, please keep in mind that ALL rotational tests are performed in a lightproof environment; that is with the lightproof booth door *closed* (or the video goggles covered in a boothless rotational suite). Videos shown on the PluralPlus companion website often show the rotation of the chair with the door open. This is for illustrative purposes only

Acknowledgments

My life's accomplishments are the culmination of my individual experiences, but one of the greatest lessons I learned in life is from my parents:

Anything is possible; but nothing will happen unless you take the first step.

This book has been a labor of love. And despite a single name on its cover, it would not have been possible without the support and encouragement from my beautiful and amazing wife Christine, and my two beautiful daughters Maddie and Katie. In a way that no words could ever convey, I wish to express my love, gratitude, and unending thankfulness to them. I also wish to thank my friends and colleagues who provided insight, motivation, guidance, and knowledge. And finally, to my students, whose curiosity continues to inspire me.

"The energy of the mind is the essence of life"
—Aristotle

To Robert Steven Ackley
For the encouragement, the opportunity, the mentorship, the support,
and most of all . . . the friendship.

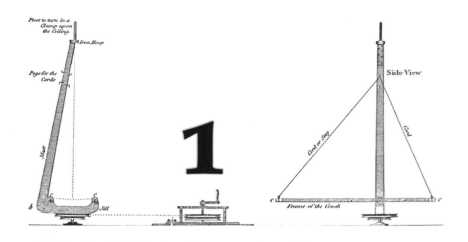

Historical Perspective of Human Rotation and Centrifugation

VERTIGO AND HERALDING OF THE SIXTH SENSE

Aristotle (384–322 BC) was the first to introduce the scientific study of the human senses, as well as provide the first written account of vertigo in 330 BC (Ross, 1927).

> Why is it that to those who are very drunk everything seems to revolve in a circle, and as soon as the wine takes a hold of them they cannot see objects at a distance? . . . objects near at hand are not seen in their proper places, but appear to revolve in a circle. (p. 892a)

Despite a growing body of knowledge and understanding of vestibular anatomy and physiology beginning in the late 1700s, and extending into the early 1800s, Aristotle's five senses remained unchanged and unchallenged until 1824 (Wade, 2003). During this time, the vestibular labyrinth was believed to assist in the localization of sound in the environment. Moreover, the perception of vertigo was attributed to animal spirits (Thomas Willis, 1621–1675), visual disturbances (Julien Offray de la Mettrie, 1709–1751; William Porterfield, 1696–1771; Erasmus Darwin, 1731–1802;

Robert Waring Darwin, 1766–1848), and even the independent rotation of the cerebellum (Jan Evangelista Purkyně, 1787–1869). It was not until 1792 when Charles Wells (1757–1817) provided the first scientific evidence that argued for the expansion of Aristotle's original five senses to include the perception of motion provided by the vestibular system (Wade, 2003). In his treatise entitled, "An Essay Upon Single Vision With Two Eyes" published in 1792, Wells provided indisputable evidence supporting a link between the patterns of eye movements in relation to the direction of post-rotary vertigo (Figure 1–1). Through his use of afterimages following rotations, Wells published the first accurate and objective account of the vestibular response, describing for the first time, the fast and slow phase of vestibular nystagmus.

A few years after Charles Wells published his essay, Erasmus Darwin (grandfather of the famous evolutionist Charles Darwin) published his pinnacle, two-volume treatise "Zoonomia; Or, The Laws of Organic Life" (Vol. 1, 1794; Vol. 2, 1796). In the second volume, Erasmus Darwin and Robert Darwin (Erasmus Darwin's son) extensively wrote on vertigo. However, in their chapter on vertigo, they retained the current thinking of the day that strongly supported William Porterfield's

AN

ESSAY

UPON

SINGLE VISION WITH TWO EYES:

TOGETHER WITH

EXPERIMENTS

AND

OBSERVATIONS

ON

SEVERAL OTHER SUBJECTS IN OPTICS.

By WILLIAM CHARLES WELLS, M. D.

L O N D O N;

PRINTED FOR T. CADELL, IN THE STRAND.

1792.

A

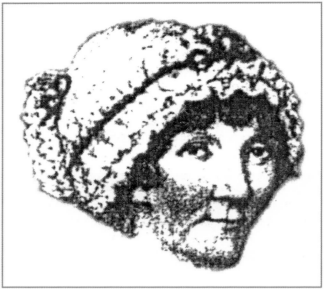

B

FIGURE 1–1. **A.** Charles Wells' treatise entitled "An Essay Upon Single Vision With Two Eyes" is the first known, detailed account of nystagmus attributed to rotation of the head. Louisa Susannah Wells (1757–1817). **B.** No known picture of Charles Wells exists; however, his sister's portrait shown here (Louisa Susannah Wells, pictured here is the only known visual reference to Charles Wells (Wade, 2003). From *Destined for Distinguished Oblivion: The Scientific Vision of William Charles Wells (1757–1817)* by Nicholas J. Wade, 2003, New York, NY, Springer. Reprinted with permission.

earlier opinion that post-rotational vertigo was *not* associated with eye movements but, rather, was due to visual disturbances (which was in direct opposition to Wells' earlier report just four years prior). Despite this opinion and growing evidence over the next decade supporting the association between vertigo and eye movements, the use of rotation for the diagnosis of vertigo and investigation of vestibular function would continue to remain absent in neurology clinics for over a century. However, secondary to Erasmus Darwin's treatise "Zoonomia; Or, The Laws of Organic Life," the application of rotation would hold a promi-nent position in the medical literature and clinical practice during the early ninetieth century. However, it was not for the investigation of dizziness, but rather, for the treatment of the mentally ill.

ROTATION IN THE EARLY NINETIETH CENTURY

Prior to heralding of the vestibular sixth sense in the early nineteenth century by Wells and others, the rotation of patients was most commonly found in psychiatric asylums rather than neurology clinics. In 1801, Erasmus Darwin introduced his concept of a "rotating couch" (Wade, 2003) as a means of inducing slumber in psychiatric patients (Figure 1–2). The idea of "medicinal slumber" was well accepted at the time and motivated many in the field of mental health to prescribe such medically induced slumber for the treatment of psychiatric disorders in the early 1800s. Well-known psychiatrists Joseph Mason Cox (1763–1818), of Fishponds Private Lunatic Asylum near Bristol, England, and William Saunders Hallaran (1765–1825), physician superintendent at the County and City of Cork Lunatic Asylum in Cork, Ireland, developed their own "circulating swings" for which they are probably best remembered (Figures 1–3 and 1–4). Clinical results were well accepted throughout

many countries by numerous physicians and psychiatrists. The success of "Hallaran's Circulating Swing" in 1818 (Breathnach, 2010) was adopted by many at the time and, in particular, by Anton Ludwig Ernst Horn (1774–1848), of the Charité-Hospital in Berlin, Germany. Horn developed his own ceiling-suspended, 13-foot rotating bed, which was capable of spinning 120 revolutions per minute (Belofsky, 2013) and producing up to four to five times the force of gravity (Harsch, 2006) (Figure 1–5). Horn's "psychiatric centrifuge" was also well accepted and widely used between 1814 and 1818 to treat mental disorders. He specifically reported excellent success for the use of his "psychiatric centrifuge" in patients with hysteria (Harsch, 2006). Medicinal slumber continued through the late nineteenth century, including the

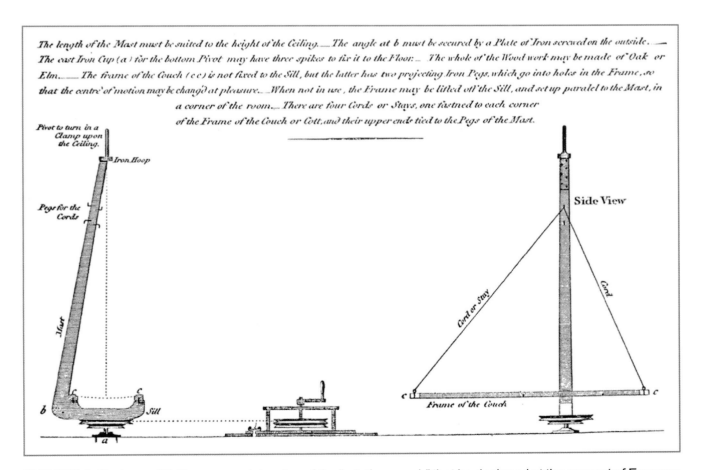

FIGURE 1–2. James Watt's proposed drawing of the "rotating couch" that he designed at the request of Erasmus Darwin. However, it is very likely the "couch" was never constructed (Wade, 2003). From *Zoonomia; Or, the Laws of Organic Life* (3rd ed.), Vol IV, by E. Darwin, 1801, London, England, Thomas & Andrews, J. T. Buckingham, printer.

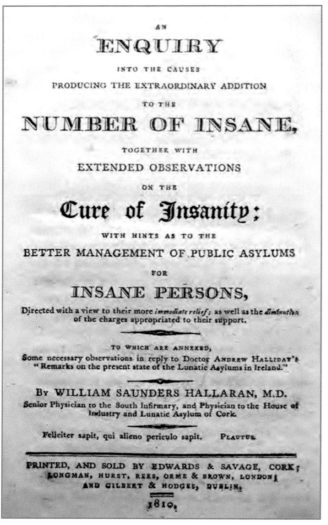

A

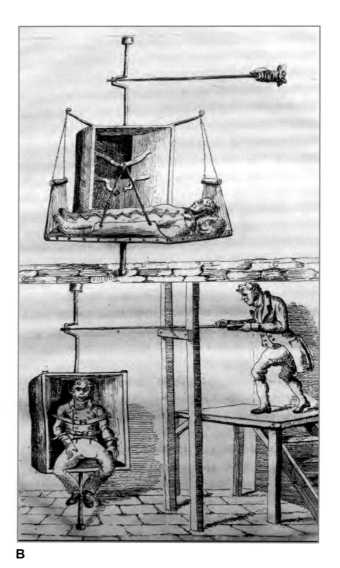

B

FIGURE 1–3. **A.** Cover of the first edition of Dr. William Saunders Hallaran's textbook entitled *An Enquiry into the Causes Producing the Extraordinary Addition to the Number of Insane Together with Extended Observations on the Cure of Insanity: with Hints as to the Better Management of Public Asylums for Insane Persons* by W. S. Hallaran, 1810, Cork, Ireland, Edwards & Savage, Cork, printer. **B.** Dr. Joseph Mason Cox's "circulating swing." From *Practical Observations on the Causes and Cures of Insanity*, (2nd ed.), by W. S. Hallaran, 1818, Cork, Ireland, Edwards & Savage, Cork, printer.

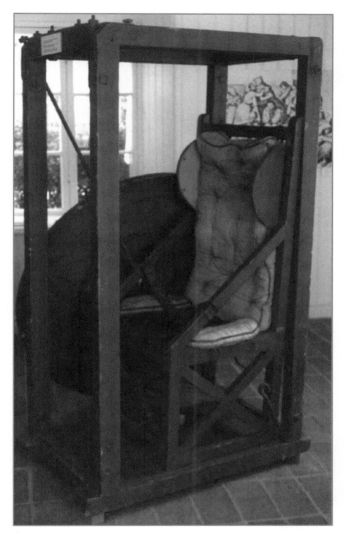

A

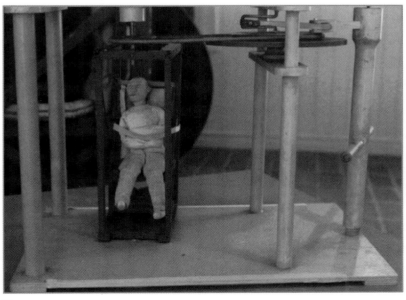

B

FIGURE 1–4. **A.** Photograph of Dr. Joseph Mason Cox's "circulating swing" in the Hospital Museum at Vadstena, Sweden. **B.** A model of the same chair. From "Cox's Chair: 'A Moral and a Medical Mean in the Treatment of Maniacs'" by N. J. Wade, U. Norrsell, and A. Presley, 2005, *History of Psychiatry*, *16*(1), 73–88. Reprinted with permission.

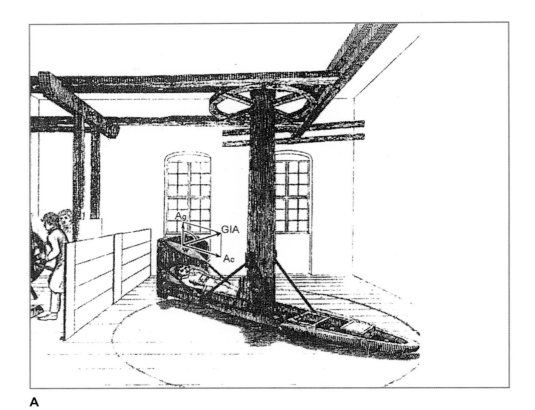

A

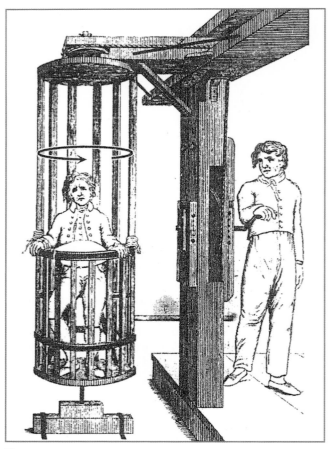

FIGURE 1–5. **A.** Dr. Horn's "Human Centrifuge" at La Charité Hospital used for psychiatric swinging for the induction of "medical slumber." Horn, 1818. **B.** Circulating Swing device possibly used by Jan Evangelista Purkyně. Hayner, 1818. From "The Physiology of the Vestibuloocular Reflex (VOR)" by B. Cohen and T. Raphan, 2004. In F. M. Fay and A. N. Popper (Eds.), *The Vestibular System,* New York, NY: Springer. Reprinted with permission.

B

use of a human centrifuge in 1898 by Dr. F. R. von Wenusch to investigate the therapeutic potential of acceleration (Figure 1–6) (White, 1964). However, the transition of using rotation for the treatment of psychiatric disease to the diagnosis of vertigo and dizziness would not take hold until the vestibular system's role was redefined from that of audition to one of motion perception. Many scientists of the time, including Jan Evangelista Purkyně, continued to believe the vestibular labyrinth's role was one of audition and sound localization, not motion perception.

In the first few decades of the nineteenth century, concurrent to the time when "ceiling swings" and "psychiatric centrifuges" were being used, the Fathers of Vestibular Science—most notably Charles Wells (1757–1817), Robert Waring Darwin (1766–1848), Jan Evangelista Purkyně (1787–1869),

and Jean Pierre Flourens (1794–1867) (Figure 1–7) —published numerous reports citing evidence for the expansion of Aristotle's original five senses to include a (vestibular) sixth sense of motion perception. Reports were frequently contentious and often provoked the well-known feud between Charles Wells and Erasmus Darwin regarding the origin of vertigo, and the exact role of the vestibular system (Wade, 2003). However, despite such feuding, there was one underlying hypothesis that almost all vestibular scientists of the time slowly began to acknowledge—that the vestibular system was likely not responsible for audition, but rather, was indeed, somehow, related to the perception of motion.

Although the early nineteenth century brought a significant amount of scientific evidence corroborating the existence of a sixth sense (most

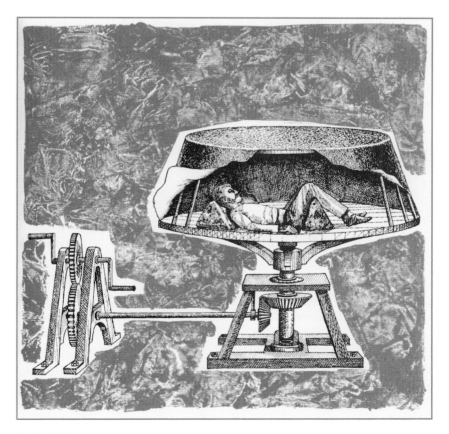

FIGURE 1–6. Dr. F. R. von Wenusch's Human Centrifuge for investigation of therapeutic potential of acceleration. From *A History of the Centrifuge in Aerospace Medicine,* by W. J. White, 1964, Santa Monica, CA, Douglas Aircraft Company, Inc.

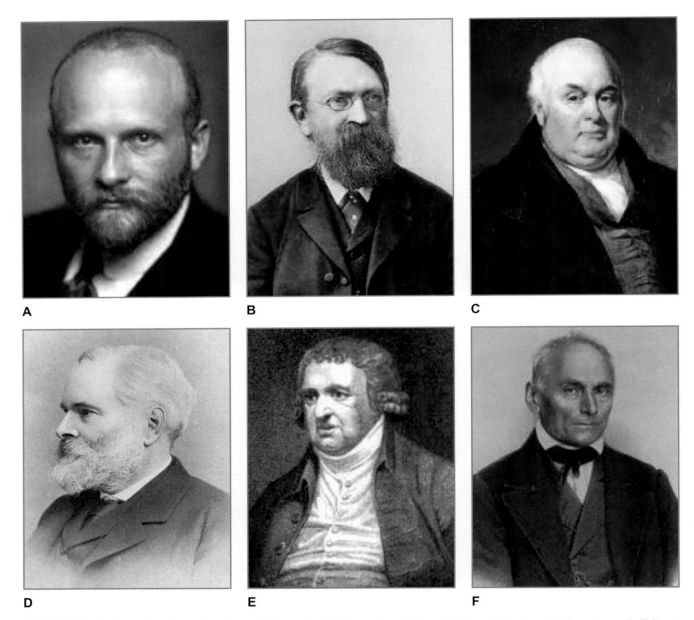

FIGURE 1–7. Portraits of prominent vestibular scientists from the eighteenth through the twentieth century. **A.** Róbert Bárány (1876–1936). **B.** Ernst Josef Mach (1838–1916). **C.** Robert Waring Darwin (1838–1916). **D.** Alexander Crum Brown (1838–1922). **E.** Erasmus Darwin (1731–1802). **F.** Jan Evangelista Purkyně (1787–1869). *continues*

notably by Charles Wells, Erasmus Darwin, and Robert Waring Darwin) (Wade, 2003), it was not until the work of Flourens in 1824 that Aristotle's five senses officially added one more. Flourens' research involving the extirpation of semicircular canals in pigeons finally provided the irrefutable evidence for the vestibular system's role in the perception of motion, thus heralding the elusive sixth sense.

The emergence of the sixth sense struggled for nearly 2000 years after Aristotle first described the five principal human senses. Therefore, it was not surprising that widespread acceptance was not appreciated by all scientists at the time, including Jan

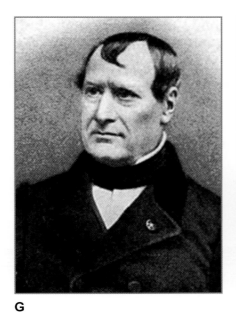

G

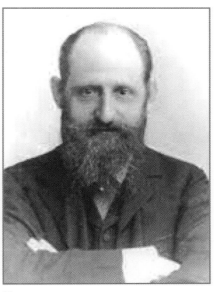

H

FIGURE 1–7. *continued* **G.** Jean Pierre Flourens (1794–1867). **H.** Josef Breuer (1842–1925).

Evangelista Purkyně, who continued to remain hesitant in acknowledging all the available scientific evidence at the time (Wade, 2003).

Despite the quiescence of reports investigating the use of rotational chairs for the clinical diagnosis and treatment of vertigo throughout the early and mid-1800s, there were significant advancements in the understanding of vestibular *physiology* in the last quarter of the nineteenth century. Ernst Josef Mach, Alexander Crum Brown, and Josef Breuer (see Figure 1–7) almost simultaneously proposed the "hydrodynamic theory of semicircular canal function" in 1874 to 1875. Ernst Josef Mach, in particular, was instrumental in this theory. During this time, Mach also published scientific reports investigating the nature of otolith responses, as well as the first reports indicating the semicircular canals responded to *acceleration*, not velocity (Cohen & Raphan, 2004). Between the years 1874 and 1875, Ernst Mach constructed a rotational chair that was mounted in a rotatable frame, and examined the perception of the visual vertical during static tilt, and also the visual aftereffects of body rotation (Figure 1–8). Mach performed such studies after observing the

vertical tilting of telegraph poles when rounding an inappropriately banked curve on a train (Cohen & Raphan, 2004). For his work on subjective visual vertical, some consider Ernst Mach the "Father of Otolith Function Testing." Despite this otological notoriety, Ernst Josef Mach, being an Austrian physicist and philosopher, is probably better known for the Mach principle, which was the precursor to Einstein's theory of relativity.

It is also worth noting that during the time of Mach's discoveries, Alexander Crum Brown also devised methods for measuring thresholds for detecting body movements on a rotating stool. He determined that thresholds were lowest when the head was positioned so that one of the semicircular canals was in the plane of rotation; a precursor to Ewald's laws of semicircular canal function. Finally, toward the beginning of the twentieth century, Lorente de Nó (1933) first described in detail the three-neuron arc that connects the peripheral vestibular end organs to the ocular muscles, thus detailing the Vestibular Ocular Reflex (VOR) pathways that Charles Wells eloquently described 140 years earlier (Cohen & Raphan, 2004).

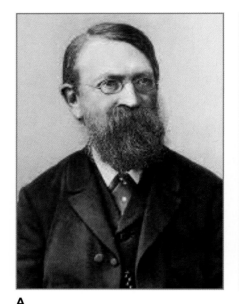

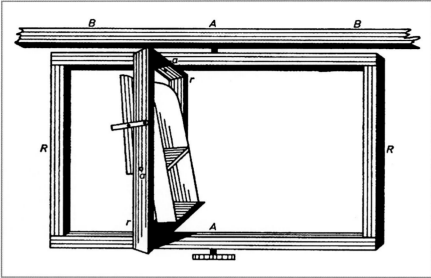

A **B**

FIGURE 1–8. **A.** Ernst Mach (1838–1916). **B.** The rotational chair that was mounted in a rotatable frame, which examined the perception of the visual vertical during static tilt, and also the visual aftereffects of body rotation. Some consider Ernst Mach the "Father of Otolith Function Testing." From *Grundlinien der Lehre von den Bewegungsempfindungen*, by E. Mach, 1875, Leipzig, Verlang von Wilhelm Engelmann.

ROTATION IN THE EARLY TWENTIETH CENTURY

Despite the scientific evidence heralding the emergence of the vestibular system as the sixth sense, the application of clinical rotation withstood a slow transition from the psychiatric treatment of mental disorders to the clinical assessment of otolaryngological disease. Toward the later part of the nineteenth century and the early part of the twentieth century, the *medicinal* evidence for Horn's "psychiatric centrifuge" finally gave way to more *scientific* evidence supporting the use of rotation as a clinical method for investigating vestibular function. Nearly a century after the well-accepted and routine use of patient rotation for the treatment of psychiatric disorders, Róbert Bárány (see Figure 1–7) introduced the application of patient rotation in 1907 as a means for the clinical assessment of the vestibular system. Bárány developed the first rotational chair that was universally adopted in otolaryngology clinics at the time (Figure 1–9). For this reason, modern

day rotational chairs are sometimes referred to as "Bárány chairs." Although modern chairs have come along way in their function, chairs similar in appearance and function to Bárány's original chair are actually still in use today in some aerospace and military motion tolerance labs.

Introduction of Rotational Testing in the Assessment of Vestibular Function

Róbert Bárány first introduced the idea of rotational testing in routine clinical assessment of the vestibular system in 1907. Bárány devised a method of impulse stimulation whereby an abrupt acceleration was applied to a rotational "Bárány chair," with the patient being given 10 rotations in 20 seconds, which was then followed by an abrupt cessation of rotation applied by a manual foot brake. Immediately following cessation of rotation, the presence of post-rotary nystagmus was visualized and timed by the examiner. It was believed that the slow decay of nystagmus reflected activity of the horizontal cupulae. The

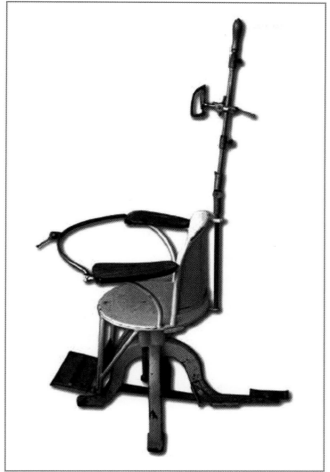

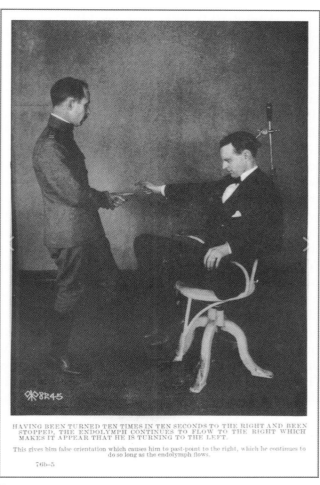

A   **B**

FIGURE 1–9. **A.** Bárány chair. From *Background and Introduction to Whole-Body Rotational Testing* by A. M. Goulson, J. H. McPherson, and N. T. Shepard, 2016. In G. P. Jacobson and N. T. Shepard (Eds.), *Balance Function Assessment and Management*, (pp. 347–364). San Diego, CA, Plural Publishing. Reprinted with permission. **B.** Use of a Bárány chair applying the past-pointing procedure following cessation of rotation. Reprinted with kind permission from http://www.goflightmedicine.com

test was then repeated in the opposite direction and the results were often compared. Although the principles of the test were believed by many early twentieth century neurologists to be very insightful into the function of the vestibular system, the administration and subsequent interpretation of this test was also recognized as problematic, as control of stimulus delivery was often inconsistent, particularly between different patients.

A few years later in 1931, Veits suggested that Bárány's method of impulse stimulation over a 20 second period was, in fact, too short to allow

for the cupulae to return to their original position after having received such brisk accelerations. Therefore, Veits suggested that the cessation of rotation during Bárány's impulse protocol likely occurred while the cupulae were still deviated. In an attempt to remedy this problem, Veits suggested delivering extremely slow accelerations until reaching a constant velocity of 180°/sec. At this velocity, Veits proposed maintaining a constant level of rotation until resetting of the cupulae were assured. He determined this by an absence of nystagmus and cessation of vertigo. Only after these criteria were met, was the brake applied to the Bárány chair and the duration of the post-rotary nystagmus recorded.

In 1948, another attempt to improve upon Bárány's impulse stimulation test was proposed by van Egmond, Groen, and Jongkees. These authors described a method similar to Veits involving the use of slow accelerations. However, van Egmond, Groen, and Jongkees slowly accelerated patients to a number of predetermined target velocities, at which time the chair was abruptly stopped and the post-rotary nystagmus and subjective vertigo was again timed. van Egmond, Groen, and Jongkees plotted each nystagmus response against the various target velocities and coined the term "cupulometry" to describe the vestibular response over a broader range of frequencies.

During the 1940s, vestibular scientists were also beginning to investigate the effects of *linear* acceleration on the vestibular system. Modified human centrifuges were used by various researchers during the mid-1900s. Graybiel and Hupp (1946), and Graybiel, Niven, and Walsh (1952) devised a method to apply centripetal force to study the effects of linear acceleration on the utricle. Aside from Ernst Mach's experiments, these are perhaps some of the earliest vestibular studies using "modern" human centrifuges and eccentric rotation. However, detailed ocular measures of nystagmus were lacking, and reports were often confined to patient reports of apparent subjective tilting of the body, as well as the ostensible visual tilting of surrounding objects in space.

Some of the earlier successor chairs to the Bárány chair were the Hallpike, Hood, and Byford chair (1952) (Figure 1–10), the Tönnies apparatus (1955) (Figure 1–11), the Frenckner and Preber chair (1956) (Figure 1–12), the Fluur chair (1960) (Figure 1–13), the Johnson and Taylor table (1961) (Figure 1–14), the "Girograph of Montandon" (Geneva, Switzerland, 1955; Montandon & Russbach, 1955), the Stille-LKB Rotating chair (Stille-Werner, Stockholm), and the Heidelberg chair (Ey & Feldman, 1964; Figure 1–15) (McNally & Stuart, 1967). For an excellent review of the rotational chairs used during the mid-twentieth century from military institutions, domestic hospitals and laboratories, as well as foreign laboratories, the

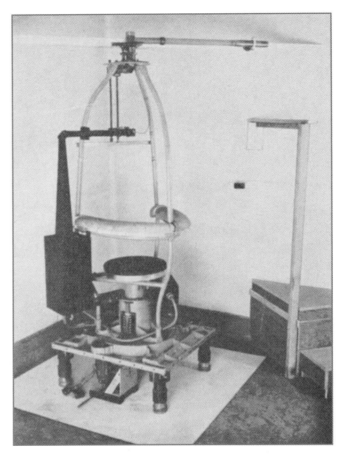

FIGURE 1–10. Hallpike, Dix, and Byford rotational chair, 1952. From "The Design, Construction and Performance of a New Type of Revolving Chair Some Experimental Results and Their Application to the Physical Theory of the Cupular Mechanism" by C. S. Hallpike, J. D. Hood, and G. H. Byford, 1952, *Acta Oto-Laryngologica*, *42*(6), 511–538. Reprinted with permission.

reader is encouraged to read Guedry and Graybiel's (1961) report entitled *Rotation Devices, Other Than Centrifuges and Motion Stimulators: The Rationale for the Special Characteristics and Use*. In general, from 1907 until the 1960s, rotational assessments using the Bárány chair and its successors were essentially confined to impulse stimulation and cupulometry protocols. Early attempts were frequently proposed in an attempt to improve testing and provide better outcome measures; however, results were plagued with unreliability and poor sensitivity at identifying vestibular pathology.

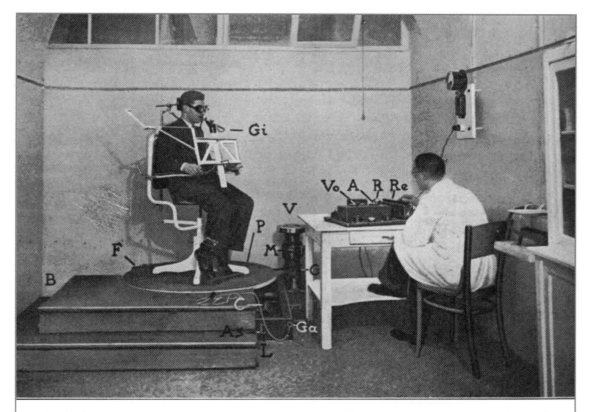

Fig. 8. TÖNNIES model of chair, consenting measuration of positive and negative angular acceleration, and of the ang. velocity.

P = Platform; M = Motor; V = Wheel; G = Friction joint; B = Basement; R = Thermoion. valve; Re = Rheostat; A = Amperometer; Vo = Voltmeter; L = Brake's lever; As = Brake's board; C = Cylinder of compressed air; Gi = Goniometer applied to the arrangement for the rigid fixation in the space of subject's head; F = Apparatus for the registration of the angular acceleration and velocity; Ga = trigger of brake's lever.

A

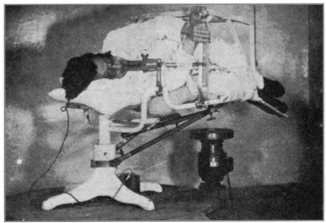

B

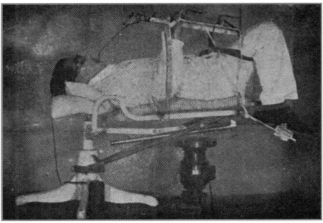

C

FIGURE 1–11. Early model of Tönnies apparatus rotational chair. Chair orientation could be modified to study horizontal nystagmus (**A**), vertical nystagmus (**B**), and torsional nystagmus (**C**). From "On Acceleratory Stimulation," 1955, *Acta Oto-Laryngologica*, *45*(Suppl. 122), 22–44. Reprinted with permission.

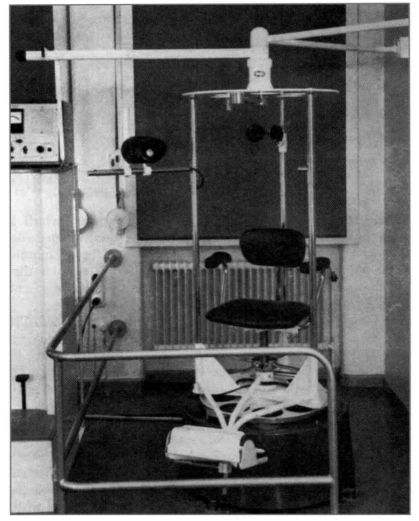

A

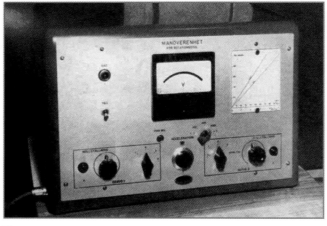

B

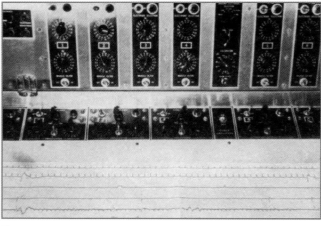

C

FIGURE 1–12. Frenckner and Preber chair. Rotational chair (**A**), computer console (**B**), and nystagmus printout (**C**). From "Relationship Between Vestibular Reactions and Vegetative Reflexes, Studied in Man by Means of a Revolving Chair of New Design" by P. Frenckner, and L. Preber, 1956, *Acta Oto-Laryngologica*, *46*(3), 207–220. Reprinted with permission.

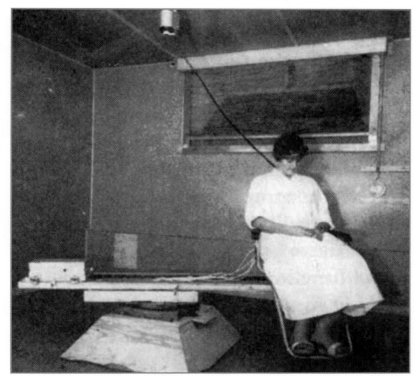

A

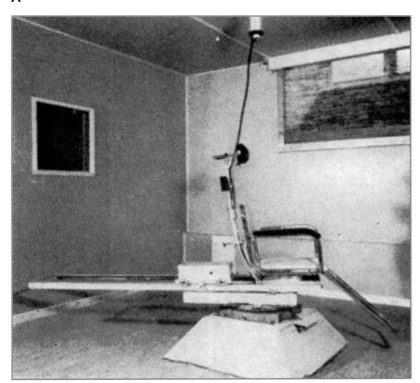

B

FIGURE 1–13. The Fluur rotational chair. **A.** Chair positioned for nasion-occipital eccentric rotation. **B.** Chair positioned for interaural axis eccentric rotation. From "A Novel Rotary Chair" by E. Fluur, 1960, *Acta Oto-Laryngologica*, *52*:1–6, 210–214. Reprinted with permission.

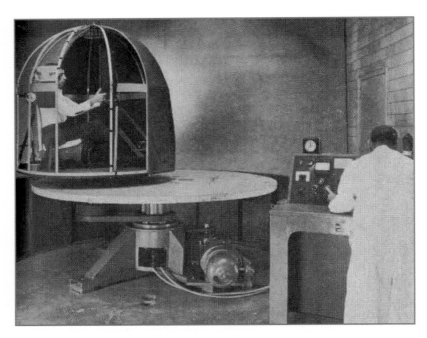

FIGURE 1–14. The Johnson and Taylor rotational chair. From "The Importance of the Otoliths in Disorientation" by W. H. Johnson, 1964, *Aerospace Medicine*, *35*, 874–877. Reprinted with permission.

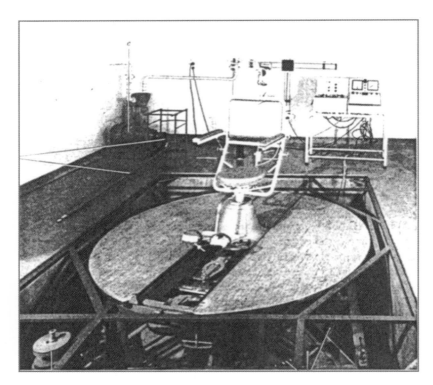

FIGURE 1–15. Heidelberg chair. From "Der Heidelberger Planeten-Drehstuhl, eine neuartige Mehrzweck-Drehstuhlanlage für Vestibular-isreflexprüfungen" by W. Ey, and H. Feldman, 1964, *Archiv Ohren-, Nasen- u. Kehlkopfheilk. 184*, 73–80. Reprinted with permission.

This was largely due to the fact that stimulus delivery was manually generated, or electrically driven through inefficient motors and turntables. It was not until the late 1960s and early 1970s, when the advent of computer-controlled precision torque motors were able to deliver more consistent and reliable stimuli, thus improving the various outcome measures.

The slow advancement of rotational research and its use in clinical assessments in the early twentieth century may have also been due to one of the most (if not *the* most) significant discovery in clinical vestibular physiology. In 1906, Róbert Bárány published, "Untersuchungen ueber den vom Vestibularapparat des Ohres reflektorisch ausgelösten rhythmischen Nystagmus und seine Begleiterscheinungen" ("Investigations of Rhythmic Nystagmus and Its Accompanying Manifestations Arising From The Vestibular Apparatus of the Ear") (Nylen, 1965). In this work, he described the caloric response for which he was later awarded the Nobel Prize in Physiology and Medicine in 1914. In fact, no other Nobel Prize has been awarded in the field of vestibular medicine (noting that George von Békésy also received the Nobel Prize in Physiology and Medicine in 1961, although this was for his work in the field of *hearing* science on the cochlear traveling wave). The caloric test became an otolaryngological breakthrough for the discovery of labyrinthine disease and identifying normal vestibular function. Given the caloric test's success and the concomitant unreliability of rotational data at the time, the rotational test was likely overshadowed by the simplicity and widespread acceptance of caloric irrigations.

ROTATION IN THE MID-TO-LATE TWENTIETH CENTURY

During the mid-twentieth century, the caloric test flourished due to its increased diagnostic sensitivity for vestibular disease, while rotational chair testing received only a moderate degree of attention, secondary to its inherently unreliable nature. However, with the advent of "personal" computing in the later quarter of the twentieth century, and the increased knowledge regarding vestibular physiology (such as the discovery of the neural integrator and the velocity storage mechanism by Raphan, Matsuo, and Cohen in 1979), research and development in the field of rotational testing was once again about to flourish and emerge as a highly specialized vestibular test, both in clinical and research settings.

The introduction of smaller (personal) computers in the late 1960s and early 1970s significantly changed the clinical canvas of nearly every physiologic test, and rotational testing was no exception. With the personal computer came significant advancements in the ability to deliver exacting stimuli through new torque motors with a higher degree of precision and low vibration noise, thus eliminating the immeasurable variability and clinical uncertainty associated with manually produced brake-rotations common with the Bárány chair. Moreover, the discovery of the corneoretinal potential by Emil du Bois-Reymond (1818–1896) in 1948 opened the door for the objective measurement of nystagmus (Brey, McPherson, & Lynch, 2008a). Recording of the corneoretinal potential through electrooculography (EOG) allowed for the quantification of nystagmus, rather than the subjective timing of the post-rotary nystagmus decay response, which introduced much needed sensitivity to rotational analyses.

The number of accounts of rotational investigations beginning in the late 1960s into the 1970s was exponential in growth. From the development and application of new linear sleds, to the development of more advanced yaw angular rotational chairs (and rooms), numerous published reports detailing the various vestibular ocular response parameters and new stimulus paradigms, occurred at a rapid pace. Niven, Carroll Hixson, and Correia (1965) devised the "Coriolis Acceleration Platform," which was able to produce 16 feet/sec linear accelerations with a peak linear acceleration of 3-gravitational forces (McNally & Stuart, 1967). This study is often cited as the first investigation to show nystagmus with linear acceleration. However, the use of linear sleds was extraordinarily expensive due to the shear size of the laboratory needed to build and use such equipment. To address the massive size requirements needed for such linear sled experiments, Johnson and Taylor (1961) devised an electrically driven turntable upon which they mounted a second counterrolling table that was eccentrically positioned 2 feet from the center axis of rotation on the main table (see Figure 1–14). Rotation of the table occurred such that, for every rotation of the main table, the second table completed one rotation, only in the opposite direction. Johnson claimed such an eccentric-driven table was capable of producing horizontal nystagmus and, given enough time and research, could eventually be adopted for use in routine vestibular laboratory testing.

With the newly discovered corneoretinal potential, the analysis of rotationally induced nystagmus also advanced at an exponential rate. Mathog (1972) is credited with one of the first reports detailing the various response parameters analyzed from the nystagmus during sinusoidal acceleration testing (Goulson, McPherson, & Shepard, 2016). In his report, Mathog described rotational analysis parameters of directional preponderance and VOR gain in response to sinusoidal rotations delivered at low-, mid-, and high-frequency accelerations. Such analyses bridged the way to current methods of sinusoidal rotational analysis. A few years prior, Wilmot (1966) was arguing for a thorough examination of the vestibular system to include rotational measures that detected *threshold* of motion perception. With a custom built rotational chair, Wilmot showed that vestibular threshold detection measures could reliably be obtained with the use of single-eye electrooculography (EOG) recordings. Electrooculography recordings were crude at that time. However, Dix, Hallpike, and Hood (1963) were improving current methods by introducing direct current amplification to record both sustained eye deviations, as well as dynamic nystagmus movements. Despite using enhanced EOG recording methods, the idea to record vestibular threshold detection responses (much like auditory thresholds) was highly novel. Wilmot (1966) is also likely the first to describe the use of rotational testing as a screening tool to detect early pathological vestibular changes. In his report, Wilmot argued for the use of angular rotations to record threshold detection measures for the early identification of vestibular disease to promote early medical intervention (McNally & Stuart, 1967).

Since the 1970s, various manufacturers have increased the level of sophistication in signal processing, both in the recording of the ocular response (EOG versus videooculography, VOG), as well as in the delivery of the various rotational stimuli. Stimuli delivery was particularly improved when rotational chairs transitioned from DC- to AC-driven torque motors. Motors were now capable of delivering highly precise stimuli with little to no vibration noise independent of patient weight.

The military and aerospace divisions have long been given credit for a great deal of research using human centrifuges. William J. White published an elaborately illustrated work entitled *A History of the Centrifuge in Aerospace Medicine* in 1964, which describes the use of rotational systems to explore the effects of various environments on the human vestibular system. As early at 1935, the military and aerospace facilities led much of the way in the development and production of human centrifuge research. The Wright Field Centrifuge located in Riverside, Ohio, (Wilbur Wright Field, now part of Wright-Patterson Air Force Base) was the first human centrifuge constructed in North American (Figure 1–16). The largest and most powerful human centrifuge (even to this day) was constructed in 1950 in Warminster, Pennsylvania, at the Johnsville Naval Air Development Center (NADC) (Figure 1–17). With a 50-foot radius, the Johnsville Centrifuge was capable of producing 40 *g* while traveling at a velocity of 175 mph. Its use significantly impacted the success of aerospace missions, and functioned up until 2004, at which time the Johnsville Centrifuge facility was decommissioned. Although the facility has since been repurposed, much of the history (as well as the original Mercury 7 Johnsville gondola) has been preserved under the care of the Johnsville Centrifuge and Science Museum. Considered to be of equal notoriety to the Johnsville Centrifuge, the Karolinska Centrifuge in Stockholm, Sweden, was equally impressive, with a 40-foot radius capable of producing 30 *g* (Figure 1–18). Finally, Guedry, Kennedy, Harris, and Graybiel (1962) reported on the absence of any psychological or physiologic effects on four servicemen during a two-week exposure in the Pensacola Slow Rotation Room in Pensacola, Florida.

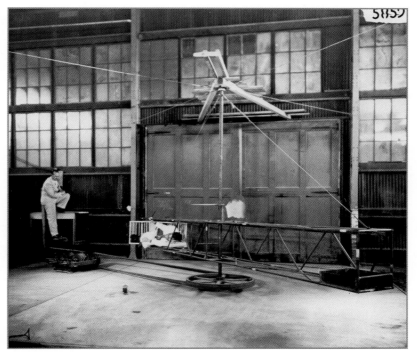

A

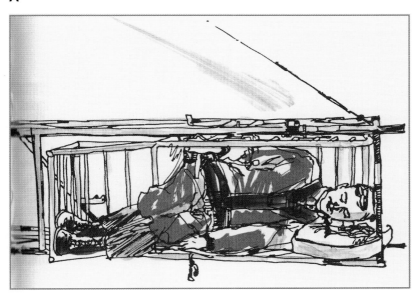

B

FIGURE 1–16. The Wright Field Centrifuge (1935). **A.** The first human centrifuge in North America by Drs. H.G. Armstrong and J. W. Heim. Consisted of a 10-foot radius tubular aluminum frame with a side-mounted adjustable seat (gondola) on one end. *Source*: Reprinted with the courtesy of Special Collections and Archives, Wright State University, Dayton, OH. **B.** Sketch of the pilot position held within the centrifuge gondola. From *A History of the Centrifuge in Aerospace Medicine* by W. J. White, 1964, Santa Monica, CA, Douglas Aircraft Company, Inc.

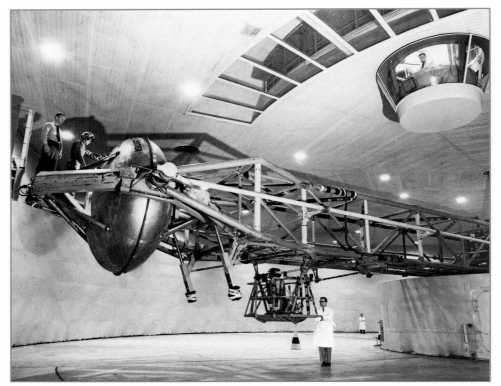

A

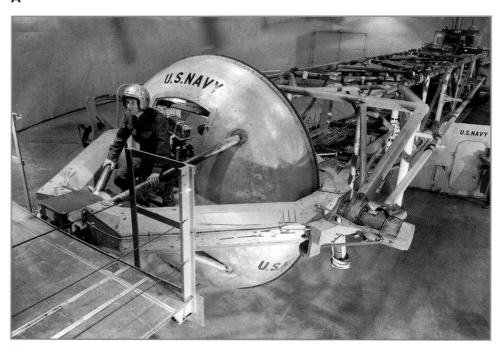

B

FIGURE 1–17. The Johnsville Centrifuge, Warminster, PA (1950–2004). Johnsville Naval Air Development Center (NADC) constructed the largest and most powerful human centrifuge ever built, even to this day, with a 50-foot radius, capable of producing up to 40 g at 175 mph. **A.** Reprinted with permission from Boeing Aircraft Company. **B.** Reprinted with permission from the Johnsville Centrifuge Science Museum.

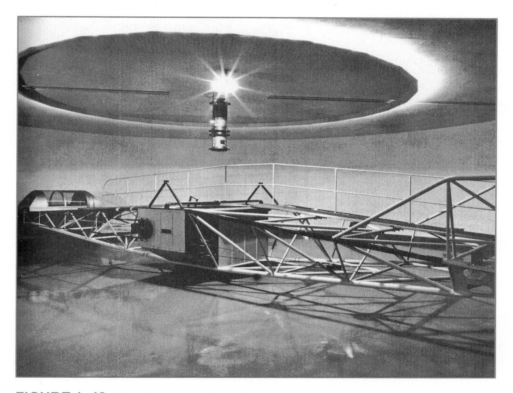

FIGURE 1–18. The Karolinska Centrifuge, Stockholm, Sweden, (1954). Swedish Committee for Aeronautical and Naval Medical Research at the Karolinksa Institute built this 40-foot radius, 30 *g* human centrifuge. *Source*: Reprinted with permission from the Karolinska Institute, Department of Physiology and Pharmacology.

Between the 1970s and 1990s, *clinical* rotation research and the application of clinical rotational assessments also grew at an exponential rate. There were a number of proprietary rotational chairs at the time, as well as some commercially available *clinical* rotational chairs, that were designed and constructed with the sole purpose of evaluating the vestibular response. Such clinical rotational chairs included the Tönnies apparatus (Figure 1–19) and the ICS, Inc. rotational chair (Figure 1–20). Although the system processors were large, (see Figures 1–19 and 1–20), and the analysis often tedious and limited, (compared to current analysis standards), the stimuli and EOG recording methods were a vast improvement over the mid-twentieth century rotational suites.

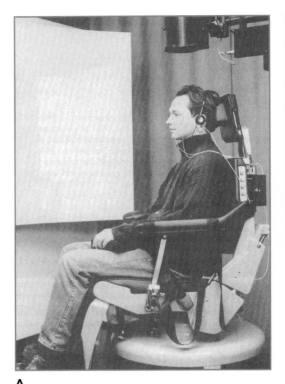

A

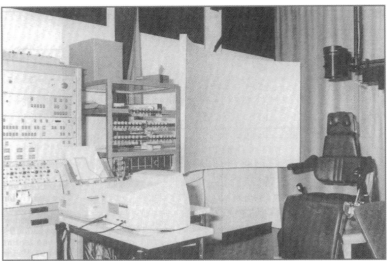

B

FIGURE 1–19. Tönnies apparatus rotational chair (**A**) and computer console (**B**). From *Normal Values of Post-Rotatory and Per-Rotatory ENG Parameters* by R. Mösges, and L. Klimek, 1993. In I. K. Arenberg (Ed.) *Dizziness and Balance Disorders: An Interdisciplinary Approach to Diagnosis, Treatment and Rehabilitation* New York, NY, Kugler Publications. Reprinted with permission.

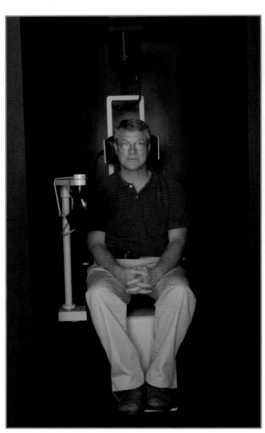

A

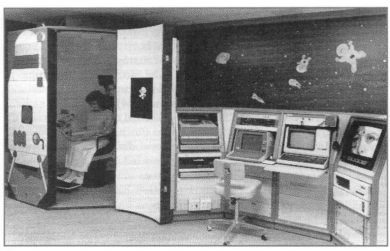

B

FIGURE 1–20. **A.** ICS rotational chair. From National Institutes of Health. **B.** ICS Rotational Chair adapted for pediatric testing. From *Vestibular Assessment* by D. G. Cyr, 1991. In W. F. Rintelmann, *Perspectives in Audiology Series: Hearing Assessment* (2nd ed., pp. 739–803). Boston, MA: Allyn & Bacon. Reprinted with permission.

ROTATIONAL TESTING IN THE PRESENT DAY

Rotational test suites and the precision of rotational stimuli have continued to develop over the past two decades. In particular, vestibular test equipment in general has seen some of the fastest development over the past decade alone. With the introduction of video head impulse testing (vHIT), as well as ocular vestibular evoked myogenic potential (VEMP) testing, the comprehensive nature of vestibular testing has flourished. Advancements in rotational testing have similarly seen increased success. Some of these successes are reviewed in the final chapter when discussing the future advancement of rotational testing.

The current state of rotational testing employs exacting stimuli with high-grade, digital videographic displays, and extremely fast infrared video goggles, with ultra-precise digital sampling rates. Advanced research MOOG platforms (Moog, Inc., Buffalo, NY) (Figure 1–21) have significantly enhanced the delivery of highly specialized stimuli that can be presented to the vestibular system. Furthermore, all data can now be recorded, measured, and analyzed using specialized software algorithms that have tremendously enhanced our sensitivity to identify even more subtle vestibular dysfunction. Finally, highly specialized research rotational chairs, capable of rotating in all axes, (both horizontal and vertically), are greatly expanding our reach into vestibular science. Rotational test suites like the "Roto Tilt

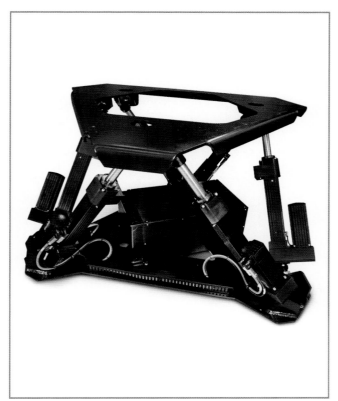

A

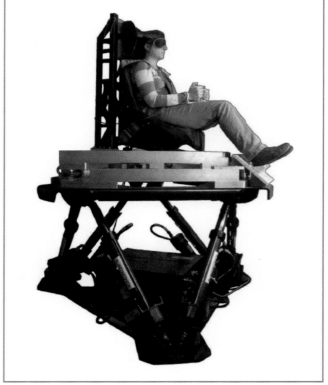

B

FIGURE 1–21. **A.** MOOG six-degrees-of-freedom motion platform©. Reprinted with permission from MOOG, Inc. **B.** Application of a MOOG six-degrees-of-freedom motion platform (6DOF2000E). From "Moving Along the Mental Number Line: Interactions Between Whole-Body Motion and Numerical Cognition" by M. Hartmann, L. Grabherr, and F. Mast, 2012, *Journal of Experimental Psychology: Human Perception and Performance. 38*(6), 1416–1427. Reprinted with permission.

Chair" at the University of Alabama (Figure 1–22) is one such device that will continue to challenge our understanding of vestibular responses for some time to come. Moreover, the advancement of human disorientation devices (HDDs), such as the GRYPHON GL-6000 at Wright-Patterson Air Force Base (Figure 1–23) continues to stretch the boundaries of what may seem humanly possible. Although designed for military and aerospace research and training, the application to medicine is never too far behind.

Although rotational chairs and human disorientation devices, such as the "Roto Tilt Chair" and GRYPHON GL-6000, respectively, likely seemed implausible during the days of the simple Bárány chair, we must continue to remind ourselves that the physiology of the vestibular system is (if nothing else) extraordinarily complex. We must be cognizant that just because a chair *can* be built, does not necessarily mean we will be able to fully understand the physiologic output. Ultimately, the complex physiologic response must still be correctly interpreted. The interpretation of such exceedingly complex results may appear to be an insurmountable challenge, particularly given the obstacles clinicians face with the interpretation of certain current rotational tests, such as OVAR testing (Chapter 8). Throughout the entire historical perspective of vestibular assessment, since the days of Ernst Mach and Robert Bárány, one thing has remained a fundamental and resolute truth—that a thorough understanding of vestibular anatomy and physiology are essential to the understanding and advancement of vestibular science.

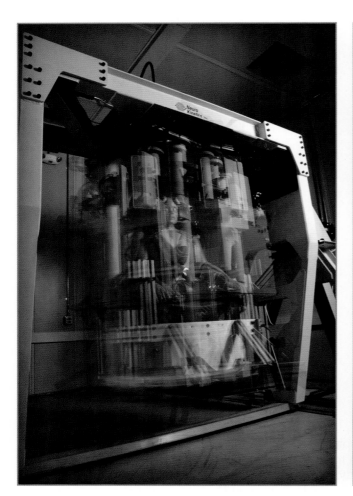 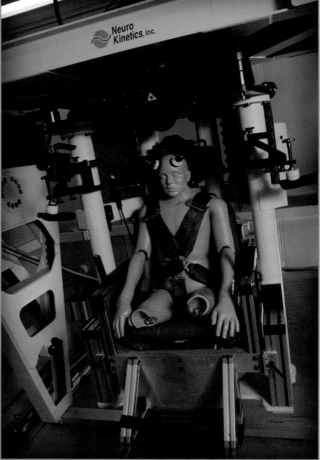

FIGURE 1–22. "Roto Tilt Chair." *Source*: Images courtesy of the University of Alabama, Tuscaloosa, AL.

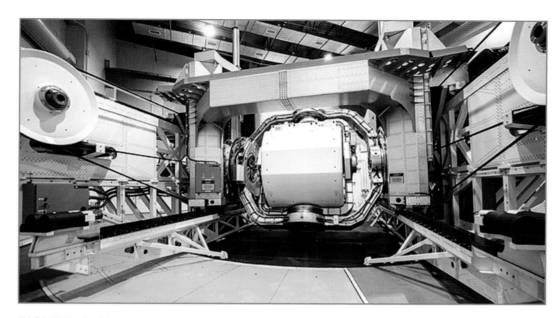

FIGURE 1–23. A Naval Medical Research Unit Dayton's (NAMRU-D) Disorientation Research Device (DRD); the GRYPHON GL-6000. Nicknamed thye "Kraken" by the U.S. Navy, the GRYPHON is a one-of-a-kind research platform capable of multi-axis motion as experienced by up to two subjects in yaw, pitch, roll, and heave while undergoing planetary and linear accelerations, up to 3 Gz. NAMRU-D's mission is to maximize warfighter performance and survivability through premier aeromedical and environmental health effects research by delivering solutions to the Field, the Fleet, and for the Future. NAMRU-D is located at Wright-Patterson Air Force Base, Dayton, OH. *Source:* https://www.etcusa.com/ribbon-cutting-ceremony-for-etcs-gryphon-gl-6000-held-by-naval-medical-research-unit-dayton-located-at-wright-patterson-air-force-base/. Reprinted with permission from VP Aircrew Training Systems Environmental Tectonics Corporation (ETC) and the Office of Public Affairs, Naval Medical Research Unit, Dayton, OH.

For it was not from complex and ultra-sophisticated rotational devices that gave us Ewald's Laws and the "hydrodynamic theory of semicircular canal function," but rather it was the result of an excellent marriage in thought between the understanding of stimuli and physiologic outcomes. The current state of vestibular science is poised to enter a new renaissance of clinical discovery. By combining unprecedented complex stimuli with a vast array of physiological understanding, new research using such highly advanced devices will undoubtedly expand our understanding of vestibular function, and dysfunction.

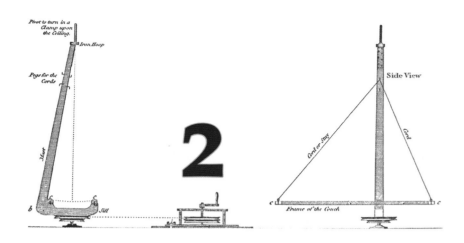

Anatomy and Physiology of the Peripheral Vestibular System

ROLE OF THE VESTIBULAR SYSTEM: AN OVERVIEW

In more highly developed mammals, the primary responsibility of the vestibular system is to provide postural orientation for basic stabilization during movement (Gacek, 2005). Although this responsibility is shared and refined by the proprioceptive, autonomic reflex, and visual systems, the central vestibular pathways are integral to the synergistic coordination of the sensory information required for effective and efficient postural stability during movement, and at rest. The vestibular system is fundamental to postural stability and control during locomotion for most multicellular organisms. In light of this, it is no surprise that the vestibular system is one of the oldest central nervous system reflex pathways, both phylogenetically, as well as otogenetically (Gacek, 2005).

In humans, a secondary, but equally important, role of the vestibular system is to provide gaze stabilization of the visual environment during brief head movements. An accurate and efficient translation of head and body movement into neural signals must effectively be represented to the central nervous system for a subjective awareness of head and body movement in space. More-over, the neural signals conveyed to the brain from the vestibular sense organs are paramount to producing compensatory eye movements during head movement in order to provide visual stability of a particular image on the retina. This is critical, because without such compensatory eye movements, a subsequent blurring and visual "jerking" of the visual field (known as oscillopsia) would occur with every movement of the head (Leigh & Zee, 2006). The vestibular system is primarily responsible for providing this effective visual stabilization during brief head movements, as well as maintaining successful posture and equilibrium.

PERIPHERAL VESTIBULAR SYSTEM ANATOMY: AN OVERVIEW

The vestibular system is located within the otic capsule, which is located within the petrous portion of each temporal bone. Within the otic capsule is the bony labyrinth of the inner ear, which is filled with perilymph, an extracellular fluid that is rich in sodium. Encased within the bony labyrinth is the membranous labyrinth where the cochlear and the vestibular sensory end organs are bathed in a potassium-rich fluid known as endolymph (Lysakowski, McCrea, & Tomlinson, 1998). The sensory end organs of the cochlear and vestibular systems are highly complex and are ultimately responsible for hearing and sensing motion, respectively. Within the vestibular membranous labyrinth are five sensory end organs responsible for sensing movement and postural orientation both during motion, and at rest. These five vestibular sensory end organs synapse directly with the eighth (VIII) cranial nerve in order to provide a neural response that can be coordinated by the central nervous system (Baloh & Honrubia, 1998). The five vestibular sensory end organs, as well as two vestibular branches of the VIII cranial nerve, are collectively known as the peripheral vestibular system (Figure 2–1). Their anatomy and physiology are highly complex. Although much is known regarding its form and function, much still

remains undiscovered. Ongoing research continues to uncover information regarding the molecular microstructure, proteomics, neural response properties, and adaptation/compensation mechanisms of the vestibular system.

Each peripheral vestibular system is comprised of five sensory end organs and two vestibular branches of the VIII cranial nerve (CN). The five sensory end organs of the peripheral vestibular system include two primary groups of vestibular sense organs; the cristae ampullari of the semicircular canals, and the otoconia-rich matrix of the otoliths, known as the maculae (Lysakowski et al., 1998). There are three semicircular canals and two maculae within each vestibular membranous labyrinth. The three semicircular canals are responsible for sensing *angular* acceleration and are identified and labeled with respect to their orientation in space: the horizontal, the anterior, and

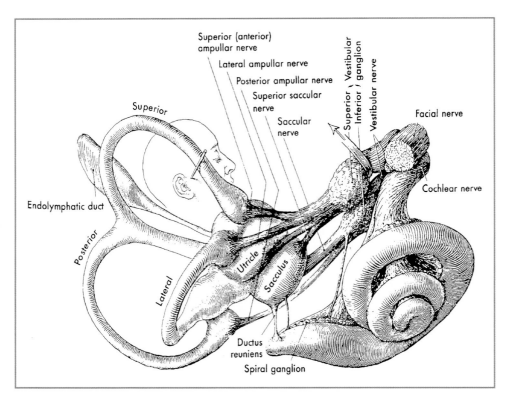

FIGURE 2–1. Peripheral vestibular membranous labyrinth showing vestibular sensory end organs (semicircular canals, saccule, and utricle) and the innervations of the superior and inferior branch of the vestibular nerve. From *Three Unpublished Drawings of the Anatomy of the Human Ear* by M. Brödal, 1946, Philadelphia, PA, W. B. Saunders. In Cummings et al. (1998), *Otolaryngology Head and Neck Surgery* (3rd ed.), St. Louis, MO, CV Mosby. Reprinted with permission.

the posterior semicircular canal (Lysakowski et al., 1998). The two maculae, the utricle and saccule, are responsible for sensing gravity, *linear* acceleration, and static head tilt (Leigh & Zee, 2006). Fundamental to the function of all vestibular receptor sensory organs is the vestibular hair cell, of which there are two types, type I and type II (Baloh & Honrubia, 2001). The hair cells produce the bioelectric response that synapses with cranial nerve VIII. Along with the cochlear nerve, there are two branches of the vestibular nerve, the superior and inferior branch. The two vestibular branches are named according to their anatomical orientation to one another.

VESTIBULAR HAIR CELL RECEPTOR

The basic element of all vestibular end organs is the hair cell. Similar to the outer and inner hair cells located within the organ of Corti, the vestibular hair cell transduces mechanical forces to nerve action potentials (Baloh & Honrubia, 2001).

Endovestibular Potential and Hair Cell Stereocilia Bundles

The apical surfaces of all vestibular hair cells bathe in the potassium-rich (K+) endolymph, which, in contrast to the +80 mV cochlear endolymph potential, is much lower at +5 to 10 mV (Baloh & Honrubia, 1998). Extending from the surface of the cuticular plate of each vestibular hair cell are the mechanosensing organelles, known as stereocilia bundles. Unlike the prestin-rich hair cells and stereocilia bundles in the cochlea that actively contract to electrical transduction, vestibular hair cells and their respective stereocilia bundles contain the protein actin, and carry out flagella-type movement (Baloh & Honrubia, 2001). The reason for this is not completely understood; however, Baloh and Honrubia (2001) offer a possible explanation.Although it remains unproven, Baloh and Honrubia indicate that it is possible that hair cells at the periphery of the vestibular organs actively pull the cupula or otolithic membrane to influence the response of the more centrally placed hair cell.

This, of course, is analogous to the cochlear amplifier and the effect of cochlear outer hair cells on inner hair cells. In addition, there is evidence to suggest that deflection of the stereocilia exhibits non-linear transduction potentials with respect to their degree of displacement (Baloh & Honrubia, 2001). Small stereocilia displacements produce a more linear response in the hair cell receptor potential, whereas large displacements produce potentials that become non-linear near saturation of the hair cell receptor response (Baloh & Honrubia, 2001). This is likely a key component of the cupular pendulum model, which is discussed in subsequent chapters of this text.

Vestibular Hair Cell Types

There are two types of labyrinthine hair cells in the vestibular system, type I and type II hair cell receptors (Figure 2–2). Type I vestibular hair cells are globular in shape and are often marked by a single afferent synapse with a terminal nerve ending known as a chalice, or calyx (Lysakowski et al., 1998). This calyx-type nerve ending completely surrounds the basal portion of the hair cell. Type II vestibular hair cells are cylindrical in shape and are often marked by multiple, and much smaller, efferent, and afferent nerve endings known as boutons (Lysakowski et al., 1998). There is a clear morphologic organization of type I and type II sensory hair cells across all sensory epithelium. In general, type I hair cells, with their large calyx nerve endings and larger diameter afferent nerve fibers, are predominantly located in the center of the various vestibular epithelia, whereas the type II hair cells are more common along the periphery (Baloh & Honrubia, 2001). This holds true for both the cristare ampullari, as well as the maculae.

In the human vestibular end organ, there are approximately 23,000 hair cells (type I and type II) in the SCC cristae, and about 52,000 in the two maculae (Baloh & Honrubia, 2001). Type I and type II hair cells are present in nearly a 1:1 ratio within the vestibular end organs (Harsha, Phillips, & Backous, 2008). The functional (physiological) differences between type I and type II hair cells occur largely because of the different afferent innervation to each hair cell type, rather than the morphological differences

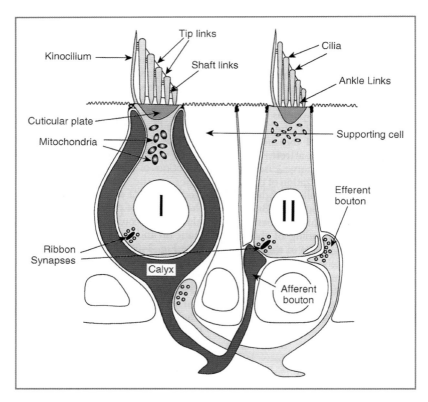

FIGURE 2–2. Type I and type II vestibular hair cells and their respective innervations. From *Baloh and Honrubia's Clinical Neurophysiology of the Vestibular System* (4th ed.) by R. W. Baloh, V. Honrubia, and K. A. Kerber, 2011, New York, NY, Oxford University Press. Reprinted with permission.

between each hair cell. These innervation differences have a significant implication with respect to the tuning of vestibular afferents, which is discussed in greater detail later.

SEMICIRCULAR CANALS

The semicircular canals (SCC), and their respective cristae ampulla, respond to *angular* acceleration. The horizontal canal, also known as the lateral canal, is responsible for sensing angular movement of the head or body in the horizontal, or yaw, plane. The anterior aspect of the horizontal SCC is inclined approximately 30° upward from the true horizontal plane, connecting the external auditory canal to the lateral canthus, known as Reid's baseline (Della Santina, Potyagaylo, Migliaccio, Minor, & Carey, 2005) (Figure 2–3). The anterior SCC, also known as the superior SCC, is primarily responsible for sensing angular movements in the roll (side-to-side) plane. The anterior SCC is oriented approximately 90° from the horizontal SCC (Della Santina et al., 2005). The posterior SCC, also known as the inferior SCC, is responsible for sensing angular movements in the anterior-posterior, or pitch, plane. The posterior SCC is oriented approximately 92° from the horizontal canal. The posterior and anterior SCCs are oriented roughly 24° from one another (Schwarz & Tomlinson, 2005).

Collectively, the SCCs exhibit an orthogonal (mutually perpendicular) relationship to one another, such that the three-dimensional orientation is similar to the meeting of two conjoining walls and floor at the corner of a room meeting, forming three surfaces at right angles to one

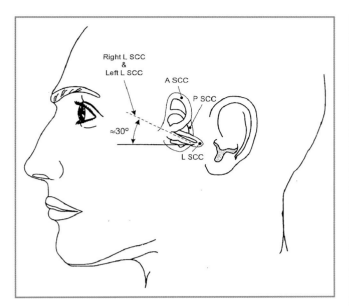

FIGURE 2–3. Orientation of the horizontal semicircular canal with respect to the horizontal plane. The horizontal canal is oriented at an approximate angle of +30° from the horizontal plane, which forms an imaginary line from the tragus to the lateral ocular canthus, known as Reid's baseline. From Barin, K. & Durrant, J. (2000). Applied physiology of the vestibular system. In P. R. Lambert & R. F. Canalis (Eds.). *The Ear: Comprehensive Otology*, Philadelphia, PA, Lippincott Williams & Wilkins. Reprinted with permission.

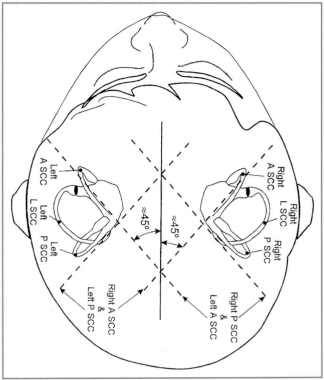

FIGURE 2–4. Orthogonal or coplanar relationship of the semicircular canals showing the orthogonal planar relationship of the right anterior and the left posterior canals (RALP plane), the left anterior and the right posterior canals (LARP), and the right and left horizontal canals. From Barin, K. & Durrant, J. (2000). Applied physiology of the vestibular system. In P. R. Lambert & R. F. Canalis (Eds.). *The Ear: Comprehensive Otology*, Philadelphia, PA, Lippincott Williams & Wilkins. Reprinted with permission.

another (Figure 2–4). Due to the slightly less than perfect orthogonal relationship between the three canals, as well as the functional implication that head or body movements occur rarely, if ever, in a single plane of motion, excitation of a single crista ampullaris from a distinct vestibular labyrinth is highly unlikely (Barin & Durrant, 2000). Therefore, it is almost certain that a neural synapse occurs from two, if not all three cristae ampullari, during normal daily activities.

Semicircular Canal Ampullaris (Cupula)

Each SCC crus arches approximately 240° (Gulya, 1997), and is marked by two distinct ends, a closed amupullar end and an open end. The open end of each SCC crus articulates with the common vestibule of each labyrinth and allows for free endolymph flow in and out of each SCC. The open

end of each *horizontal* SCC articulates directly with the vestibule, however, the open ends of the *anterior* and *posterior* SCCs first form a common crus before communicating with the vestibule. The opposite end of each SCC crus, known as the ampulla, is a distended or bulbous portion and is approximately twice the diameter of each SCC arching crus (Gulya, 1997). Each ampullated end is "occluded" by a fluid-tight partition known as the cupula (Figure 2–5). The cupula is a gelatinous mass with approximately the same density as the surrounding endolymph. The cupula is held tight against the entire ampullar lumen, forming a fluid-tight diaphragm. Although the cupula is

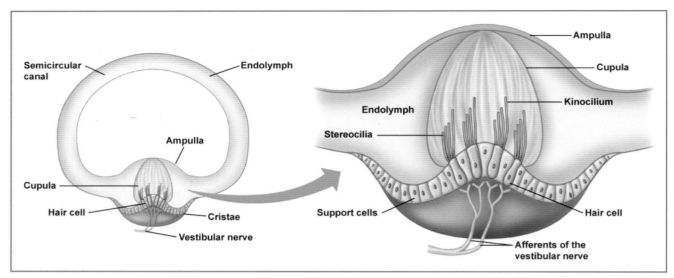

A

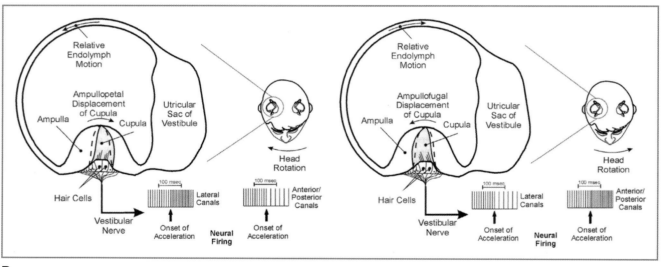

B

FIGURE 2–5. **A.** Semicircular canal cupula forms a fluid-tight partition against the surrounding walls of the ampullar ending of each semicircular canal. Embedded within each cupula are a number of stereocilia bundles that deflect in response to angular acceleration of the head in space. From *Principles of Human Physiology* (6th ed.) (p. 323) by C. L. Stanfield, 2017, Pearson Education. Reprinted with permission. **B.** Deflection of the fluid-tight cupula and underlying stereocilia bundles via head rotation creates either an excitation or inhibition response. From Barin, K. (2009). Clinical neurophysiology of the vestibular system. In Katz et al. (Eds.). *Handbook of Clinical Audiology* (6th ed.). Baltimore, MD: Lippincott Williams & Wilkins.

not structurally attached to the ampullar lumen, the opening is "sealed" by the cupula due to cellular turgor pressure (Lysakowski et al., 1998). The density matching of the cupula to the surrounding endolymph is critical so as not to exert a resting force on the sensory epithelium embedded within the cupula due to a potential negative gravity vector that could be applied during certain orientations of the head in space.

Crista Ampularis and the Semicircular Canal Neurosensory Epithelium

Beneath the cupula, and forming the floor of the ampulla, is the crista ampullaris, which houses the neurosensory epithelium containing the sensory hair cells and stereocilia bundle that are ultimately responsible for creating the neural synapse to the VIII CN (see Figure 2–5). Stereocilia bundles project through the cuticular plate of each sensory hair cell, and are embedded into the gelatin mass of the surrounding cupula. A single stereocilia bundle is comprised of approximately 100 to 200 stereocilia and a single kinocilium that are linked together with microtubules known as tip-links (Gacek, 2005). Orientation of the kinocilium, in relation to the stereocilia bundle, is dependent on each SCC. The kinocilium of the horizontal SCC is located on the side of the crista closest to the vestibule, whereas the kinocilium of the anterior and posterior SCC is located on the side of the crista closest to the canal (Lysakowski et al., 1998). Orientation of the kinocilium is critical, as deflection of the kinocilium toward or away from the stereocilia will determine the type of polarization, or bioelectric response that is applied to the underlying vestibular hair cell (see Figure 2–6). Deflection of the stereocilia bundle toward the kinocilium causes a depolarization of the underlying hair cell and results in a transduction of potassium cations into the hair cell. As described by Harsha, Phillips, and Backous (2008), this influx causes a positive deflection of the resting membrane potential of the hair cell, and a subsequent opening of the voltage-gated calcium channels at the basal-lateral aspect of the cell. Subsequently, there is an influx of calcium and an increase in

the release of excitatory neurotransmitter glutamine, which leads to an increase in the firing rate of the afferent vestibular neurons. Deflection of the stereocilia bundle away from the kinocilium causes a hyperpolarization of the underlying hair cell and results in an inhibitory bioelectric response (Barin & Durrant, 2000). A subsequent decrease in the action potentials of the synapsing afferent vestibular nerve fibers ensues (Figure 2–6).

Stereocilia deflection toward or away from the kinocilium occurs in response to angular accelerations within the plane of a particular SCC. Free-flowing endolymph lags behind and exerts a hydrodynamic pressure against the cupula. Consequently, the cupula is deflected by the lagging endolymph flow in the direction opposite head rotation. The resulting displacement of the embedded stereocilia bundle, either toward or away from the kinocilium, polarizes the underlying sensory hair cells. Depending on the induced polarization, an excitatory or inhibitory neural synapse is applied to the afferent vestibular nerve fibers (see Figure 2–6).

Coplanar Semicircular Canal Physiology

Each of the three semicircular canals is oriented in such a way that the polarization of a particular crista ampullaris from one otic capsule has an antagonistic, yet *complementary*, polarization from a SCC in the opposing otic capsule. As a result, when depolarization (excitation) of a particular SCC occurs from the right otic capsule, hyperpolarization (inhibition) occurs from the complementary SCC in the left otic capsule (Baloh & Honrubia, 1998) (Figure 2–7). The horizontal semicircular canals are complements of one another. However, due to the orthogonal relationship of the SCCs, the posterior and anterior canals of opposing otic capsules are complements of one another. The anterior canal in one otic capsule is oriented in the approximate plane as the posterior canal in the opposite otic capsule. This orientation is often referred to as coplanar (Baloh & Honrubia, 1998) (see Figure 2–4). Specifically, the right anterior semicircular canal is aligned with the left posterior canal, which is often referred to as the

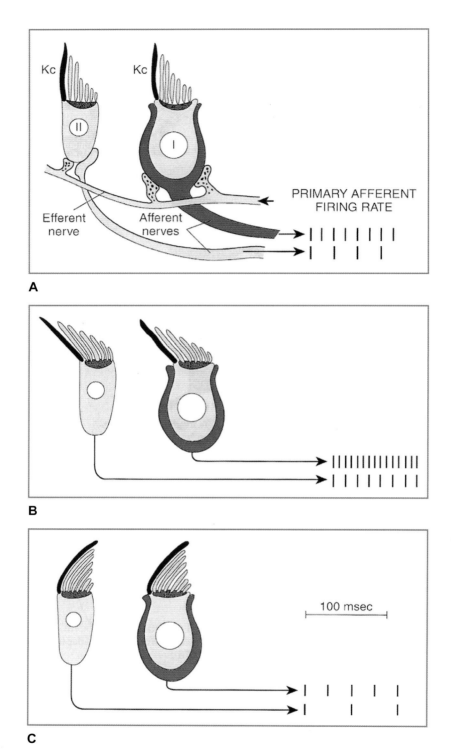

FIGURE 2–6. Semicircular canal cupular deflection causes a subsequent deflection of the underlying stereocilia embedded within the cupula. **A.** At rest (no head movement) the underlying resting neural potential (firing rate) is approximately 90 spikes per second. **B.** Deflection of the kinocilium away from the stereocilia bundle causes depolarization of the hair cell and a subsequent increase in the resting neural firing rate above the resting neural rate of 90 spikes per second (excitation). **C.** Deflection of the kinocilium toward the stereocilia bundle causes polarization of the hair cell and a subsequent decrease in the resting neural firing rate below the neural resting rate of 90 spikes per second (inhibition). From *Baloh and Honrubia's Clinical Neurophysiology of the Vestibular System* (4th ed.) by R. W. Baloh, V. Honrubia, and K. A., Kerber, 2011, New York, NY, Oxford University Press. Reprinted with permission.

34

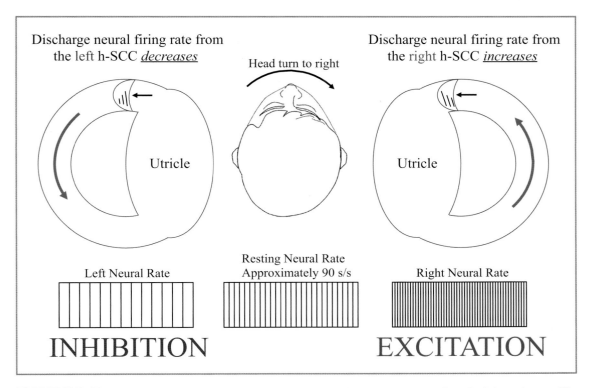

Discharge neural firing rate from the left h-SCC *decreases*

Head turn to right

Discharge neural firing rate from the right h-SCC *increases*

Utricle

Utricle

Left Neural Rate

Resting Neural Rate
Approximately 90 s/s

Right Neural Rate

INHIBITION

EXCITATION

FIGURE 2–7. Image depicting left and right deflection of the cupulae and underlying stereocillia within the horizontal semicircular canals in response to a right head turn. Green arrows depict the direction of endolymph flow. Deflection of the right cupula is toward the utricle (ampullopetal stimulation), which causes deflection of the stereocilia toward the kinocilium, and a subsequent increase in the neural firing rate. Deflection of the left cupula is away from the utricle (toward the canal (or ampullofugal stimulation), which causes deflection of the stereocilia away from the kinocilium, and a subsequent decrease in the neural firing rate. Adapted from Barin, K. & Durrant, J. (2000). Applied physiology of the vestibular system. In P. R. Lambert & R. F. Canalis (Eds.).

RALP plane of excitation/inhibition. Conversely, the left anterior semicircular canal is aligned with the right posterior canal, which is often referred to as the LARP plane of excitation/inhibition. The same is true of the opposing right and left horizontal semicircular canals (see Figure 2–4). It is this coplanar orientation that is often referred to as a push-pull arrangement insomuch that one SCC is always excited as its opposing complement is always inhibited (see Figure 2–7). The advantages of this push-pull arrangement are threefold: (1) It allows for a more effective functional recovery, or compensation, if damage is to ever occur in one labyrinth, (2) It also allows for a greater neural disparity between the two labyrinths than if each were operating independent of one another or

with similar polarizations, and (3) It offers a physiological redundancy that allows for detection of head movement despite a diseased labyrinth due to the inhibition (decrease) of neural activity from the intact labyrinth (Gacek, 2005). Each of these is discussed in greater detail later.

Cupular Physiology and the Cupular Pendular Model of Semicircular Canal Function

The primary function of the cupula and the embedded neural sensory epithelium of the semicircular canals are to mechanically integrate angular head movement, specifically acceleration, into an afferent neural response, which will ultimately be encoded into an eye velocity response. The mechanical properties of the cupula have been likened to a dampened torsional pendulum within the ampulla whose displacement from the hydrodynamic pressure form the free-flowing endolymph within the membranous canal can be mathematically described and predicted (by the pendular model of cupular mechanics) (Baloh & Honrubia, 1990; Leigh & Zee, 2006). In response to head accelerations, the viscoelastic cupula is displaced (deflected) within the ampulla, and subsequent shearing of the embedded stereocilia occurs. Any changes in head acceleration will continuously alter the mechanical properties of the "pendular" cupula, causing a continuously changing neural signal being delivered to the afferent nerve fibers. Because of this, the cupula has often been referred to as an accelerometer, as it detects and monitors changes in head or body accelerations. It has been reported that the SCCs are exquisitely sensitive to head accelerations as small as 0.1° per second squared. This equates to the completion of a single 360-degree rotation in approximately 90 seconds (Harsha et al., 2008). In addition, the operating frequency range of the sensory epithelium of the semicircular canals is between 0 to 20 Hz, which is well beyond the 1 to 6 Hz functional range of everyday life activities (Schubert & Shepard, 2008). Under constant and sustained velocity (*unchanging* acceleration), however, the viscoelastic properties of the cupula become significant and cause it to return to its resting position with an exponentially decaying time course (in accordance with the pendular model). Although cupular time decay has not directly been measured in humans, it is estimated to be around 6 seconds (Leigh & Zee, 2006). In other words, it takes approximately 6 seconds for the viscoelastic cupulae to return to their resting position following an abrupt acceleration, despite ongoing constant velocity. This pendular model of cupular mechanics is well known and reflects how the vestibular system responds to accelerations and not velocity. Consequently, the pendular model of cupular mechanics also forms the mathematical prediction construct for understanding normal vestibular physiology, as well as vestibular pathology (Leigh & Zee, 2006).

OTOLITH RECEPTORS

The otolith sensory receptors, collectively known as the maculae, are comprised of the utricle and the saccule. The utricles are located directly behind the ocular orbits, whereas the saccules are positioned essentially behind the maxillary sinuses (Figure 2–8). The orientation of the utricle and saccule within each otic capsule is roughly in the horizontal and vertical planes, respectively (Figure 2–9). The maculae are anatomically oriented such that each otolith's epithelium is positioned at approximately 90 degrees (or right angles) to one another. As the semicircular canals are responsible for sensing angular acceleration, the otolith sensory receptors are responsible for sensing translational accelerations in the linear plane. Specifically, each otolith receptor is described as being a curved-shaped sac that senses gravitational, linear, tangential, and centripetal forces during head movement (Leigh & Zee, 2006).

Utricle Anatomy

The utricle is an oddly shaped elliptical tube that is tilted backward and downward by 25 to 30 degrees, and laterally by about 10 degrees (Figure 2–10). This orientation is nearly identical to the orientation of the horizontal SCC. Since normal head position tilts the stereotactic plane by about 25 degrees with the chin downward, both of these structures are normally positioned in the plane of their maximum sensitivity during daily life activities (Schwarz & Tomlinson, 2005). This is in accordance with Ewald's first law, which states that maximum afferent excitation (and inhibition) will occur in the spatial plane of the particular semicircular canal being stimulated. Although Ewald's law describes semicircular canal function, a similar (although more complex) pattern can be derived from utricular stimulation.

The utricle contains the sensory epithelium that transduces horizontal linear accelerations into neural afferent signals. Also located within the utricular sac is the open end of the h-SCC crus, as well as the common crus opening of the a-SCC/

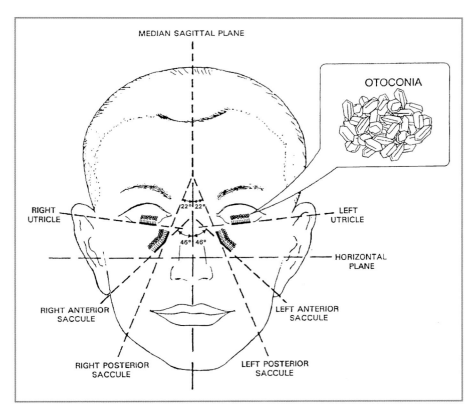

FIGURE 2–8. Anatomical location and orientation of the maculae with respect to the head in the upright position. Dashed lines further indicate the relative orientation of each semicircular canal. Inset image depicts the otoconial layer with respect to the surface of each maculae. From *The Physiology of the Vestibuloocular Reflex (VOR)* by B. Cohen and T. Raphan, 2004, New York, NY, Springer. Reprinted with permission.

p-SCC. Here, endolymph flows freely between the nonampullated ends of each SCC crus and the utricle. Within the utricular space on the anteroinferior wall lays the utriculo-endolymphatic valve from which extends the endolymphatic duct, which terminates in the endolymphatic sac. The valve is believed to act in a passive manner to release excess endolymphatic pressure (Gulya, 1997).

Saccule Anatomy

The saccule is a flattened sac that lies in the vertical parasagittal plane, with its lower end deflected laterally by about 18° (Schwarz & Tomlinson, 2005). It lays inferiorly and at an approximate right-angle to the utricle (see Figures 2–8 and 2–10). Of particular note to saccular anatomy is its proximity to the cochlea. Of all the vestibular sensory end organs, the saccule endolymphatic space is the only one to communicate directly with the cochlea via the ductus reuniens (see Figure 2–1). The saccule and utricle are connected via the utricular and saccular duct. The saccule contains the sensory epithelium that transduces vertical linear accelerations into neural afferent signals.

Otolith Orientation

The orientation of the otolith receptors in space is critical to understanding their physiological

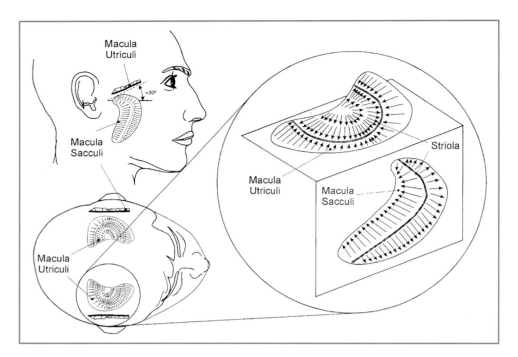

FIGURE 2–9. Anatomical location and orientation of the maculae with respect to the horizontal plane. Arrows indicate the direction of the kinocilium with respect to the stereocilia bundle, as well as the direction of linear force responsible for hair cell excitation. From *The Ear: Comprehensive Otology* by Barin, K. & Durrant, J. (2000). Applied physiology of the vestibular system. In P. R. Lambert & R. F. Canalis (Eds.). Philadelphia, PA, Lippincott Williams & Wilkins. Reprinted with permission.

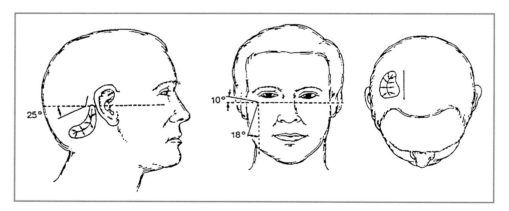

FIGURE 2–10. Planar orientation of the maculae with respect to the horizontal plane. Respective degrees of anatomical position are detailed in sagittal and coronal view. From *Physiology of the Vestibular System* by Schwarz, D. W. F., and Tomlinson, R. D., 2005. In Jackler and D. E. Brackman, (Eds.), *Neurotology* (2nd ed.) (p. 96), Philadelphia, PA, Elsevier Mosby. Reprinted with permission.

function. Given each end organ's orientation in space, the saccule is positioned in such a way that it responds to the omnipresent presence of grav-ity, craniocaudal motion of the head, and linear acceleration in the inferior-superior (vertical) vector. The utricle is oriented nearly horizontally, and thus detects head tilt, anterior-posterior (horizontal) head acceleration, and lateral-linear (side-to-side) head acceration (Harsha, Phillips, & Backous, 2008). Simply put, the saccule responds to vertical linear accelerations and the utricle responds to horizontal linear accelerations.

Otolith Sensory Epithelium

The microstructure and sensory epithelium of the otolith receptors found in both the utricle and saccule are extremely complex. It is similar to that of the semicircular canals insomuch that each contains a network of sensory hair cells containing tip-linked stereocilia bundles and a single kinocilium (Harsha et al., 2008). In addition, each otolith receptor contains a gelatinous mass extending from the cuticular plate, known as the otolithic membrane. Similar to the cupula, the kinocilium and stereocilia are embedded within this gelatinous membrane. This gelatinous mass, however, differs greatly from that of the cupula located within each SCC. The otolithic membrane is a complex tri-membrane layer that is approximately 35 µm thick (Harsha et al., 2008) and contains superficial gravity-sensitive calcium deposits on the upper-most layer, known as otoconia (see Figure 2–11). Harsha and colleagues (2008) provide a detailed description of the otolithic membrane. In their report, they indicate that the bottom gel layer is roughly 10 µm in thickness and contains the embedded cilia of the vestibular hair cells. The middle layer of the membrane, also approximately 10 µm thick, is a mesh layer that is hypothesized to disperse the local shearing forces of the otoconia. The uppermost otoconial layer is approximately 15 µm thick. The otoconia are calcite (or calcium carbonate) salt crystals of varying sizes (0.5 to 30 µm) and shapes that have a density of 2.7 g/cm^3, twice the specific gravity of endolymph (Harsha et al., 2008). Specifically, otoconia are made of calcium carbonate ($CaCO_3$) combined with several ear-specific glycoproteins, known as otoconins (Söllner & Nicolson, 2000). The most common glycoproteins associated with calcite (calcium carbonate) are known as otoconin-90 (Wang et al., 1998) and otoconin-95 (Verpy, Leibovici, & Petit, 1999).

The otolithic membrane and its otoconial layer provide the means by which mechanical translational forces are ultimately transduced into afferent vestibular neural signals. The gravity-sensitive, otoconia-rich membrane, having roughly twice the density of the surrounding endolymph, creates an inertia-responsive environment (Harsha et al., 2008). As a result, the membrane effectively lags behind any gravitational, linear, tangential, or centripetal forces produced during head movement (Figure 2–11). This lag in response to "linear" acceleration creates a shearing force in the direction of gravity, or opposing inertia, which, in turn, produces a shearing force of the underlying mesh and gel layer of the otolithic membrane, and a consequent displacement of the embedded stereocilia and kinocilium. Subsequent displacement of the stereocilia bundles create a hyperpolarization (inhibition) or depolarization (excitation) of the underlying sensory hair cell and a resultant change in the action potential of the afferent neural fibers of CN VIII (Harsha et al., 2008).

Macular Kinocilium Arrangement

The maculae do not exhibit the exact push-pull, orthogonal co-planar arrangement that exists between the vertical semicircular canals. That is, the right utricle does not have a complementary, whole-organ polarization that is opposite to the left saccule. However, there is evidence to support a complementary functional relationship between similar-maculae; that is between the right and left utricles or similarly between each saccule (Leigh & Zee, 2006). Each macula is regionally "divided" into two halves, or hemimaculae, the medial and lateral hemimaculae. The hemimaculae are demarcated by an area of smaller dense otoconia that traverse along the center of each macular sensory epithelium known as the striola (see Figures 2–9 and 2–12). Strong evidence supports a complementary "coplanar" arrangement of opposing hemimaculae between like-otolithic organ receptors (Leigh & Zee, 2006). The distinct advantages of this hemimaculae "coplanar" arrangement are complex and significant, and are discussed in detail later.

Kinocilium arrangement within each hemimacula is oriented with respect to the striola for

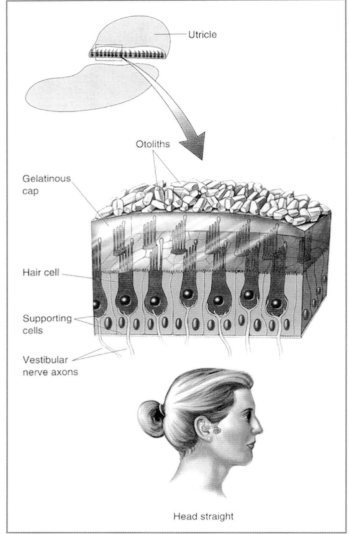

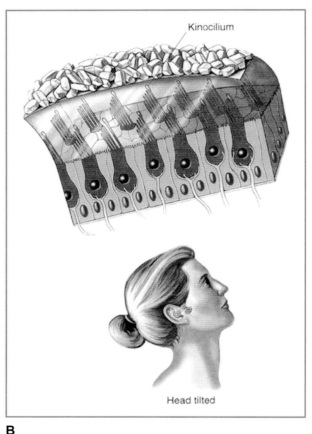

A   **B**

FIGURE 2–11. A. Cross-section of the utricle showing the tri-layer matrix containing the supporting cell layer, the gelatinous layer, and the uppermost otoconial layer. Embedded within the supporting cell and gelatinous layer are vestibular type I and type II hair cells. **B.** Macular physiology depicting the shearing of underlying stereocilia bundles secondary to the gravity-sensitive otoconial matrix. A similar displacement of the utricular epithelium will occur in response to forward and lateral linear displacement. From *Neuroscience: Exploring the Brain* (4th ed.) by M. F. Bear, B.W. Connors, and M.A. Paradiso, 2016, Philadelphia, PA, Wolters Kluwer. Reprinted with permission.

each otolith receptor. In the utricle, the kinocilium is oriented toward the striola, as opposed to the kinocilium in the saccule, which is oriented away from the striola (see Figure 2–9). One primary advantage of this hemimacular arrangement is that each otolith receptor has a sensory epithelium arrangement and kinocilium orientation that allows for both hyperpolarization (inhibition) and depolarization (excitation) within a *single* macula

receptor. Subsequently, any linear force and subsequent uniform displacement of the kinocilium and stereocilia across the entire surface of each otolith receptor causes both an excitatory and inhibitory response within each labyrinth (Leigh & Zee, 2006). This arrangement not only allows for redundancy within the vestibular system, but also facilitates effective macular compensation (Leigh & Zee, 2006). This is because each otolith macula

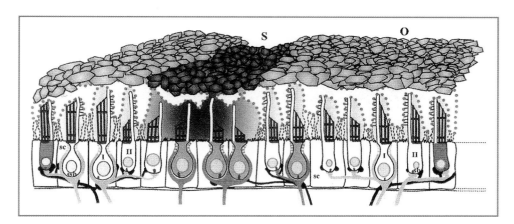

FIGURE 2–12. Transverse section of the mammalian utricle. The utricle is centrally divided by the striola (S), and is flanked by hair cell bundles with opposite polarization. Central striolar hair cells are dominated by type I hair cells (*blue*), whose kinociliae are not embedded within the otoconia cellular matrix (*red dotted line*). The peristriolar and extrastriolar regions are dominated by type II hair cells (*red*), whose kinociliae are embedded within the otoconia matrix. Otoconia saturate the epithelial surface, and are smaller and more dense in the striolar region. From *The Mammalian Otolith Receptors: A Complex Morphological and Biomechanical Organization* by A. Sans, C. J. Déchesne, and D. Demêmes, 2001. In P. Tran Ba Huy and M. Toupet. (Eds.), *Otolith Function and Disorders* (p. 10), New York, NY. Karger Publishers. Reprinted with permission.

is able to function independently, regardless of the status of the opposing receptor.

Otolith Hair Cell Receptor Properties

The anatomical and physiological properties that exist in the maculae are far more complex than those of the cupulae (see Figure 2–12) (Gretsy, 1996).

First, each macula's sensory epithelium contains an inverse polarization of stereocilia bundles. Second, there exists a morphologic segregation of type I and type II hair cells across the neurosensory epithelium (Figure 2–13). Third, there exists a secondary segregation of nerve endings and subsequent neural firing patterns across the neurosensory epithelium (Gresty, 1996). Fourth, it has also been shown that the stereocilia located in the medial and peripheral extrastriolar regions are significantly longer than those located directly within the striola (Sans, Dechesne, & Demémes, 2001). Fifth, there is almost no subcupular meshwork in the striola, creating an environment where the shorter stereocilia bundles are free, and subsequently lack any coherence with the otoconia membrane (Lim, 1984). These findings

led Lim (1984) to conclude that [type I] hair cells in the striolar region are likely highly specialized insomuch that their response (deflection) would be predicated more so from endolymph drag, rather than the sheering force of the otoconia matrix. In light of this, the striolar type I hair cells would, therefore, be more sensitive to velocity rather than displacement. Finally, Raymond and Demémes (1983) provide evidence to support that a greater number of efferent synapses are located in the medial and peripheral zones of the utricle than those found in the striolar region (see Figures 2–12 and 2–13). They concluded that this likely represents a greater degree of efferent "sensory control" that occurs in the extra-striolar zones than those [afferent] synapses located in the striolar zones. Sans et al., (2001) further summarize the complex macular physiology. They highlight the fact that the more centralized hair cells located in the striolar zone would be greatly sensitive to the displacement of endolymph that would result in the sensory cells rapidly sending a phased message to the central nervous system, via large-caliber (type I) fibers. Sans and colleagues (2001) continue to indicate that,

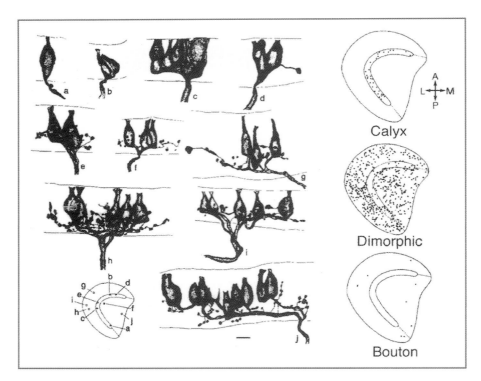

FIGURE 2–13. Morphological organization of the different afferent neural fibers and synapses for the utricle. Large calyx nerve endings synapse with type I hair cells in the striolar region, whereas smaller bouton endings synapse with type II hair cells that are more commonly located in the extrastriolar regions. Medium-sized dimorphic endings are located throughout the striolar and extrastriolar regions. Location of each hair cell type and nerve ending type are not exclusive to each region, but rather more commonly found within each region. There exist more pronounced physiological differences between the large irregular type I afferents, located in the striolar region, than those type I afferents found in the periphery of the epithelium. From *Morphophysiology of the Vestibular Periphery* by A. Lysakowski, and J. M. Goldberg, 2004. In A. M. Highstein, R. R. Fay, and A. N. Popper (Eds.), *The Vestibular System* (p. 97), New York, NY, Springer-Verlang. Reprinted with permission.

this message would be extensively refined and regulated by feedback controls originating from the short loops involving both the type I sensory cells and the calyces, and the intraepithelial afferent networks carrying messages between the neighboring macular units. The extrastriolar zones would be sensitive to the relative displacement of the otoconial membrane with regard to the hair bundles. The sensory cells contacted by fibers of medium or small diameter would send an essentially tonic message to the central nervous system, mostly regulated by a long loop involving the central efferent neurons. (p. 12)

Macular Epithelial Physiology

There are distinct differences in morphologic and physiologic properties across various epithelial regions within each macula. This is particularly relevant when one considers the sensitivity and responsibility that each epithelial region has with respect to the detection and vectors of specific types of linear accelerations. Collectively, the different anatomical properties of the medial, lateral, and central striolar regions of each macula would undoubtedly process the same linear acceleration differently (Sans et al., 2001). Therefore, one could assume that the regional differences, defined by the striola within each macula, would dictate distinct functional differences. This is, in fact, true. The opposing kinocilium arrangement between the medial-lateral hemimaculae delineated by each striola creates a distinct and complex division of physiological response properties specific to each hemimaculae (Leigh & Zee, 2006). Moreover, given the curvature of the striolae, one could also consider how the striola not only delineates a medial and lateral hemimaculae, but also creates a frontocoronal plane, that is sensitive to linear accelerations in the dorsoventral (front to back) plane. For example, each utricle is characterized by a striola that traverses dorsal-ventrally before turning medially toward midline (Figure 2–14) (Barin & Durrant, 2000). Furthermore, it is also well known that the anterior portion of the utricle is bent upward in order to optimize sensitivity in the supine or prone position (Schwarz & Tomlinson, 2005) (Figure 2–14). This upward deflection in the epithelium would likely contribute to additional, and unique, response properties of the utricle that have yet to be fully elucidated. This would be particularly true for sheer forces in the dorsoventral plane of excitation, especially during upright (seated) posture such as those experienced during many amusement park rides. Overall, it is important to understand that, because of this distinct hemimaculae arrangement, concomitant with the fact that the maculae, themselves, are not perfectly aligned elliptical end-organs that are not oriented in purely a vertical or horizontal plane, any linear force will likely cause highly complex sheering patterns across each maculae.

In light of the asymmetrical non-planar surface of the maculae, in combination with the non-linearity (curvature) of the striolae and the differentiated hair cell type morphological arrangement across the epithelium, one can begin to grasp the complexities of the macular neurophysiological response. This complexity undoubtedly produces hair cell activation along multiple linear vectors within the horizontal, and vertical planes, that inevitably would lead to extremely complex neural and ocular responses (Barin & Durrant, 2000). This would likely include linear sensitivity to forces in not only the medial sagittal plane, but also in the dorsoventral plane that may polarize specific hair cell groups located within the anterior and posterior sections of the utricle. Overall, the neural response from the various epithelial regions across each macula (as well as the extrastriolar versus striolar regions) of the saccule and utricle would differ greatly depending on the direction and type of (clinical) force applied to the head. Understanding these differences and how each macula responds to different linear accelerations and head tilts is critical when assessing and interpreting macular-ocular reflexes. Clearly, it becomes imperative for clinicians to understand the morphological and physiological differences of the maculae if one is to effectively and accurately administer, as well as interpret, tests of otolithic function. In Chapter 4, we will detail the discrete maculo-ocular responses (VOR) that are produced from

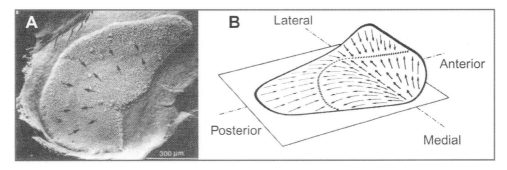

FIGURE 2–14. Utricle epithelial layer (**A**) and anatomical plane of the utricle in relation to the horizontal plane (**B**). From *Biomechanics of the Semicircular Canals and Otolith Organs* by R. D. Rabbitt, E. R. Damiano, and J. W. Grant, 2004. In S. M. Highstein, R. R. Fay, and A. N. Popper (Eds.), *The Vestibular System* (p. 181), New York, NY, Springer-Verlang. Reprinted with permission.

each hemimaculae (medial and lateral). Let us now consider some of the specialized afferent neural properties associated with the maculae.

Macular Afferent Neural Properties

The various afferent properties of the maculae further add to the complexity of the otolith system. Intracellular recordings from individual otolith receptor hair cells indicate a preferential response to precisely defined directional forces (Halmalgyi & Curthoys, 2007). Each otolith hair cell receptor is selectively tuned to a preferred direction of linear force, and any deviation from this vector causes a progressive degradation of the neural response. This morphology produces a polarization differential across each macula to assist in refinement of linear force detection from all directions. Halmagyi and Curthoys (2007) explain the complex nature of the microenvironment of the maculae. Across the epithelium of each macula,

> . . . receptor hair cells are arranged in a regular fashion across each macula so that the direction of the kinocilium of each cell shifts in direction by only a small amount relative to its neighbors, with the result that there is a highly ordered arrangement of polarization vectors across each macula. (p. 146)

Ultimately, such directional sensitivity is afforded by the arrangement of the kinocilium, which is governed by the striolae, which, in and of themselves, are not linear displaced along the maculae, but rather curved (see Figure 2–9).

Otolith hair cell receptor afferents exhibit three additional physiological properties that further refine their response characteristics. First, the hair cell receptor afferents show a polarization preponderance such that the afferent firing rate in the excitatory direction is inherently more robust than in the inhibitory direction. Second, the hair cell receptor afferents show a directional preponderance such that a greater number of otolith afferents respond to ipsilateral directed forces than contralateral directed forces. This is particularly true of the utricle where a 3:1 ratio exists to better refine ipsilateral directed linear forces (Halmagyi & Curthoys, 2007). Third, otolith hair cell receptor afferents exhibit either a regular or irregular firing rate (even at rest). The response

characteristics of each are unique such that regular afferents respond best to maintained forces and then slowly adapt. Conversely, irregular afferents respond best to abrupt forces and then quickly adapt (Goldberg & Fernandez, 1982). The opposite is, therefore, true; irregular afferents respond poorly to maintained forces, (such as sustained head tilts or eccentric rotations), and regular afferents respond poorly to abrupt linear forces. The various response characteristics and specific relationships between afferent response rates and hair cell properties are discussed in greater detail toward the end of this chapter when discussing *tuning of vestibular afferents*. For now, it is important to understand that these particular response characteristics offer a tremendous advantage such that functional specialization to different linear forces are occurring at the *peripheral* level, even prior to further refinement by the central nervous system (Goldberg & Fernandez, 1982). This functional and neurophysiological specialization further contributes to the complexities and challenges associated with the clinical assessment and interpretation of maculae responses.

The Role of the Otolith Receptors in the Detection of Linear Forces

The otolith receptors are responsible for a variety of important postural, ocular, and autonomic reflexes. First, and most notably, the otoliths are responsible for the perception of linear acceleration and gravitational tilt (Gresty & Lempert, 2001). The otolith receptors continuously and collectively integrate the omnipresent gravitational vector upward with linear accelerating forces to determine the new "uprightness" about which a body must balance, both at rest and in motion. An example of this occurs in response to the maintenance of one's balance on an accelerating platform, such as that of a departing train. The degree of body weight thrust forward is dependent on the direction and speed of platform acceleration, as well as the perceived upward acceleration vector that the otoliths must account for due to gravity. The body must be brought into parallel with the vector sum of gravity, plus the exact platform acceleration via vestibulospinal reflexes. A second role of the otolith receptors is the coordination of a series of autonomic reflexes, particularly the regulation of respirations, as well as blood pressure, and heart rate (Yates, Aoki, & Burchill, 1999). This autonomic reflex is known as the pressor response. Finally, the otoliths are responsible for compensatory eye and head movements in relation to specific postural changes (Gresty & Lempert, 2001). Together, these compensatory reflexes provide a sense of spatial orientation. However, the perception of spatial orientation involves more than just the otolith receptors. The somatosensory and visual systems have also been shown to exhibit a significant influence on the integration of otolith signals (Berthoz & Rousié, 2001; Lackner, 1988; Van Nechel, Toupet, & Bodson, 2001). The influence from these systems is significant to postural stability and will now be briefly discussed.

Role of the Otoliths in the Perception of Transduction Forces (Linear Acceleration and Gravitational Tilt)

The otolith system is responsible for the detection of three distinct types of motion perception, as well as the coordination of appropriate compensatory eye movements in response to these motions. Depending upon the transduction vector, a particular macula is responsible for the perception of linear acceleration of the head and/or body in the vertical and/or horizontal planes. Second, the maculae are responsible for the perception of static displacement or tilting of the head in the roll, pitch, or yaw axes. Finally, the otolith receptors are responsible for the perception of gravity, which creates an ever-present downward pull on the maculae. However, the sheering of the maculae hair cell receptors in response to this downward pull of gravity is equivalent to an ever-present linear acceleration in the upward direction (Tran Ba Huy & Toupet, 2001). The sensitivity of the maculae to detect changes in linear acceleration and head tilt has been determined to be as low as a fraction of one centimeter per second squared (Berthoz & Rousié, 2001), to as much as five centimeters per second squared (Gretsy & Lempert, 2001; Gianna, Heimbrand, & Gretsy, 1996). The latency of detection is dependent on the perception of a linear acceleration versus a dynamic head tilt; 20 ms to as great as 300 ms, respectively. Most perceptions of linear or tilt changes generate a compensatory response of the head or eyes to maintain postural or gaze stability. These compensatory responses occur in the form of automatic reflexes known as macular ocular reflexes, which is the third fundamental role of otolith function. The maculo-ocular reflexes are discussed in Chapter 4.

Effect of the Otolith Neurophysiology on Autonomic Reflexes

It is known that the vestibular system has a direct influence on the body's autonomic system. The vestibular system's ability to induce a visceral response is noted throughout the literature. Clinically, this may be best exampled by the nausea that is associated with the onset of vertigo, or by a subsequent migraine that is clinically provoked during vestibular testing. Such visceral responses have also been shown to be associated with otolith stimulation. Yates and colleagues (1999) demonstrated a provocation of a pressor response in individuals receiving brief linear accelerations. These authors documented an elevation in blood pressure and heart rate for approximately 10 seconds following a 1- to 2-second linear acceleration. They determined that the observed pressor response was likely otolith in origin because it was largely diminished in patients with bilateral vestibular loss. Yates and his colleagues conjectured that this response is vital to an autonomic response, which is critical when preparing the body for appropriate countermeasures when a quick linear acceleration occurs. In addition, Yates and colleagues (1999) hypothesized that this may be the reason that bilateral vestibular-loss patients feel faint when they quickly move, or suffer vertigo because they lack the autonomic preparatory response from the otoliths that would trigger the appropriate change in blood pressure and heart rate needed to counteract the abrupt change in linear acceleration.

Effect of the Somatosensory System on Otolith Receptors

It has been shown that the somatosensory system has a significant influence on the otolith system's ability to accurately integrate linear accelerations and static head tilts. Ross (1989), and Ross, Crickmar, and Sills (1969), determined that the presence of somatosensory cues is highly dependent on the otoliths to provide an accurate perception of spatial and vector orientation. In these studies, the masking of somatosensory cues proved to be highly detrimental to the accurate perception of spatial and linear perception. In addition, Aoki, Ito, and Burchill (1999) demonstrated a significant increase in tilt perception, by as much as 10°, when vibrations were introduced to the somatosensory system. Finally, Lackner (1988) showed an aberrant perception of subjective tilt when simple pressure was applied to subject's feet. In these experiments, vision-denied subjects perceived a change in their body orientation to that of earth-vertical axis (upright) rotation when pressure was applied to their feet, even though the subjects remained rotating about the earth-horizontal axis.

Effect of the Visual System on Otolith Receptors

It has also been shown that the visual system has a significant influence on the otolith system's ability to accurately represent linear accelerations and static head tilts. Bischof (1974) demonstrated that, the degree to which an image is viewed in relation to a background's representation of true-vertical, can significantly increase the variability associated with one's perception of *subjective* visual vertical. In addition, Berthoz and Rousié (2001), and Van Nechel and colleagues (2001) reported on the significant influences and integration of visual and vestibular memory on one's ability to accurately represent linear acceleration and static tilt perception.

Effect of the Smooth Pursuit Neural Substrate on Otolith Receptors. There is some evidence to suggest that a robust otolith response may show a dependence on a visual stimulus, and may in fact, be routed through the smooth pursuit neural substrate (Gresty & Bronstein, 1992). Evidence shows that patients with lesions of the brainstem and cerebellum, causing localized smooth pursuit deficits, exhibit reduced otolith VOR sensitivity (gain). In fact, the reduced gain in such patients is similar to otolith gain measured in the absence of any visual signal, providing evidence to support that neural "tuning" of the otolith VOR is likely regulated by similar brainstem pathways that

govern ocular smooth pursuit (Gresty & Bronstein, 1992). Gresty and Bronstein suggested that this correlative evidence, supporting a neural substrate codependency between otolith and smooth pursuit pathways, could be critical to understanding the relationship between disorientation (and even vertigo) reported by patients with CNS findings and a concomitant isolated otolith disorder. Anastasopoulos, Haslwanter, Fetter, and Dichgans (1998) discuss the relative importance of the nodulus and uvula of the cerebellum as a possible anatomical governing "link" that connects the otolith to the smooth pursuit pathways. Waespe, Cohen, and Raphan (1985) offered some of the first evidence that lesions of the cerebellar nodulus and uvula in primates abolishes the otolithic process of velocity storage 'dumping' of postrotatory vestibular nystagmus, as well as the elimination of steady-state otolith nystagmus during off-vertical-axis rotation. Both of these outcomes measures are discussed in greater detail in Chapter 7 and Chapter 8, respectively. Although other research has corroborated that the smooth pursuit pathways are integral to the proper functioning of the otolith response, the extent of codependency and synergistic influence continues to remain uncertain (Hashiba, 2001; Hashiba et al., 1995; Meng, Green, Dickman & Angelaki, 2005).

CRANIAL NERVE VIII

The eighth cranial nerve is comprised of the cochlear nerve and the vestibular nerve (see Figure 2–1). On its most basic anatomical level, CN VIII innervates the cochlea and vestibular end organs and, from there, course medially through the internal auditory canal (IAC) and cerebellar pontine angle (CPA) cistern before innervating brainstem structures. As it courses through the IAC, it is accompanied by cranial nerve seven (CN VII), which is also known as the facial nerve.

The Internal Auditory Canal

The internal auditory canal lies in the medial aspect of the petrous portion of the temporal bone and is an osseous opening through which the seventh and eighth cranial nerves, as well as the labyrinthine artery and vein, enter and exit the posterior cranial fossa. It lies medial to the vestibule and roughly in the same plane as the external auditory canal, with an average length of 8 mm (Guyla, 2007). Prior to entering the lateral aperture of the IAC, the anatomical position of the vestibular nerve is such that it occupies the posterior half, whereas the cochlear nerve occupies the anteroinferior portion, and the facial nerve occupies the remaining anterosuperior quadrant (Baloh & Honrubia, 2001). The coursing of the vestibular, cochlear, and facial nerves medially through the IAC is more complex as the various cranial nerves are noted to twist and fuse during their migration through the internal auditory canal and into the posterior fossa. Guyla (2005) further details that such rotation and fusion of the VII-VIII CN-complex results in the facial nerve assuming a position superior to the cochlear nerve. Such information of the medial IAC anatomic locus of the VII-VIII CN-complex is useful, particularly during vestibular nerve section surgeries. However, Guyla (2007) indicates that such morphological distinctions are less reliable in tumor work, where considerable displacement can distort the expected anatomy. Overall, the implications of the "twisting" of each respective nerve can be significant, particularly when considering the precise location of any neoplastic pathology that could originate within the IAC and impact neural function, such as from vestibular schwannomas.

The Vestibular Nerve

The vestibular nerve is comprised of bipolar neurons with peripheral and central processes. The ganglia cells of these bipolar neurons are located in Scarpa's ganglion, surrounded by cerebral spinal fluid in the internal auditory canal (Gacek, 2005). These bipolar neurons are first-order neurons that connect the vestibular sensory end organs with the central vestibular nuclei located within the brainstem. The vestibular nerve is estimated to have anywhere between 15,000 and 25,000 nerve fibers (Schubert & Shepard, 2008). The vestibular nerve is further identified as having two distinct divisions: the superior branch, and the inferior branch (see Figure 2–1). These two branches are

responsible for innervating the five vestibular sensory end organs: three SCCs and two otolith receptors. The superior branch of the vestibular nerve innervates the crista of the anterior and horizontal SCC, as well as the macula of the utricle and the superior portion of the saccular macula. The inferior branch of the vestibular nerve innervates the crista of the posterior SCC and the inferior portion of the saccular macula (Guyla, 2005).

The coursing of vestibular afferent nerve fibers is well known. From each sensory end organ's basal epithelium, a group of singular (afferent and efferent) unmyelinated nerve fibers innervate the type I and type II hair cells. Just prior to crossing through the lamina cribrosa, the singular nerves become myelinated and fuse into their respective branch of the vestibular nerve at Scarpa's ganglion, just inside the medial end (fundus) of the internal auditory canal.

Vestibular Nerve Spontaneous Firing Rate

One of the most significant discoveries regarding vestibular nerve physiology occurred in 1932. At the Physiological Laboratory of Clark University in Worcester, England, Dr. Hudson Hoagland measured a spontaneous neural activity from the afferent nerve fibers from the lateral line of the fish (Baloh & Honrubia, 2001). This spontaneous resting neural activity of the vestibular nerve was later confirmed in all hair cell systems and is particularly fundamental to the understanding of vestibular physiology. A spontaneous resting neural firing rate allows for an increase (excitation) in neural firing rate secondary to depolarization of the sensory hair cell, as well as a decrease (inhibition) in the neural firing rate secondary to hyperpolarization of the sensory hair cell. Spontaneous resting neural discharge rates of the vestibular nerve vary in humans, but have been measured from as few as 10 spikes per second to as many as 100 spikes per second (Goldberg & Fernandez, 1975). The mean firing rates in the nerve supplying the cristae are somewhat higher than those of the maculae; 90 and 60 spikes per second, respectively (Gacek, 2005). Because of the spontaneous neural firing rate, angular acceleration in any direction causes both an excitatory and inhibitory response due to the coplanar relationship of the SCCs. Thus, in response to a single head turn, a depolarization of type I and type II vestibular sensory hair cells occurs from the *leading* vestibular labyrinth, which creates a subsequent increase in afferent vestibular nerve firing rate. Conversely, a concomitant hyperpolarization of type I and type II sensory hair cells occurs in the opposing (coplanar) labyrinth, which causes an opposite but complementary decrease in vestibular nerve firing rate in the trailing labyrinth. As a result, the overall difference between opposing afferent vestibular neural activity is significantly larger than it would be if inhibition were not possible. The maximal excitatory afferent neural drive is approximately 400 to 500 spikes per second, whereas the maximal inhibitory neural drive is a complete saturation to 0 spikes per second (Gacek, 2005). This difference represents a nearly threefold higher excitatory drive than inhibitory drive. Although this physiological design intentionally creates a larger and more effective vestibular afferent imbalance during natural head movement, the existence of such a high spontaneous resting potential is not without a consequence. Specifically, such a high spontaneous firing rate creates an opportunity for an inconsequential pathophysiologic neural imbalance following unilateral labyrinthine insult. The deleterious implications of such a unilateral destructive event are significant and will be discussed later.

Tuning of Vestibular Afferents

Tuning of vestibular afferents exist within the vestibular nerve; however, the tuning of these fibers is different from that of the cochlear nerve. Evidence shows that vestibular afferents are broadly tuned to acceleration stimuli and respond similarly over a wide range of angular and linear frequencies (Leigh & Zee, 2006). Evidence also shows afferent response gain and phase to be relatively equal across a broad mid-frequency range (e.g., from 0.1 to 1.0 Hz), with an increase in sensitivity at higher frequencies and a decrease at lower frequencies (Highstein, 1996). This sensitivity is likely governed by the type of firing rate generated by the different types of afferents. Calyx nerve endings, associated with type I hair cells and large diameter afferent fibers, exhibit predominantly *irregular* discharge rates and often show no firing while at rest (Baloh &

Honrubia, 2001). Bouton nerve endings, associated with type II hair cells and small afferent diameters, predominantly have *regular* discharge rates with little variability in their tonic neural discharge rate (Baloh & Honrubia, 2001). These regular afferents appear to be fundamentally important to vestibular-ocular reflexes (VOR) because ablation of irregular afferents cause little, if any, effect on the VOR (Minor & Goldberg, 1991; Goldberg, 2000). Irregular afferents, however, may be pertinent to an effective and efficient functioning of the vestibulospinal reflexes (VSR), as well as responding to abrupt acceleration stimuli (Gresty & Lempert, 2001; Hain & Helminski, 2007). A summary of the various properties associated with each type of afferent nerve ending can be seen in Table 2–1.

Vestibular Afferent Neural Projections

Three sizes of afferent vestibular nerve fibers have been identified. Some of the largest afferent nerve fibers in the body (10 µm in diameter) are known to terminate with the larger calyx nerve endings that synapse with type I vestibular hair cells (Baloh & Honrubia, 2001). The smallest afferent nerve fibers (<2.5 µm in diameter) terminate with the smaller bouton nerve endings and synapse primarily with type II vestibular hair cells. Medium-sized afferent nerves (2.5 to 4.5 µm in diameter) terminate on both calyx and bouton nerve endings, and synapse with both type I and type II vestibular hair cells (Baloh & Honrubia, 2001).

Independent of sensory epithelium (cristae ampullari or maculae), the location of each type of afferent nerve fiber is also morphologically dependent (see Figure 2–13). Large fibers terminate predominantly in the center of the cristae, or toward the striola in the maculae, as well as course centrally within each vestibular nerve (Baloh & Honrubia, 2001). Small fibers terminate predominantly in the periphery of the sensory epithelium, and synapse with multiple type II hair cells with smaller bouton nerve endings. Small afferent nerve fibers are also noted to course more peripherally within and along the perimeter of the vestibular nerve (Baloh & Honrubia, 2001). Medium-sized fibers are dispersed evenly throughout the surface of the sensory epithelium and throughout the diameter of the nerve (Baloh & Honrubia, 2001) (see Figure 2–13).

Table 2–1. Differences Between Vestibular Hair Cell and Afferent Nerve Types

Type of Hair Cell	Type I	Type II	Type I & Type II
Type of Nerve Ending	**Calyx Nerve Ending**	**Bouton Nerve Ending**	**Dimorphic Nerve Ending**
Diameter of Afferent Fiber	Large	Medium to Small	Intermediate
Firing Rate	Irregular	Regular	Irregular (central & peripheral) & Regular (peripheral)
Loci of Innervation on End-Organ Epithelium	Central Region	Periphery	Throughout sensory epithelium
Afferent Neural Fiber Organization	Central fibers within the vestibular nerve	Peripheral fibers of the vestibular nerve	Central and peripheral
Sensitivity to Linear Stimulation (Otolith)	Responsive to quick linear translations	Responsive to sustained centrifugal force or head tilt	Quick linear (Type I) Sustained (Type II)
Sensitivity to High Acceleration Angular Stimuli (SCC)	Increased sensitivity to high/abrupt angular acceleration stimuli	Decreased sensitivity to high/abrupt angular acceleration stimuli	Variable sensitivity from central irregulars to peripheral regulars
Contributions to VOR	Minimal (ablation of irregular type I hair cells/ afferent nerve fibers has little impact on VOR response)	Significant	Type I—low sensitivity in central zone; high sensitivity in peripheral zone Type II—significant
Adaptation to Prolonged Stimuli	Fast	Slow	Fast (Type I); Slow (Type II)
Overall Gain	Higher	Lower	
Overall Phasic Responsiveness	More phasic in response	Less phasic in response	
Linearity	Non-Linear	Linear	Non-Linear (Type I); Linear (Type II)
Spontaneous Rate	Low	High	
Second-Order Neuron Innervation	Innervate Large 2nd-order neurons	Innervate Small 2nd-order neurons	
Suppressed by Galvanic Stimulation	Yes	No	
Role(s) of TYPE I Irregular Afferents: VOR adaptation and compensatory responses, especially for high Hz and high velocity rotational stimuli. Modulation of VOR during eccentric rotation. Cancellation of the VOR. Generation of low-Hz, velocity storage component of the VOR. Extend the linear range of the VOR at high rotational accelerations		Role(s) of TYPE II Regular Afferents: Compensatory responses to unilateral labyrinthine lesions for low rotational stimuli. High-Hz, high-velocity, t-VOR.	

Source: Adapted from Baloh & Honrubia, 2001; Goldberg, 2000; Gresty & Lempert, 2001; Leigh & Zee, 2006; Minor & Goldberg, 1990; Ödkvist, 2001.

Superior Branch of the Vestibular Nerve

The superior branch of the vestibular nerve (SBVN) innervates the horizontal and anterior SCC, the utricle, and the anterosuperior portion of the saccule (see Figure 2–1). Upon entering the fundus (medial end) of the IAC, the SBVN begins its course in the posterosuperior position in relation to the cochlear, facial, and superior/inferior branches of the vestibular nerve. Upon exiting the porus oticus, (lateral end of the IAC) the SBVN is oriented in the anterosuperior position (Gulya, 2007).

Innervation of the Horizontal Semicircular Canal. Type I and type II hair cells located in the crista of the horizontal semicircular canal (h-SCC) synapse with afferent projections of the SBVN (Gacek, 2005). Secondary to the arrangement of the kinocilium in both types of hair cells (located on the utricular side of the crista), endolymph flow toward the utricle (also know as ampullopetal flow) causes a depolarization of the sensory hair cells and a subsequent increase in the afferent neural firing rate. Conversely, endolymph flow away from the utricle (also known as ampullofugal flow) in the h-SCC causes a hyperpolarization in the underlying hair cells and a subsequent decrease in the afferent neural firing rate (Lysakowski et al., 1998) (see Figure 2–7).

Innervation of the Anterior Semicircular Canal. Type I and type II hair cells located in the cristae of the anterior semicircular canals (a-SCC) synapse with afferent projections of the SBVN (Gacek, 2005). Secondary to the arrangement of the kinocilium in both types of hair cells, (located on the canalicular side of the crista and opposite that of the h-SCC and utricle), endolymph flow away from the utricle (also known as ampullofugal flow) must occur to cause a depolarization of the sensory hair cells and a subsequent increase in the afferent neural firing rate. Conversely, endolymph flow toward the utricle in the a-SCC causes a hyperpolarization in the underlying hair cells and a subsequent decrease in the afferent neural firing rate (Lysakowski et al., 1998).

Innervation of the Utricle. Type I and type II hair cells located in the macula of the utricle synapse with afferent projections of the SBVN (Gacek, 2005). As cited earlier, due to the co-arrangement of the kinocilium on the utricle epithelium toward the striola, a single translational force subsequently produces both hyperpolarization, as well as depolarization of the underlying hair cells within a single utricular sensory end organ. Therefore, both excitatory and inhibitory signals are sent via the afferent nerve fibers from both utricles during a single translational vector (Leigh & Zee, 2006).

Inferior Branch of the Vestibular Nerve

The inferior branch of the vestibular nerve (IBVN) innervates the posterior SCC and the inferior portion of the saccular macula (Gacek, 2005) (see Figure 2–1). Upon entering the fundus of the IAC, the IBVN begins its course in the posteroinferior position in relation to the cochlear, facial, and superior/inferior branches of the vestibular nerve. Upon exiting the porus oticus, the SBVN is oriented in the anteroinferior position (Gulya, 2007).

Innervation of the Posterior Semicircular Canal. Type I and type II hair cells located in the crista of the posterior semicircular canals (p-SCC) synapse with afferent projections of the IBVN (Gacek, 2005). Secondary to the arrangement of the kinocilium in both types of hair cells, (located on the canalicular side of the crista and opposite that of the h-SCC and utricle), endolymph flow away from the utricle (also known as ampullofugal flow) must occur to cause a depolarization of the sensory hair cells and a subsequent increase in the afferent neural firing rate. Conversely, endolymph flow toward the utricle in the p-SCC causes a hyperpolarization in the underlying hair cells and a subsequent decrease in the afferent neural firing rate (Lysakowski et al., 1998).

Innervation of the Saccule. Type I and type II hair cells located in the inferior macula of the saccule synapse with afferent projections of the IBVN (Gacek, 2005). As previously discussed, due to the arrangement of the kinocilium on the saccule epithelium away from the striola, a single translational force subsequently produces both hyperpolarization, as well as depolarization of the underlying hair cells within a single saccular sensory end organ. Therefore, both excitatory and inhibitory signals are sent via the afferent nerve fibers from both sacculae during a single translational vector.

Vestibular Efferent Neural Projections

Peripheral vestibular efferent nerve fibers originate in the vestibular nuclei within the brainstem and accompany the cochlear efferent fibers within the olivocochlear bundle. From Scarpa's ganglion, the vestibular efferent fibers join each division of the vestibular nerve and innervate type II sensory hair cells within the sensory epithelium of the cristae and maculae. Although speculation exists as to the exact function of the efferent system, its primary role remains elusive (Schwarz & Tomlinson, 2005).

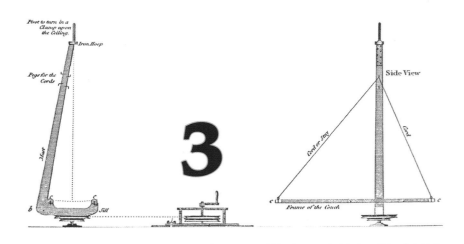

Anatomy and Physiology of the Central Vestibular System, Velocity Storage, and Central Compensation

ROLE OF THE CENTRAL VESTIBULAR SYSTEM: AN OVERVIEW

The central vestibular system is complex in form and in function. It is comprised of some of the largest nuclei in the central nervous system, and collectively integrates millions of neural signals from the peripheral vestibular system, visual system, somatosensory system, cerebellum, and postural reflex system every second of the day. It is responsible for generating and coordinating key postural and visual reflexes for the maintenance of balance and visual fixation. In addition, it has an integral and complex sub-network of commissural neural fibers, known as the velocity storage mechanism, which augments weak peripheral inputs, and assists in the adaptation of peripheral vestibular damage. This central mechanism also allows for the compensation of vestibular pathology and rebalancing of asymmetric vestibular inputs.

TRANSITION BETWEEN PERIPHERAL AND CENTRAL VESTIBULAR ANATOMY

The transition zone between the peripheral and central vestibular system occurs at the neuroglial-neurilemmal junction within the IAC near the lateral aperture (or otic porus) (Nager, 1993). This transition zone is significant as myelination converts from peripheral neuroglial cells, known as Schwann cells, to central neuroglial cells, known as oligodendrocytes. Upon exiting the medial aperture of the IAC, the now fused superior and inferior braches of the vestibular nerve course through the cerebellar pontine angle cistern where most afferent nerve fibers enter the brainstem at the rostral medulla (Gacek, 2005). The vestibular nerve courses medially, passing between the inferior cerebellar peduncle and the descending tract of the trigeminal nerve prior to entering the vestibular nuclei (Lysakowski et al., 1998). Here, ascending and descending vestibular neural fiber tracts innervate the central vestibular nuclei. A smaller subset of afferent fibers directly innervates the cerebellum (Gacek, 2005). From the vestibular nuclei, an extremely complex arrangement of afferent and efferent projections coordinates postural stability and visual stabilization. Projections from the vestibular nuclei are numerous and innervate many central nervous system ganglia and neural centers. On a gross anatomical level, the vestibular nuclei integrate signals form the peripheral vestibular end organs with those from the spinal cord, cerebellum, visual system, and the contralateral vestibular nuclei. More specifically, the vestibular nuclei project to the ocular motor nuclei (oculomotor, abducens, and trochlear nuclei), reticular and spinal centers concerned with skeletal movement, the vestibular regions of the cerebellum (flocculus, nodulus, ventral paraflocculus, and ventral uvula), as well as the thalamus and hippocampus. In addition, each vestibular nucleus has major projections to the opposing contralateral vestibular nuclei (Goldberg & Hudspeth, 2000). An overview of the vestibular nuclei and the key central structures involved in vestibular processing is illustrated in Figure 3–1.

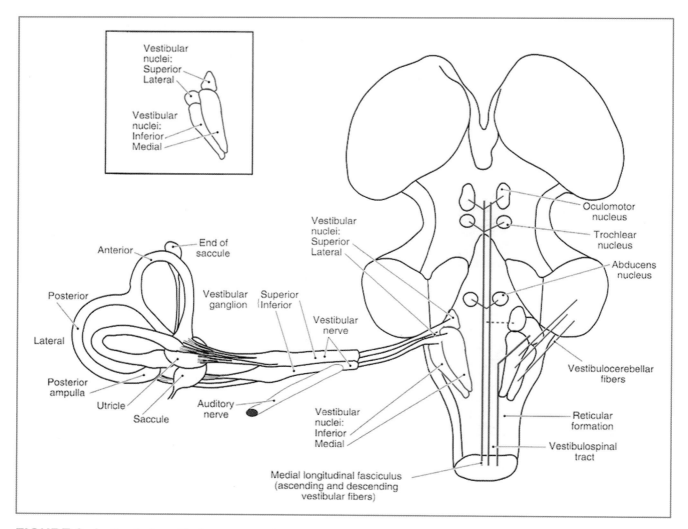

FIGURE 3–1. Central vestibular system, showing the four vestibular nuclei (*inset box*) and their respective orientation within the brainstem. The primary ocular motor nuclei (Oculomotor, Trochlear, and Abducens) are also respectively identified, in addition to the primary vestibular brainstem tracts (Vestibulospinal Tract and the Medial Longitudinal Fasciculus or MLF). The superior and inferior branches of the vestibular nerve are seen innervating the vestibular nuclei. From *Neuroscience for the Study of Communication Disorders* (4th ed.) by A. C. Bhatnagar, 2013, Baltimore, MD, Lippincott, Williams & Wilkins. Reprinted with permission.

FUNDAMENTAL ROLE OF VESTIBULAR NUCLEI

The fundamental role of the vestibular nuclei is the integration of head, neck, and trunk movements in order to coordinate an appropriate and compensatory eye movement or postural response (Lysakowski et al., 1998). The coordinated eye movement occurs in the *opposite* direction of head movement, but at a velocity that is (ideally) equal to head movement. This ensures that the visual system can maintain stabilization of an image on an extremely small area of the retina known as the fovea. In fact, clarity of an image significantly deteriorates even if the intended image was to "slip" 1° to 2° from the center of the fovea (Wong, 2008). For best visual clarity, it is imperative that images be held stable within 0.5° of the center of the fovea (Wong, 2008). If this process does not occur, or fails to occur efficiently, an inadvertent slip of the image will occur on the retina and cause significant blurring or even "visual jumping" of the image and visual scene during active head movements (this is known as oscillopsia) (Leigh & Zee, 2006). A primary and fundamental basis of vestibular anatomy and physiology is critical to the understanding of this compensatory process. The neural foundation of the compensatory eye movement is a three-neuron reflex pathway known as the vestibular-ocular reflex (VOR) (Leigh & Zee, 2006). This reflex is discussed in length in Chapter 4. The importance of understanding the VOR in association with its peripheral and central structures is vital for understanding and interpreting most vestibular testing. Three primary central vestibular structures are essential to generating the VOR, namely the vestibular nuclei, the cerebellum and central commissural neural tracts.

VESTIBULAR NUCLEI

The vestibular nuclei are subdivided into four distinct large nuclei, which are anatomically segregated with respect to their functionality and labeled with regard to their mutual anatomical position with respect to one another (Figures 3–1 and 3–2). The vestibular nuclei complex encompasses the superior nucleus (of Bechterew), the lateral nucleus (of Deiters), the medial nucleus (of Schwalbe), and the inferior nucleus (or descending nucleus) (Leigh & Zee, 2006). Several other minor nuclei cell groups, most notably the Y-group, have also been identified as being a part of the vestibular nuclei complex.

Superior Vestibular Nucleus

The superior vestibular nucleus (SVN) is located dorsally and rostrally in the vestibular complex (Lysakowski et al., 1998). The SVN is topically organized. That is, most first-order afferent nerve fibers of large to medium diameter innervate the center, whereas smaller diameter fibers innervate the periphery of the SVN (similar to the innervation pattern of the peripheral end organs and vestibular nerve branches) (Lysakowski et al., 1998). The majority of afferent fibers within the SVN originate from the crista of the SCCs (see Figure 3–2). A few fibers from the otolith macula have been identified in the lateral aspect of the SVN. Other than vestibular afferents, another major group of fibers terminating in the SVN originate from the cerebellum. (Baloh & Honrubia, 2001).

Efferent second order neurons from the SVN predominantly ascend through the medial longitudinal fasciculus (MLF) and the ascending tract of Dieters to innervate the ocular motor nuclei (Leigh & Zee, 2006). In light of these innervations, the SVNs primary role is that of maintaining and coordinating visual stabilization (ocular reflexes) in response to head movement, thus forming a critical neural center to the VOR arc.

Lateral Vestibular Nucleus

The lateral vestibular nucleus (LVN) is located inferior to, and at the caudal end of the SVN. Primary afferents that terminate within the LVN originate primarily from the cerebellum, predominantly the vermis and fastigial nuclei (Lysakowski et al., 1998). Few neurons within the rostroventral portion of the LVN receive vestibular afferents from the cristae as well as the maculae, suggesting some involvement in maintaining the VOR (Leigh & Zee, 2006) (see Figure 3–2). A lesser number of

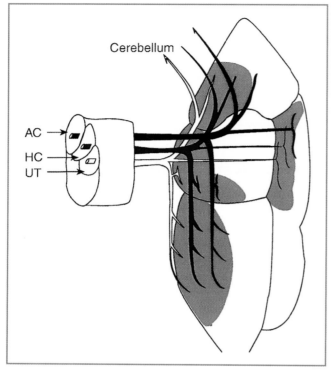

A

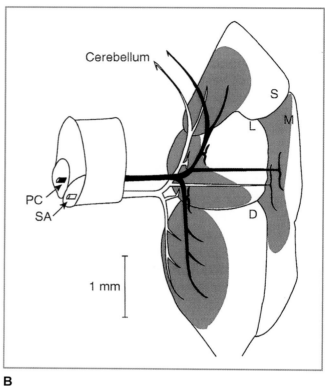

B

FIGURE 3–2. Central vestibular nuclei (VN), showing the four vestibular nuclei [Superior VN (S); Lateral VN (L); Medial VN (M); Descending or Inferior VN (D)]. The primary afferent vestibular nerve branch divisions are differentiated between the Superior Nerve Branch (**A**), and Inferior Nerve Branch (**B**). The Superior Nerve Branch carries neural information the vestibular nuclei from the Anterior SCC (AC), the Horizontal SCC (HC), and the Utricle (UT). The Inferior Nerve Branch carries neural information from the Posterior SCC (PC) and the Saccule (SA). The superior and inferior branch of the vestibular nerve are seen innervating the vestibular nuclei. From *Baloh and Honrubia's Clinical Neurophysiology of the Vestibular System* (4th ed.) by R. W. Baloh, V. Honrubia, and K. A. Kerber, 2011, New York, NY, Oxford University Press. Reprinted with permission.

afferent fibers have been identified to originate from the spinal tract as well as the contralateral vestibular nucleus through commissural fiber tracts (Barin & Durrant, 2000; Leigh & Zee, 2006).

Most of the efferent fibers from the LVN project primarily through the lateral and medial vestibulospinal tracts, suggesting, "an important station for control of vestibulospinal reflexes, particularly those involving the forelimbs" (Baloh & Honrubia, 2001, p. 56).

Medial Vestibular Nucleus

The medial vestibular nucleus (MVN) is located beneath the floor of the fourth ventricle, caudal to the SVN and medial to the LVN (Baloh & Honru-

bia, 2001). The MVN is the largest and most complex nucleus within the vestibular nuclei complex. Its anatomical separation from the SVN is less distinct than any other neighboring nuclei within the complex. It is here where small and medium afferent vestibular fibers from the cristae of the SCCs (see Figure 3–2) as well as from the fastigial nucleus and flocculus of the cerebellum have been identified (Baloh & Honrubia, 2001). Moving ventrally within the MVN, small and medium fibers from both otolith maculae (saccule and utricle) are also found (Lysakowski et al., 1998). Within the caudal and ventral portion, a preponderance of afferent fibers from the fastigial nuclei and nodulus of the cerebellum have been identified. Other afferents of lesser number are found to originate from the contralateral MVN as well as the reticular formation and nucleus prespositus hypoglossi (NPH) (Baloh & Honrubia, 2001; Leigh & Zee, 2006). The MVN-NPH complex plays a critical role in the transformation and maintenance of spatial eye position known as the neural integrator (Hain & Helmisnki, 2007).

Primary efferent fibers from the MVN project through the MLF, the spinal cord, the contralateral MVN, and the cerebellum. In light of these projections, it is suspected that the MVN is a critical center for the coordination of the VOR, central compensation, as well as head and neck movements (Leigh & Zee, 2006).

Inferior Vestibular Nucleus

The inferior vestibular nucleus (IVN) is located lateral to the MVN and inferior to the LVN. Primary afferent fibers from the cristae and maculae terminate in the lateral aspect of the IVN whereas afferent fibers from the cerebellum (flocculus, nodulus and uvula) terminate throughout the IVN (Baloh & Honrubia, 2001) (see Figure 3–2). The IVN has been identified as being a primary receptor of vestibular afferents from the otolith maculae (Lysakowski et al., 1998).

The majority of efferent fibers from the IVN terminate in the cerebellum and the reticular formation with secondary projections to the vestibulospinal pathways (Baloh & Honrubia, 2001; Lysakowski et al., 1998). In light of these efferent projections, the IVN is likely critical for the coordination of postural control through the vestibulospinal reflexes, and the cervicocollic (neck) reflexes.

Y-Group

The Y-group is located caudal and lateral to the SVN, and is bound dorsally by the LVN and ventrally by the inferior cerebellar peduncle (Lysakowski et al., 1998). Many of the afferents originate from the cerebellar flocculus and the saccular macula. Efferent projections from the Y-group nuclei predominantly innervate the cerebellar flocculus and appear to mediate and coordinate vertical eye movements (Lysakowski et al., 1998).

CEREBELLUM

A discussion of vestibular physiology without detailing the cerebellum's relevant contributions would be a significant shortfall. The cerebellum is well known to be a major recipient and propagator of neural fibers both from and to all four vestibular nuclei (Gacek, 2005). In fact, the cerebellum even receives a group of afferent fibers directly from the periphery without first innervating the vestibular nuclei (Barin & Durrant, 2000). The cerebellum is foremost an adaptive processor that monitors vestibular input and readjusts central vestibular processing (output) if necessary (Hain & Helminski, 2007). Interestingly, if the cerebellum were removed, vestibular responses (reflexes) would still occur; however, the responses would be poorly calibrated, ineffective, and extremely inefficient (Hain & Helminski, 2007).

Cerebellar Divisions

The cerebellum consists of the cerebellar cortex and the cerebellar white matter. The cerebellar cortex is comprised of ten distinct lobules that extend outward from the apex of the roof of the fourth ventricle and medially from the midline of the cerebellum known as the vermis; a narrow midline zone coursing the entire sagittal cerebellar plane (Arslan, 2001). These ten lobules are categorized into three primary lobes; the anterior lobe, the posterior lobe, and the flocculonodular lobe. The anterior lobe is comprised of lobules I to V and the posterior lobe is comprised of lobules VI to IX (Figure 3–3A). The flocculonodular lobe is separated by the posterolateral fissure and is comprised solely of lobule X (Figure 3–3B). Beneath the cerebellar cortex is the cerebellar white mat-ter from which axons project ventrally to innervate four deep, bilaterally paired cerebellar nuclei; most important of which are the fastigial nuclei. All ten lobules of the cerebellar cortex project axons to the deep cerebellar nuclei with the exception of the flocculonodular lobe, whose nerve fiber projections course directly to the vestibular nuclei (Brodal, 2004). The axonal projec-

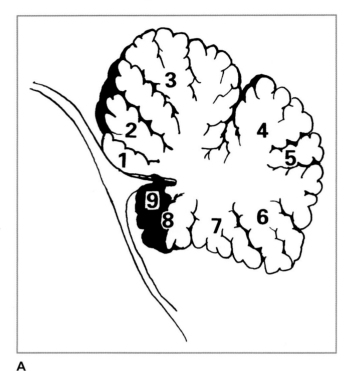

A

FIGURE 3–3. Cerebellum. **A.** Individual labeling of the cerebellar lobules (1 to 9) (sagittal plane). (1) Lingula Cerebelli, (2) Lobulus Centralis, (3) Culmen, (4) Declive, (5) Folium Vermis, (6) Tuber Vermis, (7) Pyramis Vermis, (8) Uvula Vermis, and (9) Nodulus Vermis. From Abolished tilt suppression of the vestibulo-ocular reflex caused by selective uvulo-nodular lesion by G. Wiest, L. Deecke, S. Trattnig, and C. Mueller, 1999, *Neurology* 52(2), 417–419. Reprinted with permission. *continues*

tions from the cerebellar cortex are exclusively handled by a layer of cells known as Purkinje cells (Brodal, 2004). Functionally, the cerebellum is classified into the vestibulocerebellum, the spinocerebellum, and the pontocerebellum with each serving a primary need and responsibility (Arslan, 2001).

Vestibulocerebellum (Lobule X)

The vestibulocerebellum is comprised solely of the flocculonodular lobe (lobule X). The vestibulocerebellum is the most primitive and smallest part of the cerebellum (Brodal, 2004) and is located anteroventrally within the cerebellum just dorsal to the fourth ventricle. The flocculonodular lobe primarily receives neural fibers from the vestibular nuclei as well as directly from the vestibular periphery (Brodal, 2004). The flocculonodular lobe is comprised of the nodulus in the midline and the two flocculi that flank either side (Figure 3–3B). The nodulus, located directly in the midline and anteroventrally within the cerebellum, is actually the inferior most portion of the vermis. Each flocculus is connected via a thin stalk that projects laterally from the nodulus, which

is known as the paraflocculus (Brodal, 2004). As previously stated, the Purkinje cells of the vestibulocerebellum do not have axonal projections to deep cerebellar nuclei, but rather send their axon projections *directly* to the vestibular nuclei (Brodal, 2004). The vestibulocerebellum is therefore critical to the vital components of vestibular physiology and function, including VOR regulation, equilibrium, as well as central compensation (Brodal, 2004). Functionally, the flocculus, the nodulus, and the vermis each have distinct responsibilities.

Cerebellar Flocculus. The overall responsibility of the flocculus is to maintain the gain of the vestibular ocular reflex (Hain & Helminski, 2007). The axonal fibers from the flocculus predominantly terminate in the superior and medial vestibular nuclei. From there, ascending tracts through the longitudinal medial fasciculus project to the ocular motor nuclei which eventually innervate various ocular motor muscles for coordination of eye movement (Arslan, 2001). Therefore, coordination between the flocculus and the vestibular nuclei provide a significant contribution to maintaining an effective and efficient vestibular ocular reflex.

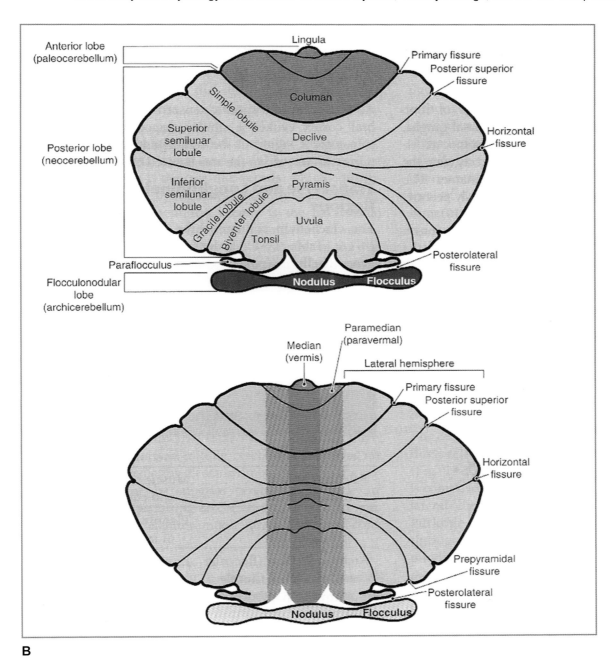

B

FIGURE 3–3. *continued* **B.** Division of lobes and fissures (flattened transverse plane). Flocculonodular lobe is also known as the vestibulocerebellum, which contains the nodulus, as well as the flocculi and paraflocculi. These structures, along with the ventral nodulus, are critical to central vestibular compensation. From *Neuroscience for the Study of Communication Disorders* (4th ed.) by S. C. Bhatnagar, 2013, Baltimore, MD: Lippincott, Williams & Wilkins. Reprinted with permission.

Cerebellar Nodulus. The overall responsibility of the cerebellar nodulus is to adjust the duration/timing of the VOR as well as to process otolith input (Hain & Helminski, 2007). Axonal projections from the nodulus are similar to that of the flocculus with the exception of a further projection to the lateral and inferior nuclei. From there, descending tracts form the vestibulospinal tracts for coordination of posture and equilibrium. In addition, strong evidence supports nodular projections to be critical for restoring and recalibrating central vestibular neural symmetry following insult during central compensation (Leigh & Zee, 2006).

Cerebellar Vermis. The overall responsibility of the cerebellar vermis is to assist in the coordination of the vestibulospinal system for effective and efficient posture and equilibrium (Hain & Helminski, 2007). Purkinje cells of the vermis as well as the anterior and posterior cerebellar lobes have prolific projections to the deep cerebellar fastigial nuclei. From there, main axonal projections bypass the vestibulocerebellum (flocculonodular lobe) and directly terminate in the lateral vestibular nuclei. From there, efferent projections descend through the lateral vestibulospinal tract and innervate the spinal cord (Arslan, 2001; Brodal, 2004). The cerebellar vermis and its efferent projections are subsequently vital for postural control (Brodal, 2004).

Spinocerebellum and Pontocerebellum

Besides the functional capacities offered by the vestibulocerebellum, the cerebellum is further divided into the spinocerebellum and the pontocerebellum (Brodal, 2004). Whereas the vestibulocerebellum is composed of the flocculonodular lobe and nodulus, the spinocerebellum is composed of the entire anterior lobe and the paravermal lobules (intermediate hemispheres) of the cerebellum (Brodal, 2004). The pontocerebellum, or cerebrocerebellum, is composed of all the lateral aspects of the cerebellar hemispheres (Timmann & Diener, 2007). Both the pontocerebellum and the spinocerebellum are named accordingly in light of the heavy axonal projections from the pontine nuclei and the spinal cord, respectively. Although neither contains heavy projections to or from the vestibular nuclei, both are believed to collectively coordinate incoming sensory data with the flocculonodular lobe in order to make continuous and fine adjustments to movement (Timmann & Diener, 2007). The spinocerebellum tracts provide essential data regarding propulsive movements (e.g., ambulation) (Arslan, 2001).

The pontocerebellum and its pontine tracts saltate neural responses from the cerebral motor areas; most notably the primary motor cortex, somatosensory cortex, supplementary motor and premotor areas, the posterior parietal lobes, as well as prefrontal and limbic areas (Timmann & Diener, 2007). Therefore, neural information is inundating the cerebellum and all its functional divisions with sensory data pertaining to the analysis, planning, integration, and initiation of gross and fine motor movements to ensure such movements are performed both smoothly and accurately.

COMMISSURAL VESTIBULAR FIBERS

Vestibular commissural fibers are a critical component to the function and efficiency of the central vestibular system (Barin & Durrant, 2000; Baloh & Honrubia, 2001). The commissural fibers play a significant role in the functioning of the velocity storage mechanism and with central compensation. Most of the commissural fibers arise and terminate within all four vestibular nuclei; however, the superior and medial nuclei receive and send most of the commissural neural tracts, with the superior nucleus comprising the majority (Gacek, 2005). Because the commissural pathways predominantly involve the superior, inferior, and medial vestibular nuclei, by default, the commissural neural activity is primarily provoked from semicircular canal neural input. As we learned in Chapter 2, the primary mechanism for this activity is afforded by the opposite polarity of peripheral hair cells in the cristae. Because maculae have an opposite polarization of the hair cells between the two halves of each sense organ (separated by the striola), commissural projections may not be necessary to produce a differential effect from activation of these sensory end organs (Gacek, 2005).

Although heavy homologous commissural projections are noted between vestibular nuclei counterparts, the existence of many more variable projections between disparate nuclei supports a more complex commissural pathway structure (Lysakowski et al., 1998). Overall, the relative importance and function of these commissural pathways should not be overlooked. The primary role of the commissural pathway is largely inhibitory and compensatory (Curthoys & Halmagyi, 1996; Raphan & Cohen, 1996). The mere existence of a commissural network largely facilitates two of the most significant physiologic attributes of the vestibular system, namely, velocity storage and central compensation (Leigh & Zee, 2006).

Velocity Storage

The following review regarding the anatomical and physiologic processes of velocity storage and central compensation has been synthesized from Curthoys and Halmagyi (1996), Barin and Durrant (2000), Baloh and Honrubia (2001), and Leigh and Zee (2006). Much of what is known regarding normal functioning of the velocity storage mechanism comes from single unit neuron recordings from animals (primarily monkeys, rats, and guinea pigs). The reader is strongly encouraged to review these sources for a complementary and complete physiological understanding of the velocity storage mechanism and its associated neural pathways.

Velocity storage is a process of integration and subsequent preservation and augmentation of afferent signals sent from the various peripheral vestibular sensory receptors. Velocity storage is particularly critical in the central augmentation of low frequency stimuli that would otherwise be too weak to effectively drive the VOR. It is mediated within the vestibular nuclei by the commissural pathways and the cerebellum (Barin & Durrant, 2000; Baloh & Honrubia, 2001). The process of velocity storage is integrated and mediated primarily by specific neuronal cells within the vestibular nuclei (Curthoys & Halmagyi, 2007). These highly specialized neuronal cells are type I and type II neurons. The activation of these central neuronal cells, however, is also heavily dependent upon the peripheral afferent signal from the SCCs and, to a lesser degree, the otoliths (Curthoys & Halmagyi, 2007). Therefore, the functional dependence of the velocity storage mechanism is reliant on adequate peripheral input. When such input is altered, such as from a peripheral vestibular lesion, the velocity storage mechanism responsibility is also modified.

Type I and Type II Vestibular Neurons

There are two types of primary neuronal cells located within the vestibular nuclei complex, type I and type II neurons, (not to be confused with type I and type II peripheral hair cells). These cell types integrate and process the peripheral vestibular sensory input (along with the cerebellum, higher brainstem, and cortical structures) prior to sending efferent responses to the appropriate ocular motor, postural motor, and vestibulocollic motor reflexes. In addition, type I and type II neurons are essential to the velocity storage mechanism as well as ensuring effective compensation for peripheral vestibular disease. Individually, each type of neuron has its own specialized function. Collectively, type I and type II neurons, in association with the commissural fibers, work together to form a complementary neurophysiologic network that is vital to the efficiency of the central vestibular system.

Type I Vestibular Neurons. Within each vestibular nuclei, there exist type I neurons that are specialized to be either excitatory or inhibitory. That is, some type I central neurons are only activated with excitation, whereas others are only activated with inhibition. This is generally dependent on the direction of head rotation, such that rotations in the yaw plane toward the right will activate primary horizontal semicircular canal afferents that project and synapse directly with the appropriate type I excitatory neurons in the right vestibular nuclei. Conversely, type I inhibitory neurons located in the left vestibular nuclei will be simultaneously activated by primary vestibular afferents driven by hyperpolarized (inhibited) hair cells originating from the crista in the left horizontal semicircular canal. Finally, type I neurons also show an indirect synaptic cleft ("connection") with type I neurons located in the contralateral vestibular nuclei through commissural projections (via contralateral type II neurons). As mentioned previously, this commissural network of decussating fibers is extensive and variable, often projecting to or away from their respective homologous contralateral nuclei division. Evidence shows that such commissural projections are inhibitory in nature (Curthoys & Halmagyi, 1996, 2007; Raphan & Cohen, 1996).

Type II Vestibular Neurons. Type II neurons differ from type I neurons is two primary ways. First, while type I neurons are either excitatory or inhibitory, type II neurons are always inhibitory and only receive synaptic projections via the commissural pathways from excitatory type I neurons located in the contralateral vestibular nuclei (Curthoys & Halmagyi, 1996; Raphan & Cohen, 1996). That is, type II inhibitory neurons are solely activated by contralateral excitatory type I neurons via the commissural pathways, (and just to be clear, *activation* of a type II inhibitory neurons refers to the neuron exerting an *increase* in inhibition). The second way type II neurons differ from type I neurons is that type II neurons always form synaptic clefts with neighboring type I excitatory neurons in the *same* vestibular nuclei (Curthoys & Halmagyi, 1996; Raphan & Cohen, 1996). Therefore, type II inhibitory neurons share a rather intimate relationship with type I excitatory neurons, insomuch that they share a direct synaptic cleft with neighboring ipsilateral excitatory type I neurons and also receive direct projections from contralateral excitatory neurons via the commissural pathways, thereby forming an indirect inhibitory "link" between excitatory type I neurons from opposing vestibular nuclei. The normal role of the type II inhibitory neurons is, therefore, to act as a facilitator between type I excitatory neurons from both vestibular nuclei in order to allow indirect inhibition (or even "silencing") of type I excitatory neurons located in the *contralateral* vestibular nuclei (Curthoys & Halmagyi, 1996; Raphan & Cohen, 1996). Of course, it goes without saying that the commissural fiber network plays an integral role in this process. This processes of "commissural inhibition" and the role of the type II inhibitory neurons holds true when referring to the process of velocity storage. However, the role of type II inhibitory neurons changes slightly during the "neural clamping" process that occurs during central compensation (discussed later).

Type I and Type II Vestibular Neurons Complementary Physiology. As previously stated, type II inhibitory neurons are activated solely via the commissural pathways from the contraversive excitatory type I neurons, which are driven by the semicircular canal afferents, (specifically horizontal canal afferents during yaw rotations). In a healthy vestibular system, contraversive type inhibitory II neurons are always activated (exert stronger inhibition) when ipsiversive type I excitatory neurons are activated (Curthoys & Halmagyi, 1996; Raphan & Cohen, 1996). This is critical when considering the relationship of type II inhibitory neurons with neighboring type I excitatory neurons in the same vestibular nuclei. At its most fundamental level, one could argue that it is this relationship that forms the foundation for the mechanism underlying velocity storage: specifically, the further inhibition of the contraversive excitatory type I neurons that are undergoing a transient reduction in the tonic resting neural vestibular firing rate from the periphery due to the activation of contraversive type I inhibitory neurons. Essentially, this serves to *further* lower the tonic neural rate within the contraversive vestibular nuclei in relation to the increased neural rate of the ipsiversive vestibular nuclei. Put simply, type I and type II neurons are complementary with respect to their inhibition and excitation. Overall, this process creates a larger tonic neural disparity between the two vestibular nuclei than would have otherwise existed if it were not for this type I–type II commissural relationship. As previously stated, this process is particularly important for low-frequency acceleration stimuli that would otherwise be too weak to effectively drive a functional VOR.

To summarize the relationship between type I and type II central neurons thus far, let us consider an example. When turning toward the right, type I excitatory neurons located in the right vestibular nuclei are activated by *right* (ipsiversive) horizontal canal afferents, which, in turn, activate type II inhibitory neurons in the contraversive left vestibular nuclei. During the same rotation, toward the right, type I inhibitory neurons in the left vestibular nuclei are activated (Barin & Durrant, 2000; Baloh & Honrubia, 2001; Curthoys & Halmagyi, 1996). Simultaneously, type I *excitatory* neurons in the *contraversive* left vestibular nuclei are *inhibited* by their neighboring type II neurons secondary to activation signals sent via commissural projections from the ipsiversive type I excitatory neurons located in the right vestibular nuclei. This "commissural inhibition" is critical to the process of velocity storage and central compensation. However, this part of the complementary process is only one-half of the "story." The commissural relationship between type I excitatory neurons and type II inhibitory neurons does not end here, and is even more dramatic and complex than presented thus far. Let us now continue to dissect how this commissural relationship forms the basis for the velocity storage mechanism in the process of augmenting a weak neural response.

Velocity Storage Central Mechanism

The complete process of velocity storage involves an intricate, complex, and *cyclical* interaction between the type I and type II neurons within and between the VN, via the commissural fiber network. It is the *cyclical* component to the velocity storage process that we must now discuss. In doing so, we must continue to consider the interaction between type I and type II neurons, and how they form the foundation for the velocity storage mechanism within each vestibular nuclei and across the commissural fiber network.

We have previously discussed how the efficiency of the peripheral vestibular system is frequency dependent. That is, because the cupulae respond to acceleration, low frequency acceleration stimuli are less apt to provoke a robust response than mid-to-high frequency stimuli (greater than 0.05 Hz). However, that is not to say that the vestibular system fails to respond to low frequency acceleration stimuli. In fact, it *is* able to respond to extremely low frequency stimuli. It just so happens that the central processing of this poorly integrated weak peripheral response requires a mechanism by which the impuissant neural response can be "amplified," (not a concept too far different than that of the cochlear amplifier). That mechanism is known as velocity storage.

Velocity storage is critical for the processing and augmentation of the weak neural response produced from low frequency stimuli (in addition to its integral involvement with central compensation). This reliance on the velocity storage mechanism for the processing of low frequency stimuli will repeatedly be highlight during our discussion of sinusoidal acceleration testing as it pertains to low-frequency stimuli in Chapter 6. Let us consider the neurophysiological response to a low frequency angular stimulus applied to the horizontal cristae. A depolarization of the peripheral vestibular receptor causes an increase in the ipsiversive

afferent vestibular neural firing rate, which activates type I excitatory neurons within the ipsilateral VN. The ipsiversive type I excitatory neurons synapse directly with the contraversive type II excitatory neurons via the commissural fibers. Meanwhile, a concomitant and opposite signaling, that originates from the contraversive hyperpolarized horizontal canal afferents, activates type I inhibitory neurons within the contraversive VN.

The activation of the type II inhibitory neurons in the contraversive VN, in combination with the activation of the type I inhibitory neurons, is critical to the augmentation of the weak peripheral input. The increased activation of contraversive type II neurons, via the commissural fibers, provides an *indirect* decrease in the activation of type I excitatory neurons on the hyperpolarization side—that is, type II inhibitory neurons exert increased inhibition on the contraversive type I excitatory neurons. This occurs because the increase in contraversive type II neuron activation (increased inhibition) serves to reduce the excitatory nature of the type I excitatory neurons on the hyperpolarization (inhibition) side, thus creating an even more inhibitory environment. This is particularly true because type I inhibitory neurons are concomitantly creating an inhibitory environment due to the decrease in resting neural tonic activity signaled by the hyperpolarized periphery.

We have now reached a critical point in the neurophysiology of the velocity storage mechanism. The next step is critical, as it pertains to a *further* reduction of the contraversive type I excitatory neurons with a concomitant "augemented" increase in the ipsiversive type I excitatory neurons. This next step in the commissural process causes the neurophysiology of the velocity storage mechanism to become highly efficient in augmenting weak neural responses. Because the contraversive type II inhibitory neurons have reduced the activity of the contraversive type I excitatory neurons, and because these contraversive excitatory neurons have an analogous direct synapse back to the type II inhibitory neurons of the *ipsiversive* side, the decrease in the excitatory activity of the contraversive type I excitatory neurons causes a subsequent *decrease* in the activation of type II *ipsiversive* neurons via the commissural pathways. This decrease in the activation of ipsiversive type II inhibitory neurons (i.e., the neurons are made less inhibitory) serves to *reduce* the inhibition of the ipsiversive type I excitatory neurons, which, in turn, allows them to further *increase* their excitatory nature beyond that which was already produced by the increase in the resting firing rate due to the depolarization of the horizontal canal crista.

Now we have come to a neurophysiologic moment that creates a repeating cycle; a velocity storage cycle (if you will) that effectively can, centrally, augment a weak peripheral afferent signal. As the ipsiversive type I excitatory neurons are centrally driven to a higher tonic level, (due to a decrease in their inhibition, complements of the inhibited contraversive type I excitatory neurons and the commissural fibers), this in turn *further* activates the contraversive type II neurons inhibitory control over the contraversive type I excitatory neurons. This process is similar to that of the start of our discussion regarding the initial commissural interaction between ipsiver-

sive excitatory type I neurons and contraversive inhibitory type II neurons. This process, in turn, creates a repeating effect of decreased activation of ipsiversive type II neurons causing a further increase in ipsiversive type I excitatory neurons, all while, concomitantly creating a centrally increased inhibitory neural-state in the contraversive vestibular nuclei. And the cycle repeats itself. And repeats itself. And repeats itself. And so on. Thereby, creating a positive neural feedback loop.

In summary, ipsiversive type I excitatory neurons increase their tonic activity level by activation from the periphery, in addition to reduced inhibitory control from neighboring ipsiversive type II inhibitory neurons, (via the commissural fibers from the inhibited contraversive type I excitatory neurons). This creates an eloquent synergism between type I and type II central neurons, and is the fundamental neurophysiological structure of the velocity storage mechanism. Figure 3–4 (A–M) complements the previous discussion and

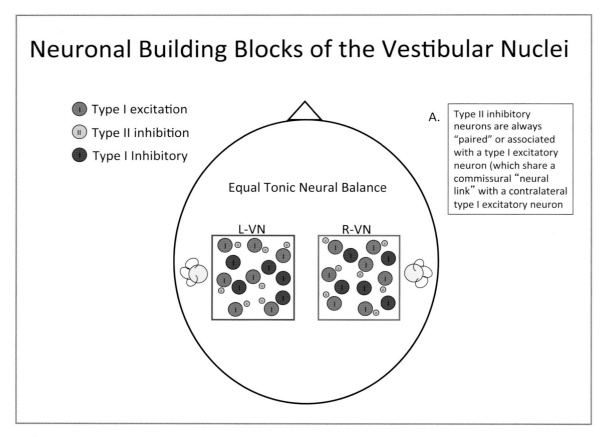

FIGURE 3–4. A–M. Progressive stages associated with process of velocity storage. Large boxes represent the right and left vestibular nuclei. *continues*

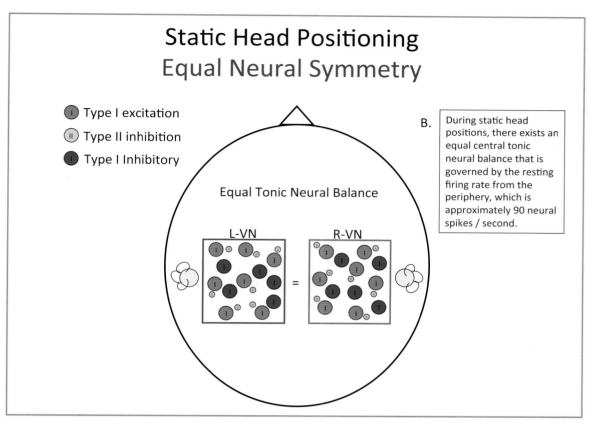

Static Head Positioning
Equal Neural Symmetry

- Type I excitation
- Type II inhibition
- Type I Inhibitory

Equal Tonic Neural Balance

L-VN = R-VN

B. During static head positions, there exists an equal central tonic neural balance that is governed by the resting firing rate from the periphery, which is approximately 90 neural spikes / second.

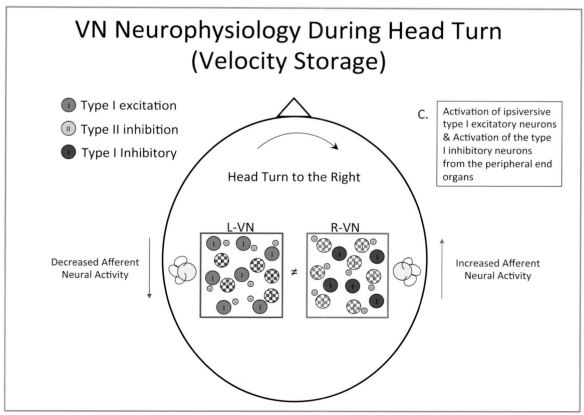

VN Neurophysiology During Head Turn
(Velocity Storage)

- Type I excitation
- Type II inhibition
- Type I Inhibitory

Head Turn to the Right

L-VN ≠ R-VN

Decreased Afferent Neural Activity

Increased Afferent Neural Activity

C. Activation of ipsiversive type I excitatory neurons & Activation of the type I inhibitory neurons from the peripheral end organs

FIGURE 3–4. *continues*

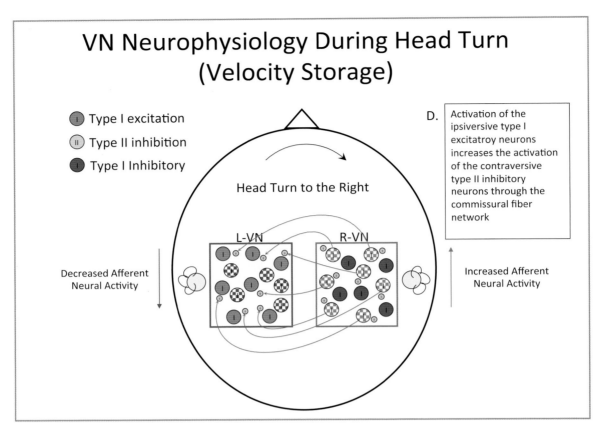

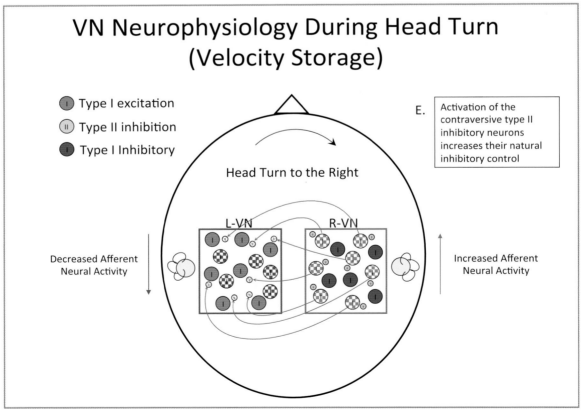

FIGURE 3–4. *continues*

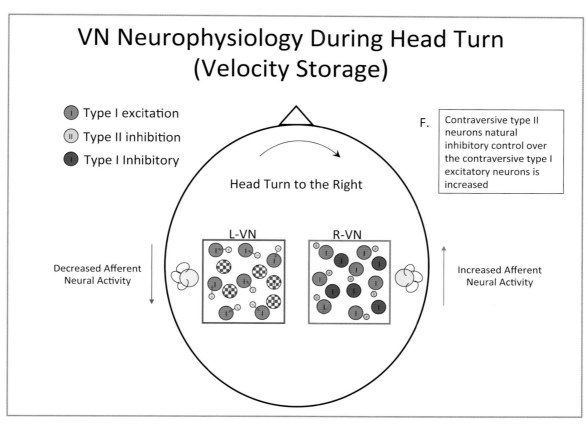

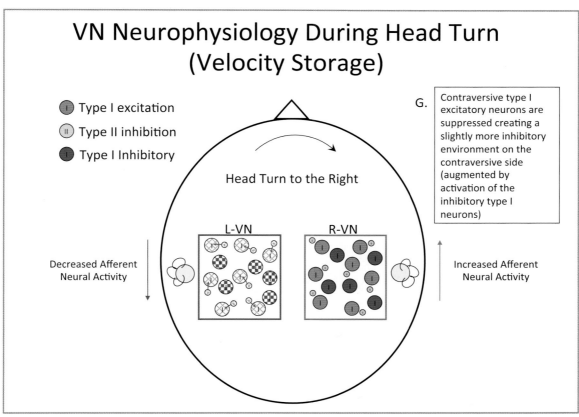

FIGURE 3–4. *continues*

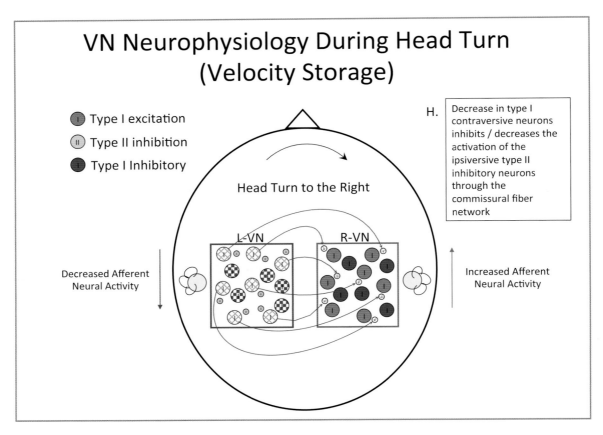

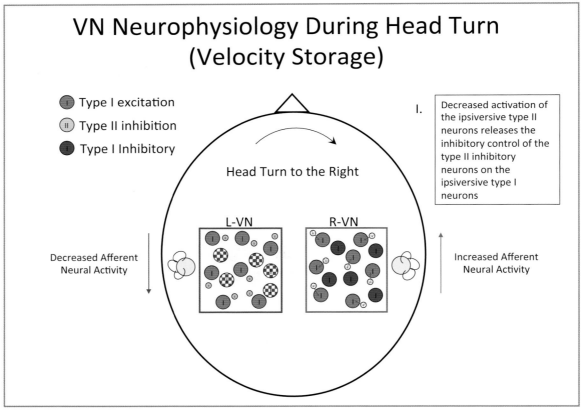

FIGURE 3–4. *continues*

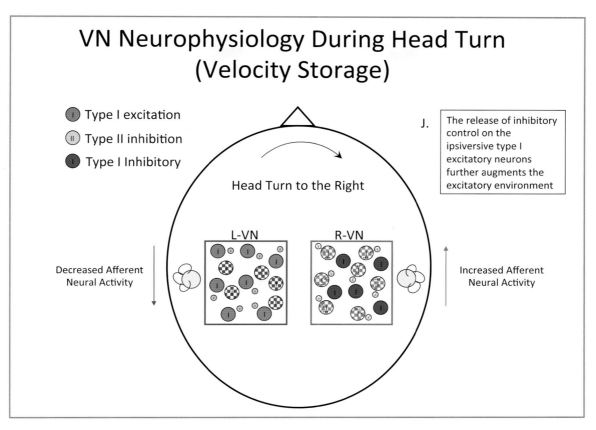

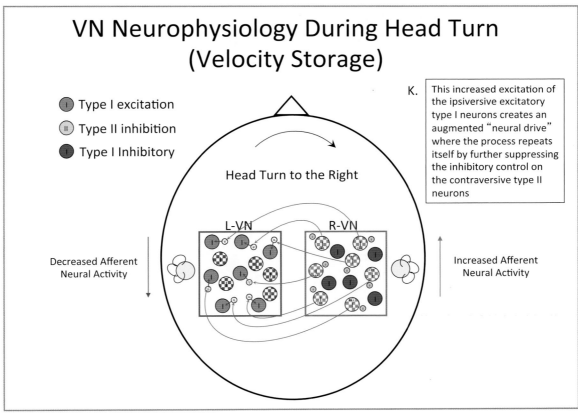

FIGURE 3–4. *continues*

VN Neurophysiology During Head Turn (Velocity Storage)

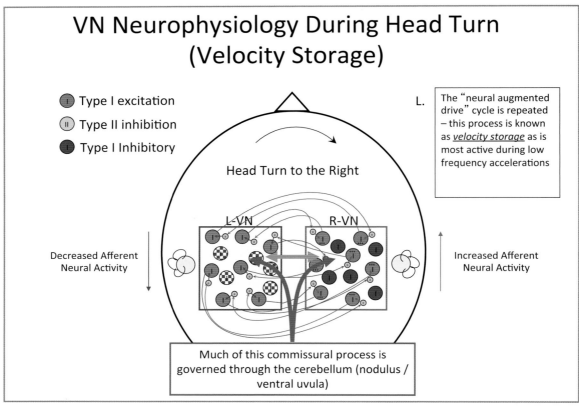

- Type I excitation
- Type II inhibition
- Type I Inhibitory

Head Turn to the Right

Decreased Afferent Neural Activity

Increased Afferent Neural Activity

L-VN   R-VN

L. The "neural augmented drive" cycle is repeated – this process is known as *velocity storage* as is most active during low frequency accelerations

Much of this commissural process is governed through the cerebellum (nodulus / ventral uvula)

VN Neurophysiology During Head Turn (Velocity Storage)

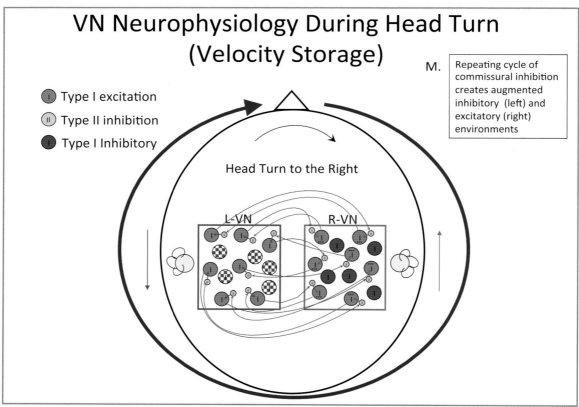

- Type I excitation
- Type II inhibition
- Type I Inhibitory

Head Turn to the Right

L-VN   R-VN

M. Repeating cycle of commissural inhibition creates augmented inhibitory (left) and excitatory (right) environments

FIGURE 3–4. *continued*

illustrates the various stages that occur during velocity storage.

Positive Feedback Loop. This process of afferent augmentation (and preservation of the neural response), however, is not limitless or self-sustaining. Rather, the positive feedback loop is heavily mediated by the nodulus of the vermis and the vestibulocerebellum (Barin & Durrant, 2000; Curthoys & Halmagyi, 1996). Of course, we now know that the net effect of this positive feedback loop effectively augments a weak afferent signal beyond the primary peripheral input and is termed velocity storage (Baloh & Honrubia, 2001; Curthoys & Halmagyi, 2007; Markham, 1996). Augmentation of weak peripheral afferent signals is vital to the accurate perception and integration of low-frequency head movement, or more specifically, low frequency accelerations that are below 0.05 to 0.1 Hz (Highstein, 1996). Fundamentally, the process of velocity storage primarily exists to extend (or increase) the sensitivity (gain) of low frequency stimuli where the effectiveness of the VOR is less efficient in transducing slow acceleration stimuli (Highstein, 1996). This loss of efficiency is primarily due to a decrease in the tuning of vestibular afferents below 0.1 Hz (as eluded to earlier in Highstein, 1996). Although there is some debate as to the degree of functional consequence that exists when the efficiency of the velocity storage no longer exists due to vestibular pathology, this concept is further discussed in Chapter 6.

The dependency on velocity storage mechanisms for stimulus frequencies greater than 0.1 Hz is essentially zero. That is because the cupulae are accelerometers and respond (deflect) well to higher frequency stimuli. As the pendular model of semicircular canal function would dictate, deflection of the cupulae and underlying hair cells for more robust stimuli (>0.1 Hz) produces an afferent neural firing rate (drive) that is sufficient, by itself, to drive the VOR. Therefore, central augmentation is not needed for such mid-to-high frequency stimuli. It is only during low frequency accelerations that velocity storage mechanisms are required to augment an impuissant neural afferent drive that is, otherwise, not an issue with higher (more robust) frequency stimuli. This concept of

the vestibular afferent drive being a frequency dependent system is discussed and detailed again when reviewing VOR outcome measures (specifically VOR phase) during sinusoidal acceleration testing in Chapter 6.

Aside from the velocity storage mechanism extending the sensitivity of low frequency stimuli, this positive feedback loop can also manage tonic neural activity during conditions of *sustained* peripheral input. Most often, the vestibular system is subjected to brief head movements similar to those that occur during ambulation or conversations. However, the peripheral vestibular system can, at times, be subjected to sustained peripheral input such as that during sustained body rotation (figure skater or playing "dizzy bats") or even during amusement park rides. This sustained peripheral afferent input must be appropriately managed by the central system, which also falls under the control of the velocity storage mechanism. As clinicians and researchers, we can also make use of this type of sustained stimulus and response scenario, which we will present in Chapter 7 when discussing velocity step testing.

Velocity Storage Dependency. The synergistic process of velocity storage is complex and highly dependent on the integrity of certain neural processes and anatomical structures. As previously noted, commissural vestibular fibers are undoubtedly essential for this process, because sectioning of commissural fibers abolishes velocity storage (Leigh & Zee, 2006). Also paramount to this process is the effective down-regulation from the cerebellum, most notably from Purkinje cells within the cerebellar nodulus and uvula (Curthoys & Halmagyi, 1996; Highstein, 1996; Leigh & Zee, 2006). Finally, velocity storage is also dependent upon afferent signals from the vestibular periphery sensory end organs. Sectioning of the vestibular nerve or peripheral sensory end organ damage (either unilateral or bilateral) essentially abates velocity storage and significantly shortens the neural output from the VN, similar to that of cupular mechanics or process alone (to be reviewed in Chapter 7 when discussing velocity step testing) (Leigh & Zee, 2006). Collectively, these mechanisms or processes are not only responsible for producing velocity storage but are also essential for ensuring effective compensation of the vestibular neural balance following unilateral vestibular insult.

Vestibular Compensation

Vestibular compensation refers to the restoration of symmetry in the central neural tone between the vestibular nuclei following unilateral peripheral vestibular insult (Barin & Durrant, 2000). On a gross level, central compensation involves a series of steps, or processes, that occur at different rates, and at different degrees and stages. Specifically, static compensation will occur at a much faster rate than that of dynamic compensation, where motion-induced activity on asymmetric labyrinths exponentially complicates the central integration required to achieve and maintain neural rebalancing (Curthoys & Halmagyi, 2007). This is particularly true for low frequency information where velocity storage heavily contributes to the VOR response. Furthermore, the success of vestibular compensation is dependent on a number of physiologic factors. Such factors include commissural efficiency between the vestibular nuclei, effectiveness of cerebellar control (i.e., clamping) of the vestibular nuclei, adaptation of disinhibited contralesional excitatory activity, orbital position, changes in neural activity due to gaze changes, reweighting of spinal inputs, synaptogenesis (slow, long-term process), and denervation sensitivity (slow, long-term process) (Curthoys & Halmagyi, 1996; Zee, 2007). In short, because neurons located within the vestibular nuclei receive so many afferent fibers other than the peripheral vestibular labyrinths (cerebellum, spinal, cortical, brainstem), the processes that modulate and regulate the recovery of neural symmetry are often complicated and sometimes slow to succeed.

Static Compensation

To understand the process of static central vestibular compensation, it is vital to understand the neurophysiologic basis of excitatory and inhibitory interactions of type I and type II neurons within the vestibular nuclei (see discussion on velocity storage). Following acute vestibular insult, the average resting neural discharge rate of the VN on the intact side increases due to the lack of inhibition from the ipsilesional labyrinth (Barin & Durrant, 2000; Curthoys & Halmagyi, 2007). Concomitantly, the higher resting rate of intact VN only serves to further "silence" or inhibit the lesioned side. This, of course, is best illustrated by using the fundamental neurophysiological constructs that we just discussed for velocity storage and the inhibitory commissural network.

Following a unilateral peripheral vestibular lesion, the ipsilesional type I excitatory neurons are substantially reduced. Recalling the direct synaptic projections to the contralesional type II inhibitory neurons, the pathologic reduction of the ipsilesional type I excitatory neurons causes a *decrease* in the activation of the contralesional type II inhibitory neurons (i.e., less inhibitory control). Given the intimate neighboring relationship between the contralesional type II inhibitory neurons and the contralesional type I excitatory neurons, the reduction in activation of the contralesional type II inhibitory neurons (decrease of inhibitory control over the type I excitatory neurons) causes a subsequent increase in the tonic excitation level of the contralesional type I excitatory neurons, *which occurs despite the lack of any head rotation or movement*. This neurophysiologic process is what primarily drives the contralesional side to a higher tonic resting firing rate, some level above the normal 90 neural spikes per second. However, the deleterious and insidious neurophysiologic process is not yet finished. Because the contralesional type I excitatory neurons have now assumed a higher level of tonic activation, they in turn project an increase in activation across the commissural network to the ipsilesional type II inhibitory neurons that are directly synapsed to their neighboring ipsilesional type I excitatory neurons, the very same type I excitatory neurons that have been negatively impacted due to the peripheral pathology. This signaling for an increase in activation of the ipsilesional type II inhibitory neurons only serves to increase their inhibitory control over the ipsilesional type I excitatory neurons, which in turn subsequently drives their tonic neural activity even lower, if this is even possible (Curthoys & Halmagyi, 2007). Of course, this cycle of further-and-further inhibition of the ipsilesional type I excitatory neurons and increase in tonic excitation of the contralesional type I excitatory neurons will continue in a vicious cycle, similar to the process of velocity storage; thus continuously driving a higher level of tonic neural firing rate in the contralesional VN concomitant to a decreasing level of tonic neural firing rate in the ipsilesional VN.

Neural Clamping. As our discussion on velocity storage would previously suggest, this cyclical commissural process, albeit pathological, would propagate and persist unless otherwise interrupted and regulated. Such regulation has been identified (at least in rats) within the cerebellum, specifically from the nodulus of the caudal vermis and the flocculi during periods of early central vestibular asymmetry (Kitahara et al., 1998; Kitahara, Fukushima, Takeda, Saika, & Kubo, 2000). This intervention has been termed "neural clamping," which involves the down regulation of neural activity within the intact VN (Barin & Durrant, 2000; Curthoys & Halmagyi, 2007). Evidence shows that a reduction in the efficiency of the neurotransmitter receptor for gamma-aminobutyric acid (GABA) on the type I excitatory neurons on the intact side would allow for greater (recovery) activity of ipsilesional type I neurons. This is because ipsilesional type I excitatory neurons would not be affected by as much inhibition from their synaptic neighboring type II inhibitory neurons due to a decrease (or elimination) of inhibition signaling from the now "stabilized" contralesional type I excitatory neurons (Curthoys & Halmagyi, 2007). In fact, this process of "neural clamping" can be clinically induced within hours of a non-pathologic vestibular asymmetry, such as that from sustained unilateral vestibular stimulation (Barin & Durrant, 2000). Within a week of a unilateral vestibular lesion, neural activity from the type I excitatory neurons can be measured within the vestibular nuclei from the *lesioned* side. Supplemental evidence has also shown this "neural regeneration" to originate not from the afferent periphery, but rather from other sources within the CNS (Barin & Durrant, 2000).

During the later stages of asymmetric central repair, a progressive increase and rebalancing in neural activity is observed as the "neural clamping" from the cerebellum is adapted and modified. Kitahara and associates (1998; 2000) have proposed that neurons in the flocculus may regulate the "hyperactive" type I excitatory neurons in the intact vestibular nucleus. In turn, and more importantly, this action would serve to regulate the inhibition of the type I excitatory neurons in the ipsilesional side, (via a reduction in the inhibition of the ipsilesional type II inhibitory neurons), thus allowing for a restoration of type I neural activity in the absence of any afferent peripheral input from the damaged labyrinth. This process likely continues and is continually modified by the cerebellum until the neural activity of the "clamped" contralesional side returns to prelesioned levels, and a symmetrical *central* neural tone is restored between the two vestibular nuclei. Figure 3–5 (A–V) complements the previous discussion on static compensation, and illustrates the various stages that occur during the compensation process.

This process of central compensation is most stable and effective when the lesion is stable and the environment (individual) is static. In fact, the process of static compensation is extremely robust, and very little appears to hasten or hinder it (Curthoys & Halmagyi, 2007). Conversely, the restoration of *dynamic* equilibrium, or the process of *dynamic* compensation, is much more complex and involves the integration of all systems involved with movement, such as the vestibulocollic reflex and the autonomic reflex system.

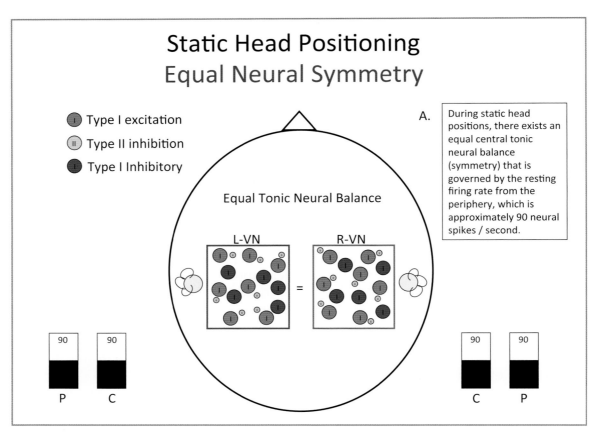

FIGURE 3–5. A–V. Progressive stages associated with process of central vestibular compensation following a unilateral vestibular lesion. Large boxes represent the right and left vestibular nuclei. Smaller vertical rectangles (two flanking each bottom side) represent the hypothetical level of neural tonic activity within the peripheral (P) and the central (C) vestibular systems. *continues*

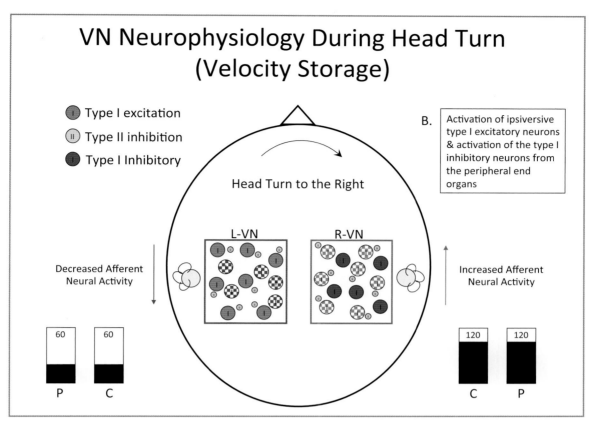

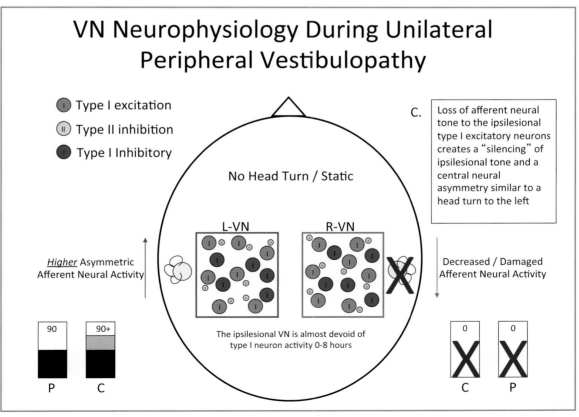

FIGURE 3–5. *continues*

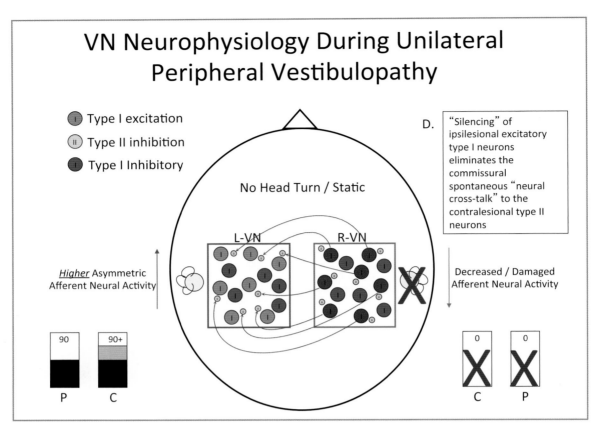

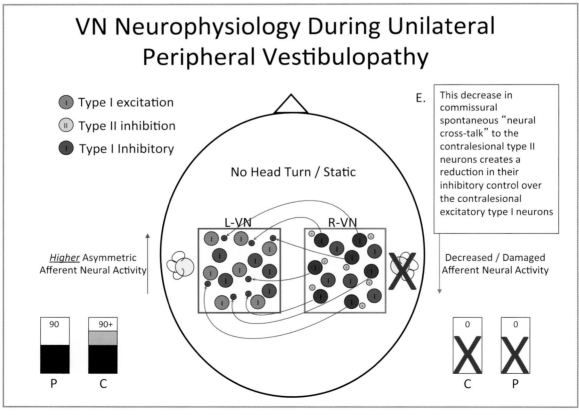

FIGURE 3–5. *continues*

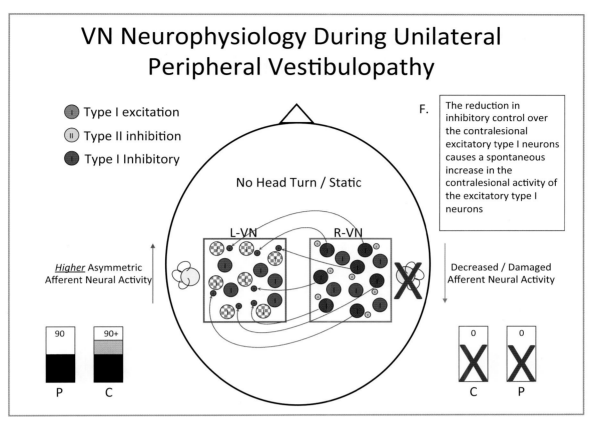

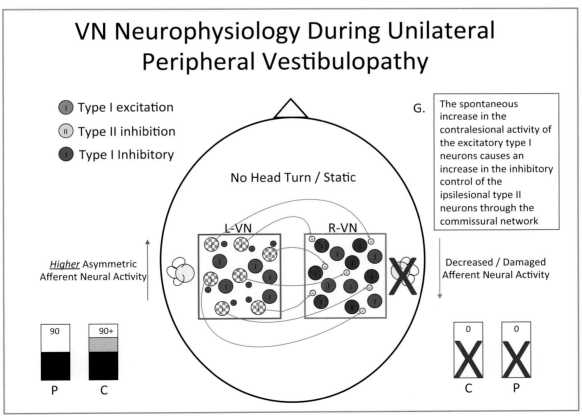

FIGURE 3–5. *continues*

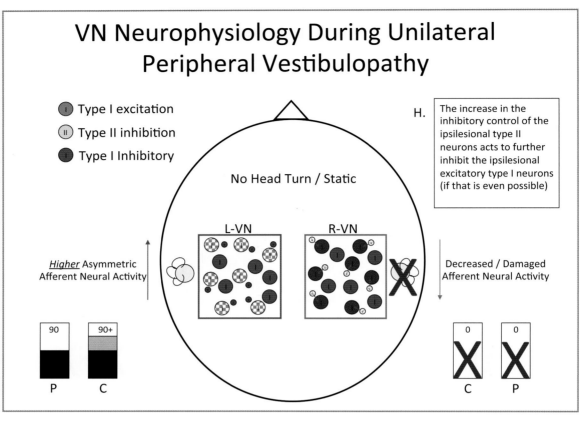

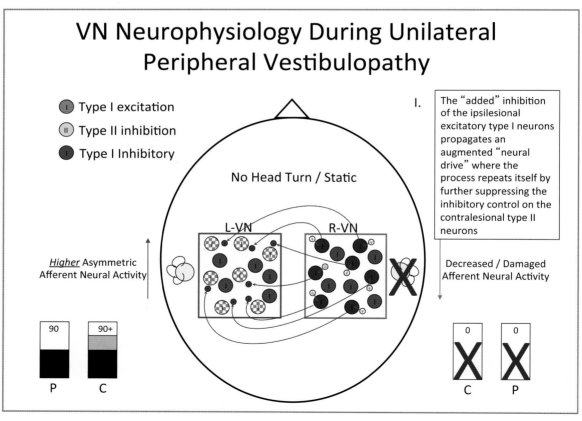

FIGURE 3–5. *continues*

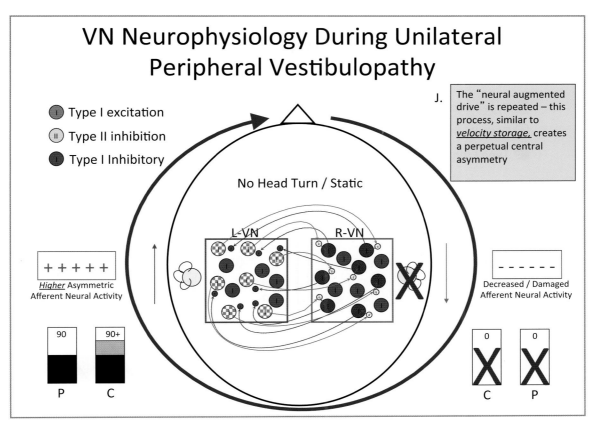

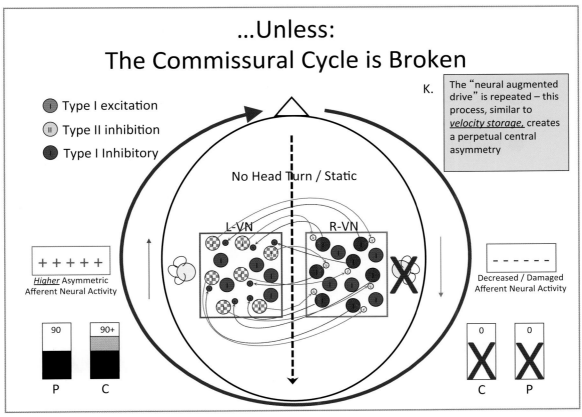

FIGURE 3–5. *continues*

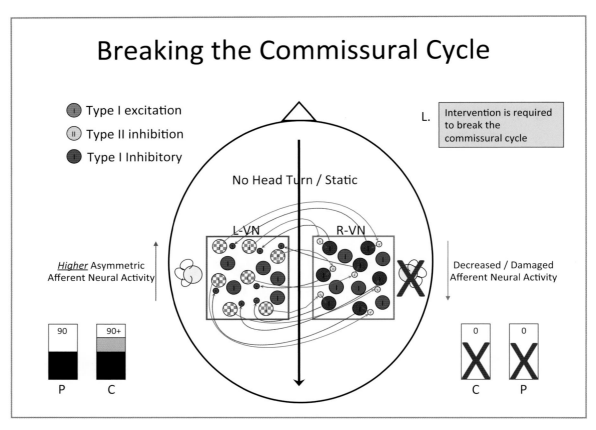

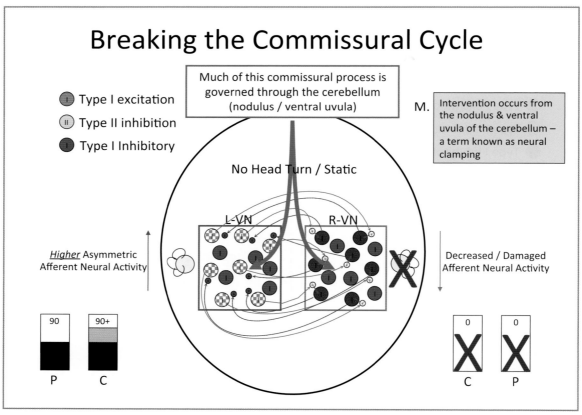

FIGURE 3–5. *continues*

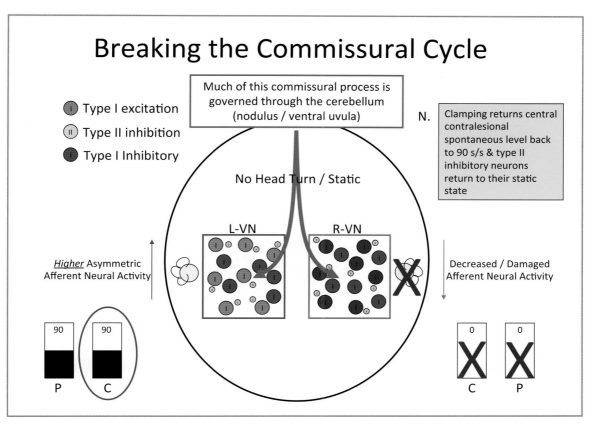

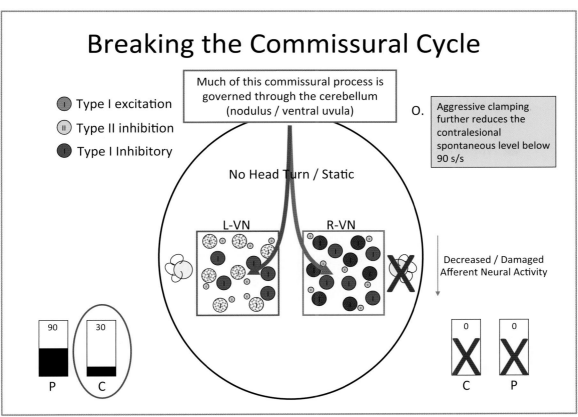

FIGURE 3–5. *continues*

81

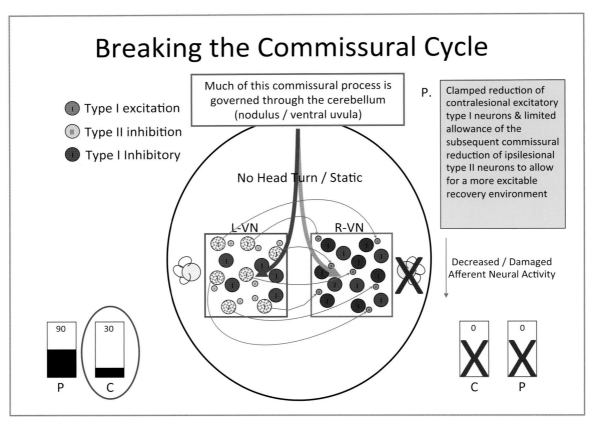

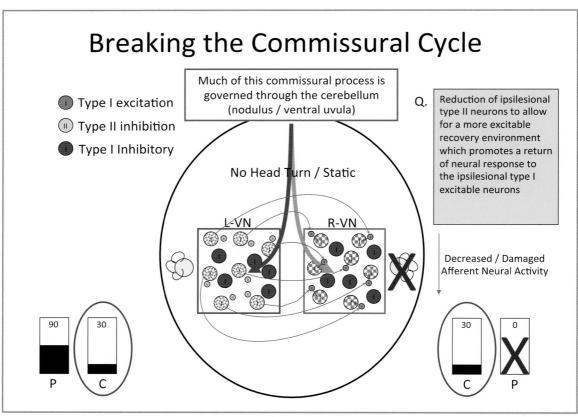

FIGURE 3–5. *continues*

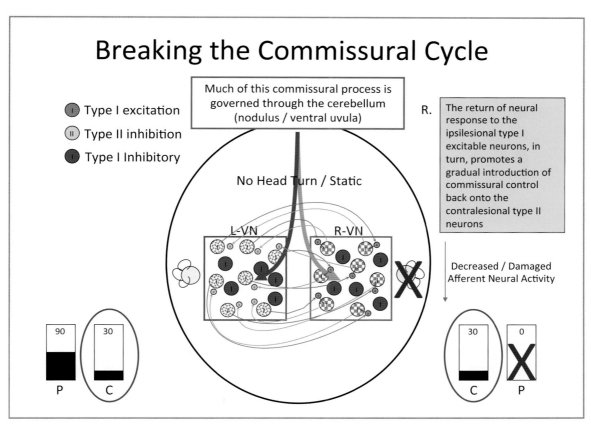

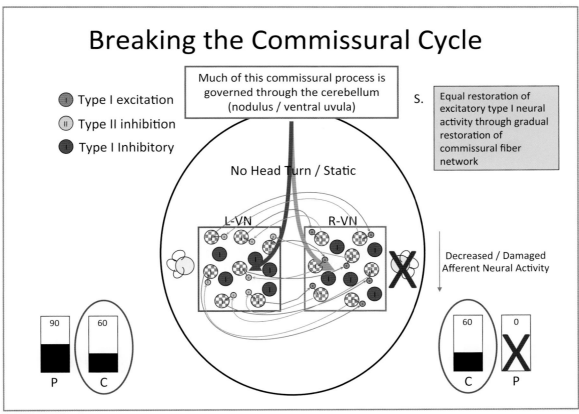

FIGURE 3–5. *continues*

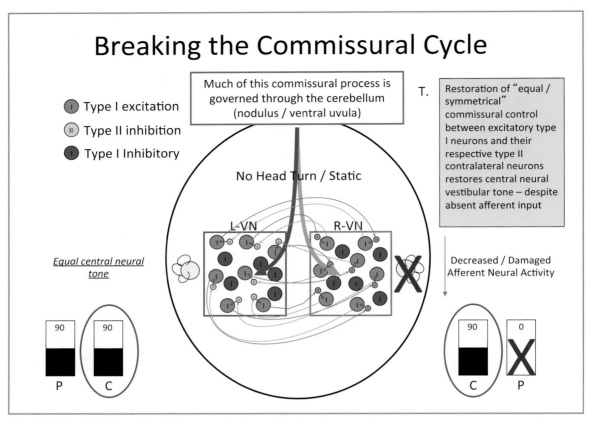

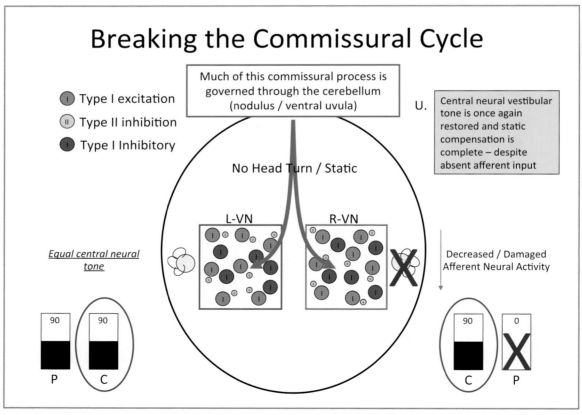

FIGURE 3–5. *continues*

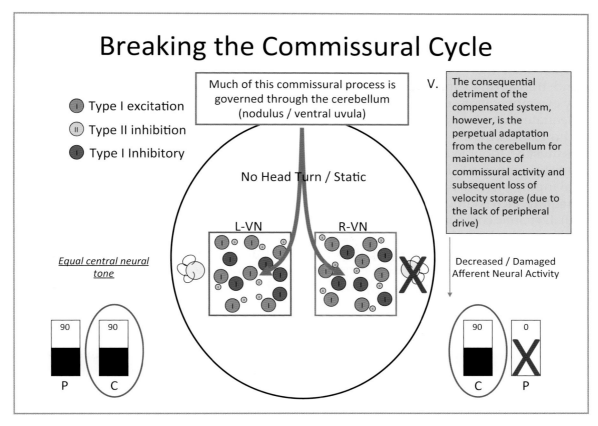

Breaking the Commissural Cycle

Type I excitation

Type II inhibition

Type I Inhibitory

Much of this commissural process is governed through the cerebellum (nodulus / ventral uvula)

No Head Turn / Static

L-VN   R-VN

Equal central neural tone

V. The consequential detriment of the compensated system, however, is the perpetual adaptation from the cerebellum for maintenance of commissural activity and subsequent loss of velocity storage (due to the lack of peripheral drive)

Decreased / Damaged Afferent Neural Activity

90   90
P   C

90   0
C   P

FIGURE 3–5. *continued*

Dynamic Compensation

Static compensation occurs at a much more efficient rate than dynamic compensation. Unfortunately, patients with unilateral labyrinthine damage exhibit difficulty integrating an accurate representation of the acceleration and velocity of head movement for some time, (even following static compensation), due to significant end organ asymmetry. Recall that the central compensation is just that, *central*. The tonic balance is within the vestibular nuclei. However, during head movement, the statically compensated central vestibular nuclei will continue to receive asymmetric peripheral input. It is this end organ imbalance that, despite effective static compensation, continues to cause considerable problems under dynamic (head movement) conditions (Barin & Durrant, 2000). Rotation of the head away from the lesioned labyrinth will quickly saturate the neural response to

zero spikes per second (if the system is not already in this state). Conversely, the excitatory afferent response from the intact side is unaffected. Consequently, integration of the asymmetric afferent neural signals from the unbalanced peripheral system, even in the presence of statically compensated central vestibular nuclei, will be ineffective in generating an appropriate central neural asymmetry necessary for detecting the precise velocity and direction required for an effective VOR.

The solution for dynamic compensation is much more complex. Consider that the absolute magnitude difference in vestibular input is approximately one-half of what it used to be prior to the peripheral insult; that is, if one peripheral labyrinth was completely lesioned only 50%, or 1/2 of the physiology remains. During dynamic compensation, the vestibular pathways need to be "recalibrated" to accept and process the new "one-half" pattern of neural firing rates. Moreover, this must be accomplished in relation to the laterality of lesion versus the direction of head movement (either toward or away from the peripheral lesion). This must then be appropriately integrated and transformed into appropriate compensatory eye movements, exhibiting a VOR gain that is adequate enough so as not to produce any perceived dizziness by the patient. Certain VOR pathways must be "doubled" during certain head movements to compensate for the one-half loss of peripheral input, whereas other head movements may not require such compensation (Barin & Durrant, 2000). Dynamic compensation often involves additional neural adaptations that facilitate the process such as vestibulocollic reflex pathways. Collectively, these processes can take a considerable amount of time, which largely depends on a variety of different factors, from the degree of severity of the peripheral vestibular lesion, to the age and overall health, as well as the activity level of the patient.

The Effects of Dynamic Compensation Is Also Frequency Dependent. Generally, the ineffective integration of neural signals during dynamic head changes, even following static compensation, is more pronounced for low-acceleration stimuli. The most efficient method of increasing the overall gain or sensitivity of the vestibular system, given that half of the system is now extinguished, is to increase the output (lessen the restriction/control) of the central system's ability to integrate and coordinate the VOR response (Barin & Durrant, 2000). This method, however, is not without significant consequence. By increasing the overall integration and output of the VOR pathways, less afferent peripheral input is effectively "stored" in the neural integrator. That is, the mechanism and efficiency of velocity storage is significantly and permanently reduced (if not completely modified by the cerebellum to "zero" storage) and the ability of the central system to propagate, extend, or augment the neural output for low-frequency stimuli is essentially disrupted or completely lost. Consequently, the processing and integration of low-frequency head movements is significantly degraded more than any other stimuli. This helps to explain why, despite effective static *and* dynamic compensation, patients with non-acute

unilateral vestibular lesions often perceive slight swaying and rocking sensations while standing and sitting still (low frequency stimulation), and feel much better upon movement (higher frequency stimulation) (Curthoys & Halmagyi, 2007). In addition, it is not surprising to see long-standing abnormalities during vestibular testing that incorporates low-frequency stimuli (i.e., prolonged low frequency VOR phase leads), as the vestibular system's ability to integrate and process such stimuli often remains significantly and, quite often, permanently modified. This is true even following effective static and dynamic compensation, because once the mechanisms for central velocity storage are damaged, such processes are seldom, if ever, restored (Barin & Durrant, 2000). Moreover, the repair of such processes (velocity storage) may not even be desired, as the consequence of returning velocity storage to its prelesion status may have consequences in VOR gain that are greater than the alternative. This idea is again discussed at greater length in Chapter 6 when reviewing sinusoidal acceleration testing.

Overall, the process of dynamic compensation is likely more complex than simply increasing the overall gain of the VOR, or modifying velocity storage. The VCR and the VSR are intimately involved in the process of signal integration, and their involvement is undoubtedly vital to effective dynamic compensation.

OTHER NON-VESTIBULAR AFFERENT / EFFERENT PROJECTIONS

The vestibular nerve and cerebellum are not the only sources of afferent input to the vestibular nuclei. Many nonvestibular afferent projections to the vestibular nuclei are known to exist; however, the function of each source of non-vestibular afferents is not always well understood. Such sources include the visual system, cervical and spinal cord neurons, as well as autonomic nervous system pathways. Many of the physiologic responses from these neural centers have been clearly shown to be affected by behaviors and stimuli not related to vestibular nerve activity (Lysakowski et al.,

1998). The more prevalent nonvestibular afferent signals delivered to the vestibular nuclei are from the visual system, as well as from cervicocollic (neck) and cervicospinal pathways.

Visual Contributions

The visual system is fundamental to posture and overall balance function (Nashner, 1997; Peterka, 2002). It is no surprise, therefore, that the visual system has independent projections to the vestibular nuclei. As previously mentioned, there exists a well-known and immensely critical efferent projection from the VN to the ocular motor system, known as the VOR. However, it is also critical that the visual system independently project afferent fibers to the VN. These fibers provide a redundancy to the vestibular system but more importantly, supplement the perception of movement for low frequencies, where the vestibular system is less efficient (Lysakowski et al., 1998). Specifically, the efficiency of the cristae and the maculae to low-frequency movements (accelerations) at or below 0.05 Hz is rather poor (Lysakowski et al., 1998). In fact, the relative inefficiency of the vestibular system to such low-frequency stimuli often creates a significant physiological problem when attempting to produce an appropriate ocular or postural reflex response, as the integration and processing of such impuissant stimuli requires supplemental mechanisms that can augment the insufficient response (i.e., velocity storage). Although velocity storage is the primary mechanism that addresses this deficiency, the visual system is another key contributor, capable of detecting extremely low-frequency movements of the visual scene and incorporating that in the VOR or postural reflex response. In doing so, the brain uses low frequency visual information to supplement the poorly integrated information obtained from the labyrinth (Lysakowski et al., 1998). In short, the inefficiencies of the vestibular system to low (and very high) frequency stimuli are compensated quite well by the visual system. Specifically, this *visual-vestibular enhancement* is largely mediated by the optokinetic system, and effectively integrates "movement" information to the vestibular nuclei when the peripheral vestibular system is unable to do so. Clinical assessment of visual-vestibular enhancement during rotational testing is discussed in Chapter 8. (Leigh & Zee, 2006). An "everday" example of such visual-vestibular interaction is the physiological perception of movement in a *stationary* car when one "perceives" the slow creeping advancement of a neighboring car at a stoplight.

One final piece of evidence to support an integral connection between the visual system and the vestibular system is motion sickness. Many people experience motion sickness, which is essentially a central conflict between the integration of visual and vestibular signals. This association provides further evidence for the existence of independent, yet integrated, sensory pathways.

Cervical and Spinal Contributions

The spinal cord, particularly the cervical spinal cord, provides another source of non-vestibular afferent and efferent signals to and from the VN (Lysakowski et al., 1998). As mentioned earlier, projections from the cerebellar vermis help to coordinate neck and postural movements within the VN. Through this network, appropriate compensatory eye movements are also coordinated in conjunction with head and neck movements via the vestibulospinal and spinocerebellar neural pathways. Without this network, effective maintenance of visual and head stabilization would not be possible. The neural tracts within the cervicospinal region where the afferent and efferent fibers travel are known as the medial and lateral vestibular spinal tracts, or simply, the MVST and LVST, respectively (Lysakowski et al., 1998). The function of each tract, however, is unique. The MVST is merely an extension of the medial longitudinal fasciculus. Its projections terminate in the cervical regions of the spinal cord and serve to stabilize and centrally position the head on the shoulders by activating neck muscles that not only resist passive movements of the head (e.g., during ambulation), but also generate active head movements during intentional body movements. The lateral vestibulospinal tract extends to the lower lumbar regions of the spinal cord and provides a persistent excitatory synaptic input to postural extensor motorneurons. This tonically active neural input to the extensor muscles is critical when resisting the persistent forces of gravity (Lysakowski et al., 1998). Without such neural input, postural control would cripple under the driving force of gravity and the body would be unable to support an upright posture. Collectively, the MVST and LVST provide a sense of postural "uprightness" that is threatened in the presence of an acute unilateral labyrinthine lesion. The lack of tonic symmetry in the presence of an acute unilateral vestibular lesion, particularly in the absence of visual cues, creates a leaning posture and tendency to fall toward the side of lesion due to a lack of tonic input on the side of the lesion. This is the underlying principle for an abnormal Rhomberg or Fakuda Stepping Test. This duality of head and ocular reflex responses becomes functionally relevant if one is to visualize how compensatory head and eye movements are critically needed when reading while walking. Not only is the head "held" stable on the shoulders with every step, due to the MVST, but concomitant compensatory eye movements are produced via the VOR in order to maintain visual stabilization, due to the "bouncing" of the head with each step. A relevant example of pathologic vestibulocollic and vestibulospinal contributions is evident in Mal de Débarquement syndrome, where a conflict is experienced between spinal and vestibular inputs.

Autonomic Non-Vestibular Projections

Although not completely known or understood, a variety of other afferent and efferent fibers project to the vestibular nuclei. The thalamus is known to have some projections known as the vestibuleophthalamocortical pathways (Arslan, 2001). Lysakowski and colleagues (1998) hypothesized that, in the absence of any visual stimulation, thalamic projections may, in fact, provide a conscious awareness of vertigo, or self-motion.

VASCULAR SUPPLY

Finally, a discussion of the peripheral and central vestibular system would not be complete without discussing the vascular supply to the vestibular system (Figure 3–6). The primary blood supply to the vestibular system and its end organs is through the labyrinthine artery, also known as the internal auditory artery. It arises from the anterior cerebellar artery, the superior cerebellar artery, or the basilar artery (Lysakowski, et al., 1998). Most commonly, the labyrinthine artery arises from the anterior cerebellar artery (Wende, Nakayama, & Schwerdtfeger, 1975). The labyrinthine artery courses through the IAC together with the labyrinthine vein (in addition to the VII and VIII cranial nerves). Shortly after exiting the IAC fundus, the labyrinthine artery branches into two distinct branches: the anterior vestibular artery, and the common cochlear artery. Despite the name of the latter, the vestibular system is supplied by both branches (Lysakowski et al., 1998). The anterior vestibular artery supplies the utricle as well as the superior and horizontal SCC. The common cochlear artery divides into the proper cochlear artery and the vestibulocochlear artery. The latter further divides into the posterior vestibular artery, which is the primary blood supply to the posterior SCC and the majority of the saccule. Interestingly, the anatomical organization of the blood supply to the peripheral vestibular end organs mimics the innervation pattern of the vestibular nerve and its afferent nerve endings (Lysakowski et al., 1998).

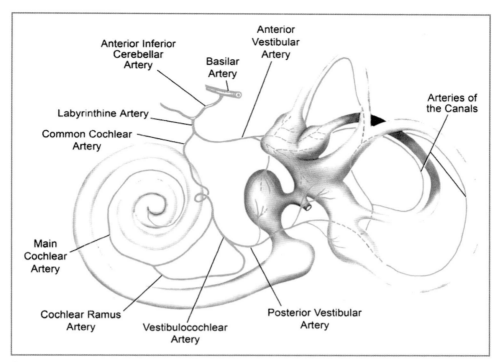

A

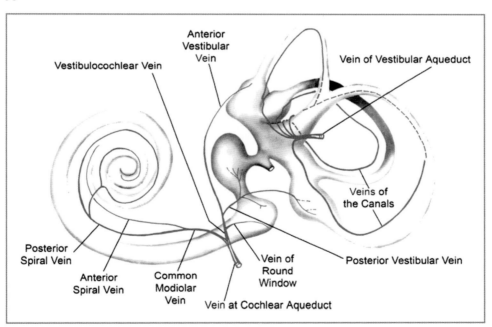

B

FIGURE 3–6. Labyrinthine vascular supply. **A.** Arterial circulation. **B.** Venous circulation. From *Schuknecht's Pathology of the Ear* (3rd ed.) by S. N. Merchant and J. B. Nadol, 2010, People's Medical Publishing House, Shelton, CT. Reprinted with permission.

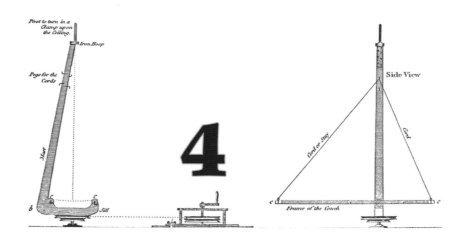

The Vestibular Ocular Reflex and Vestibular Nystagmus

THE VESTIBULAR OCULAR REFLEX (VOR)

The VOR is the best-understood reflex in human physiology (Schwarz & Tomlinson, 2005). It is an automatic reflex requiring no cognitive thought or intent. It is an extremely fast-acting reflex that occurs hundreds of thousands of times each day. Often, it is a reflex we take for granted. That is, until it goes missing or is damaged. In short, the VOR is the compensatory eye movement that occurs in the opposite direction to that of head movement so as to maintain visual fixation on an intended target during head movement. It is the reason you can read while walking or running. It is the reason you can see steady while driving on a cobblestone road. It is (partly) the reason an athlete can clearly focus on a target while exerting a high level of active head movement (recall, the visual system also compliments the VOR for high frequency head movements where it becomes less efficient). Ultimately, an effective VOR is possible due to the afferent and efferent projections between the vestibular periphery, the vestibular nuclei, the cerebellum, the ocularmotor nuclei, and the extraocular muscles.

Purpose and Properties of the Vestibular Ocular Reflex

The purpose of the VOR is to stabilize images on the retina during head movement. This is accomplished by effectively and efficiently generating extremely quick compensatory eye movements in the equal and opposite direction to that of head movement. That is, in order to maintain visual fixation on a traffic sign as your head is moved from left to right, an eye movement that is equal in velocity and opposite in direction of head movement (from right to left) must occur. The VOR is capable of generating effective vestibular-generated eye movements for head movements up to 350° per second (Leigh & Zee, 2006; Schwarz & Tomlinson, 2005). For velocities higher than this, up to approximately 500° per second, the sensitivity (gain) of the VOR deteriorates (Schwarz & Tomlinson, 2005). For velocities near or above 500° per second, the visual system attempts to compensate via the optokinetic system. The VOR must also occur with extremely short latency so as not to create any slip or blur of the image on the retina immediately following the onset of every head movement. The latency of the VOR is extremely short and measured in humans to be approximately 10 to 12 msec

(Schwarz & Tomlinson, 2005). This latency is quick enough so as not to create any temporal lag during brainstem integration that would lead to visual blur.

The *direction* of the VOR response is always opposite that of the head turn, and is integrated by the periphery. Conversely, the *velocity* of the response is primarily integrated within the VN (Gacek, 2005; Leigh & Zee, 2006). The amplitude and timing of the reflex, (that is the gain and phase of the VOR), varies greatly with respect to the velocity of the stimulus. A more equally "matched" eye velocity response occurs for mid-to-high frequency stimuli (<350° per second) (Highstein, 1996; Leigh & Zee, 2006). This suggests that the VOR is less efficient for low head velocities and more efficient for higher frequencies. This is indeed the case; however, the inefficiency of the VOR (in the absence of any supplementing visual information, or in a vision-denied condition) for low velocity stimuli is "augmented" or supplemented by an internal "neural drive" of the system known as velocity storage (discussed earlier).

The Vestibular Ocular Reflex and Ewald's Laws

The calculation of head velocity and direction are integrated by the vestibular system with respect to the specific vector and angular/translational acceleration in space. Each semicircular canal (SCC) is most sensitive to angular accelerations in the plane of their respective orientation (Lysakowski, McCrea, & Tomlinson, 1998). That is, equal and opposite compensatory eye movements occur in the same plane of the SCCs sharing the same orientation. Specifically, the h-SCC is most sensitive to producing compensatory eye movements (VOR) in response to head movements in the horizontal (yaw) plane, and vertical compensatory eye movements occur as a result of vertical SCC activation from head movements in the pitch or roll plane. This property of compensatory eye movements being produced by activation of SCC excitation and inhibition in the same plane as the occurring head movements is known as Ewald's first law (Baloh & Honrubia, 2001; Leigh & Zee, 2006). Ewald's first law specifically states that

maximal stimulation of eye movements always occurs in the plane of the canal being stimulated (Leigh & Zee, 2006). Use of this law can be very useful, not only during physiologic assessment of the vestibular system, but also when diagnosing locations of insult within the vestibular system. In addition, it is also important to be cognizant that, aside from the VOR produced by the SCCs, the otolith maculae also produce a VOR. Because of the difference between the two sensory organs' physiology, the SCC VOR is also sometimes referred to as the angular VOR (a-VOR), where the maculae VOR is sometimes referred to as the translational VOR (t-VOR). We review the physiology of the VOR for both sensory end organs in this chapter.

Aside from Ewald's first law, Ernst Julius Richard Ewald (1855–1921) also proposed two additional laws of semicircular canal function. Ewald's second and third laws grossly state that vestibular excitation provokes a stronger neural response than inhibition. This is primarily due to the fact that inhibition of the resting neural vestibular firing rate is limited to zero, whereas the excitation of the resting neural firing rate is essentially "limitless", with an actually ceiling likely around 400 to 500 spikes/second. Specifically, Ewald's second law states that ampullopetal endolymph flow (toward the utricle) in the horizontal canal causes a greater response than ampullofugal endolymph flow (away from the utricle). Moreover, Ewald's third law pertains to the vertical canals, and states that ampullofugal flow (away from the utricle) produces a better response than ampullopetal flow (toward the utricle) when the anterior and posterior canals are stimulated.

SEMICIRCULAR CANAL VESTIBULAR OCULAR REFLEX

Each of the semicircular canals forms a three-neuron-reflex pathway from the peripheral sensory end organ (cristae ampullaris) to a set of distinct ocular motor muscles. As mentioned in Chapter 1, Lorente de Nó (1933) first detailed the various three-neuron arcs that connect each peripheral vestibular end organ to their respective ocular muscles (Cohen & Raphan, 2004). The distinctive three-neuron arc for each semicircular canal is depicted in Figure 4–1. As a general rule, excitatory connections travel along the contralateral pathways, and inhibitory connections travel along the ipsilateral pathways for all three semicircular canal pathways.

Horizontal SCC VOR

The most frequent head movement, both in everyday life activities as well as during vestibular assessment, occurs in the horizontal plane. Secondary to this, a detailed discussion will be

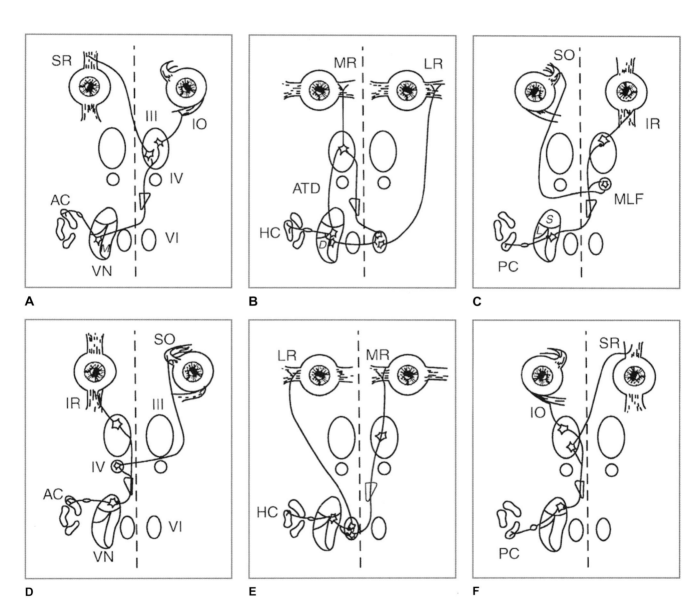

FIGURE 4–1. Vestibular Ocular Reflex (VOR) neural pathways for each semicircular canal. As a general rule, excitatory connections (**A**, **B**, and **C**) run in the contralateral medial longitudinal fasciculus (MLF), and inhibitory connections (**D**, **E**, and **F**) in the ipsilateral (MLF). AC (anterior canal); HC (horizontal canal); PC (posterior canal); ATD (Ascending Tract of Deiters); III (Oculomotor Nucleus); IV (Trochlear Nucleus); VI (Abducens Nucleus); IR (Inferior Rectus Muscle); MR (Medial Rectus Muscle); LR (Lateral Rectus Muscle); SR (Superior Rectus Muscle); IO (Inferior Oblique Muscle); SO (Superior Oblique Muscle). From *Baloh and Honrubia's Clinical Neurophysiology of the Vestibular System* (4th ed.), by R. W. Baloh, V. Honrubia, and K. A. Kerber, 2011, New York, NY: Oxford University Press. Reprinted with permission.

given primarily to this reflex, keeping in mind that the anterior and posterior canals have their own distinct angular orientation and thus, have their own distinct three-neuron VOR arc (Leigh & Zee, 2006).

The horizontal canal VOR (h-VOR) produces compensatory eye movements in the equal and opposite directions to that of head movements within the horizontal (yaw) plane. Again, because natural head movements in space rarely, if ever, occur purely within a *single* plane of orientation, it is important to realize that the resultant eye movements are likely more a representation of the VOR produced by *all* the SCCs (and otoliths). However, during vestibular physiologic testing, specifically rotational testing, great care is taken to place the head in such a plane of orientation that the h-SCC is isolated and maximally stimulated, thus producing compensatory eye movements that are largely representative of only the h-VOR. Therefore, the discussion here concentrates on the h-VOR.

Excitatory h-VOR Physiology

The h-VOR is a three-neuron arc that originates from the crista of the h-SCC and terminates on the medial and lateral rectus ocular motor muscles (Leigh & Zee, 2006). For a detailed description of the excitatory and inhibitory three-neuron-arc pathway, the reader is encouraged to review Leigh and Zee (2006) and Gacek (2005). During head rotations in the horizontal plane, both the right and left h-SCC cristae provide an afferent response. For the h-SCC, the leading ear (right ear during a rightward rotation and vice versa) displaces the stereocilia toward the kinocilium and depolarization of the underlying hair cell ensues (Ewald's second law) (Baloh & Honrubia, 2001) (Figure 4–2). Subsequently, an increase in afferent neural activity is produced on the ipsiversive side, whereby first-order vestibular neurons saltate the response through the IAC and terminate in the MVN and SVN. [For low-frequency stimuli, interneurons work to sustain the afferent responses

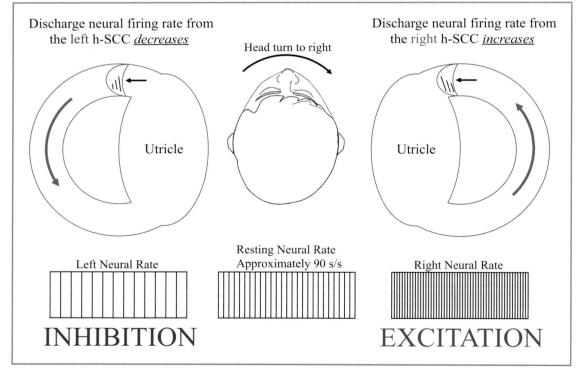

FIGURE 4–2. Image depicting left and right cupulae deflection and underlying stereocillia deflection of the horizontal semicircular canals in response to a right head turn. Green arrows depict the direction of endolymph flow. *Source:* Adapted from Barin, K., & Durrant, J. (2000). Applied physiology of the vestibular system. In Canalis, R. F. & Lambert, P. R. (Eds.).

through the process of velocity storage, a process facilitated by the cerebellum and the commissural pathways] (Curthoys & Halmagyi, 1996). From here, a group of interneurons within the ipsiversive MVN cross the midline and terminate in the contralateral abducens nucleus (VI) in order to innervate the contralateral lateral rectus motor units. Excitation of these motor units creates a muscle contraction of the contralateral eye in the opposite direction, with a peak eye velocity that is (ideally) equal to the velocity of head movement. A second group of interneurons within the SVN sends the excitation response ipsilaterally through the ascending tract of Dieters (ATD) to terminate

on the ipsilateral medial rectus muscles motor units via the ipsilateral ocular motor nucleus (III). Excitation of these motor units causes a conjugate contraction of the ipsilateral medial rectus muscle in the opposite direction, also with a peak eye velocity that is (ideally) equal to head velocity. A smaller, third group of neurons also cross the midline from the contralateral abducens nucleus, through the MLF and eventually innervate the ipsilateral medial rectus motor units via the ipsilateral ocular motor nucleus (joining the ascending fibers from the ipsilateral ATD). The excitation neural pathway for the horizontal semicircular canals is summarized in Figure 4–3.

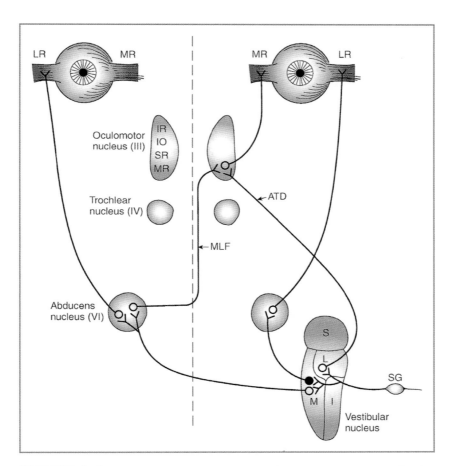

FIGURE 4–3. Vestibular Ocular Reflex (VOR) neural pathways for the horizontal semicircular canal. Medial longitudinal fasciculus (MLF); ATD (Ascending Tract of Deiters); IR (Inferior Rectus Muscle); MR (Medial Rectus Muscle); LR (Lateral Rectus Muscle); SR (Superior Rectus Muscle); IO (Inferior Oblique Muscle); SG (Superior Nerve Branch Ganglia). From *Baloh and Honrubia's Clinical Neurophysiology of the Vestibular System* (4th ed.), by R. W. Baloh, V. Honrubia, and K. A. Kerber, 2011. New York, NY: Oxford University Press. Reprinted with permission.

Inhibitory h-VOR Physiology

In light of the complimentary and antagonistic ocular muscle arrangement that maintains eye position in the center of the viscous environment within the ocular orbit, an inhibitory response must be provided to the antagonistic ocular muscles to facilitate the VOR muscle contraction in the opposite direction (Leigh & Zee, 2006). The contraversive (trailing ear) h-SCC periphery generates this inhibitory response (Barber & Stockwell, 1980). Bending of the stereocilia in the trailing ear away from the kinocilium hyperpolarizes the underlying hair cell and produces an inhibitory afferent response to eventually terminate in the contraversive MVN and SVN. Through similar pathways, as previously described for the excitatory response, second and third-order neurons eventually terminate on the contralateral medial rectus muscle and the ipsilateral lateral rectus muscle. This pathway provides an inhibitory (relaxed) muscle response, which facilitates the opposing (excitatory) contraction of the eyes in the opposite direction (Figure 4–4).

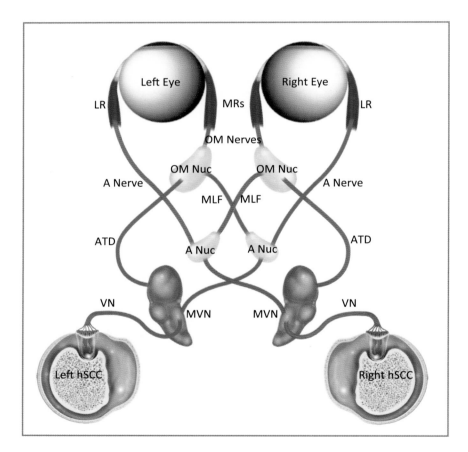

FIGURE 4–4. Vestibular Ocular Reflex (VOR) neural pathways for the horizontal semicircular canal. Excitatory pathways depicted in red and inhibitory pathways depicted in blue for a head turn toward the right. MR (Medial Rectus); LR (Lateral Rectus); OM Nerve (Ocular Motor Nerve); OM Nuc (Ocular Motor Nucleus); MLF (Medial Longitudinal Fasciculus); A Nerve (Abducens Nerve); A Nuc (Abducens Nucleus); ATD (Ascending Tract of Dieters); MVN (Medial Vestibular Nucleus); VN (Vestibular Nerve); hSCC (Horizontal Semicircular Canal). From *Electronystagmography and Videonystagmography: ENG/VNG* by D. L. McCaslin, 2012, San Diego, CA: Plural Publishing. Reprinted with permission.

Complementary and synergistic excitation *and* inhibition pathways are critical for effective operation of the h-VOR (as well as for any of the SCC or maculae VOR pathways). These separate neural pathways fundamentally provide the capability of applying varying amounts of contraction and "displacement" of each eye, independent from one another (Wong, 2008; Schwarz & Tomlinson, 2005). This becomes important as it permits fixation of targets at varying distances (vergence), or at various angles within the periphery in coordination with the VOR, by independently regulating muscle contractions from each eye (Schwarz & Tomlinson, 2005). This concept is critical when considering pathologic processes in view of the fact that documenting abnormal movement of one, or both eyes, can be different from one another. In addition, this reflex should occur within 10 to 12 ms of head movement. Any increase in the latency or amplitude (gain) of either, or both eyes, can be significant and diagnostically useful, as with internuclear ophthalmoplegia (INO).

Anterior SCC VOR

Excitation of the anterior semicircular canal produces an excitatory and compensatory eye response that is in the same roll (side-to-side) plane as the anterior canal (Ewald's first law). This response is governed by the specific muscles innervated by the three-neuron arc of the anterior VOR (a-VOR) (see Figure 4–1). Although the general aspects of the a-SCC three-neuron arc are similar in myeloarchitecture to the h-VOR, the exact neural centers, pathways, and ocular muscle innervations are slightly different (Schwarz & Tomlinson, 2005). The specific eye movements of the a-VOR can be described as a synchronized (conjugate) *upward* deviation of both eyes concomitant with a counter-rolling of the eyes, such that the upper poles of both eyes move toward the contralateral side (i.e., the ipsilateral eye intorts and the contralateral eye extorts) (Schwarz & Tomlinson, 2005). Of note, it is important to recall that the stereocilia and kinocilia arrangement on the a-SCC is opposite that of the h-SCC. That is, the kinocilium is located on the canalicular side of

the cupula. This orientation is significant because it allows the leading ear to displace the stereocilia toward the kinocilium, whereby depolarization of the underlying hair cell ensues (Ewald's third law). With respect to the anterior canals, the *leading* ear would apply to the right ear during a *forward* pitching of the head over the right shoulder (i.e., the RALP plane as described in Chapter 2), and a *forward* pitching of the head over the left shoulder for the left ear (LARP plane).

Posterior SCC VOR

Excitation of the posterior canal produces an excitatory and compensatory eye response that is in the same pitch (front-to-back) plane (Ewald's first law). This response is governed by the specific muscles innervated by the three-neuron arc of the posterior VOR (p-VOR) (see Figure 4–1). Like the a-VOR, the general aspects of the p-VOR three-neuron arc are similar in myeloarchitecture to the h-VOR, with the exact neural centers, pathways, and ocular muscles innervations also being slightly different (Schwarz & Tomlinson, 2005). The specific eye movements of the p-VOR are very similar to that of the anterior semicircular canal, and can be described in much the same fashion. With the p-VOR pathway, synchronized (conjugate) *downward* deviation occurs in both eyes concomitant to counter-rolling, such that the upper poles of both eyes move toward the contralateral side (i.e., the ipsilateral eye intorts and the contralateral eye extorts) (Schwarz & Tomlinson, 2005). While both the a-VOR and p-VOR share the same torsional vestibular slow-phase component of the nystagmus (always toward the contralateral, or inhibitory, ear), the primary distinction between the anterior and the posterior semicircular canal VOR lies the vertical component of eye movement, as the anterior canal vestibular slow-phase deviation is *upward* and the posterior canal vestibular slow-phase deviation is *downward*. This distinction actually becomes critical when considering the differential diagnosis between anterior versus posterior canal benign paroxysmal positional vertigo (BPPV).

As with the a-SCC, it is important to recall that the stereocilia and kinocilium arrangement on the p-SCC is opposite that of the h-SCC. That is, the kinocilium is also located on the canalicular side of the cupula. This orientation is significant because it continues to allow the leading ear to displace the stereocilia toward the kinocilium, and depolarization of the underlying hair cell ensues (Ewald's third law). With respect to the posterior canals, the *leading* ear would apply to the right ear during a *backward* pitching of the head over the right shoulder (i.e., the LARP plane as described in Chapter 2), and a *backward* pitching of the head over the left shoulder for the left ear (RALP plane).

OTOLITH (MACULAR) VESTIBULAR OCULAR REFLEX

Otolith Maculae VOR

Because the maculae of the otolith receptors sense linear accelerations in the horizontal and vertical plane, it can be expected that the otolith VOR would displace the eyes in the equal and opposite translational vector to that of head movement. This is, in fact, the case and is referred to as the translational-VOR (t-VOR) (Leigh & Zee, 2006). The measurement of the t-VOR, however, is fraught with complexities, because each macula's stereocilia organization produces both an excitatory and inhibitory response (Chapter 2). In light of this multi-vector epithelial organization, compensation for unilateral peripheral macula damage is often extremely quick and void of persistent or even short-term clinical effects (Gresty, Bronstein, Brandt, & Dieterich, 1992). Furthermore, the precise neural pathways from the otolithic maculae to the ocular motor system are much more difficult than they are for the semicircular canals. This is primarily due to the kinocilium arrangement of the maculae epithelium and the subsequent fact that the macular nerves communicate information about all conceivable directions of linear movements (Schwarz & Tomlinson, 2005). Because of this, clinical investigation of otolith receptor function has proven to be difficult, and remains a challenge to this day.

Effective and efficient clinical investigations into otolith receptor function remain elusive. A simple lateral head tilt should excite the macula and, in fact, does generate an opposite torsional/rotational compensatory eye movement within each orbit, known as ocular counter-rolling (Baloh & Honrubia, 1998; Gresty & Bronstein, 1992; Ödkvist, 2001; Tran Ba Huy & Toupet, 2001). These compensation eye movements, however, are highly inefficient in counteracting the effect of head tilts. This is primarily because the amplitude (gain) of induced eye torsion, even for large head tilts, is only around 10% of the amplitude of the actual head tilt (Barin & Durrant, 2001). A centripetal force applied to a single, off-centered macula of the utricle also produces a counter-rolling of the eyes equal to the gravitational inertial forces with respect to the velocity of the stimulus (Baloh & Honrubia, 1998). This induced ocular counter-rolling produces an increased subjective perceptual tilt with respect to true vertical (normal perception within 2° to 4° of true gravitational vertical) (Baloh & Honrubia, 1998). Evidence for this is secondary to lateral forces applied to the maculae (utricle) during off-center axis (centrifugation) rotational testing (Böhmer & Mast, 1999). The degree of counter-roll measured can be applied clinically; however, the cost of equipment needed to investigate the t-VOR counter-roll during centrifugation testing is expensive and, often prohibitive, beyond a research setting. Off-axis centrifugation testing is discussed in great detail later in Chapter 8.

Types of Compensatory Maculo-Ocular Reflexes

Stimulation of the maculae causes two primary reflexes that assist in the stabilization of the head and eyes during linear acceleration and static head tilt. First are maculo-spinal reflexes that assist in the stabilization of the head during postural changes. Second, are the maculo-ocular reflexes. Similar to the vestibuloocular reflexes generated by the SCCs, these otolith-generated ocular reflexes assist in the stabilization of gaze during movement (Tran Ba Huy & Toupet, 2001). Both reflexes are fundamental in the stabilization of gaze and posture during rapid translational accelerations and/or static head tilts. First to be discussed are the maculo-ocular reflexes.

Maculo-Ocular Reflexes

Compensatory maculo-ocular reflexes are generated by the otoliths in association with the ocular motor system in order to maintain gaze stability during abrupt intra-aural linear translations and/or static head tilts. Similar reflexes have been discussed with respect to maintaining gaze during angular accelerations by the SCCs. During bilateral vestibulopathies impacting the SCCs, ocular stabilization is less efficient or non-existent during angular accelerations, and oscillopsia ensues. One would assume that similar processes contributing to SCC-engendered oscillopsia would also occur in response to rapid translational accelerations if the otoliths were equally damaged. This is, in fact, true. Experimental evidence shows that, in the presence of complete bilateral vestibulopathies, a loss of visual acuity occurs when trying to fixate on targets during abrupt linear accelerations (Lempert, Gianna, & Gresty, 1997). This evidence sup-

ports the presence of a linear or translational VOR, and its relative importance in maintaining VOR gaze fixation. Two primary maculo-ocular reflexes occur: the linear or translational VOR (t-VOR) and the ocular counterrolling VOR (c-VOR).

Maculo-Ocular Reflex Pathways. The anatomical bases for the two distinct maculo-ocular reflexes (t-VOR and c-VOR) have been well studied. Each utricular macula can be subdivided into two hemimaculae, separated by the striola: the medial and lateral halves (Figure 4–5) (Leigh & Zee, 2006). As noted earlier, the kinocilium and associated stereocilia hair cell bundle orientation between the two hemimaculae are arranged such that the polarities are in opposition to one another. Moreover, there is evidence to suggest that this oppos-

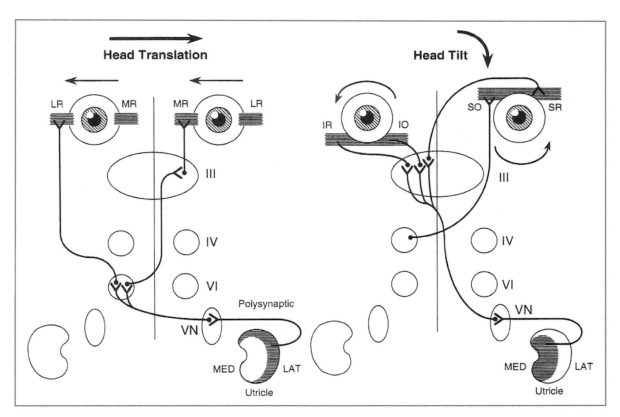

FIGURE 4–5. Utricular Vestibular Ocular Reflex pathways for tilt and translation. The medial hemimaculae (MED) contributes to counterrolling of the eyes by innervating the vertical torsional muscles. The lateral hemimaculae (LAT) contributes to a contraversive horizontal slow phase by innervating the horizontal muscles. LR (Lateral Rectus Muscle); MR (Medial Rectus Muscle); IR (Inferior Rectus Muscle); IO (Inferior Oblique Muscle); SO (Superior Oblique Muscle); SR (Superior Rectus Muscle); III (Ocular Motor Nucleus); IV Trochlear Nucleus); VI (Abducens Nucleus). From *The Neurology of Eye Movements* (5th ed., p. 75) by R. J. Leigh and D. S. Zee, 2015, New York, NY: Oxford University Press. Reprinted with permission.

ing polar relationship between one hemimacula to its contralateral complement shares a semi-coplanar relationship, similar to that of the SCCs (Tran Ba Huy & Toupet, 2001). That is, the medial half of one utricle is a complement of the lateral half of the opposing utricle in the opposite ear. As it pertains to the *utricle*, each hemimacula is responsible for either the translational (t-VOR), or the counterrolling (c-VOR) compensatory ocular reflex (see Figure 4–5). The *lateral* half of the utricle is likely responsible for generating the t-VOR, thus making it sensitive to translational accelerations (Leigh & Zee, 2006). The *medial* half is likely responsible for the ocular counterrolling reflex (c-VOR), thus making it sensitive to static head tilt (Leigh & Zee, 2006). This subdivision of responsibilities within a single macula provides a redundancy in the perception of translation versus static head tilt, and may account for varied symptoms of vestibular dysfunction, depending upon the location of macular insult. This functional subdivision also adds further evidence to highlight the complex differences in the regional morphology and physiology of the maculae cited earlier (Leigh & Zee, 2006). In addition, the semicoplanar relationship ensures that *both* a translational VOR as well as a counterrolling VOR would occur in response to a single vector linear acceleration. These subdivisions of responsibilities can also provide diagnostic insight into which macula(e), (or portion of a macula), is pathologic depending on whether the t-VOR or the c-VOR is deficient, given a known linear acceleration or static head tilt. This becomes clinically relevant insomuch that simple tests of sustained static head tilting or abrupt linear accelerations in the intra-aural vector can provide insight into the laterality of (unilateral) utricular damage.

Translational Maculo-Ocular Reflex (t-VOR).

The t-VOR is a complementary horizontal nystagmus to the c-VOR that occurs in response to rapid translational accelerations of the head. The precise compensatory t-VOR is inversely proportional to the distance of the visual target (Bronstein, Gresty, & Rudge, 2004; Gresty & Lempert, 2001). That is, as the target distance decreases, the size of the t-VOR increases. In fact, linear compensation is only needed when the visual target is fairly

close since targets viewed from a distance require negligible shifts of gaze to maintain visual acuity (Gresty & Lempert, 2001). Although these data would suggest that the t-VOR is seldom requisite, in instances where such a compensatory reflex is essential, the latency of the t-VOR has been recorded to be as fast as 20 ms in humans (Gresty & Lempert, 2001).

The anatomical connections for the maculo-ocular reflexes are less well known than those of the angular-VOR generated by the SCCs (Leigh & Zee, 2006), largely due to the complexities of developing lateral acceleration sleds that could easily be used during clinical testing. As the maculo-ocular reflex pathways pertain to the utricle, the t-VOR involves polysynaptic connections that arise from the *lateral* portion of the macula, with central connections that traverse to the contralateral vestibular nuclei possibly via the cerebellum (Leigh & Zee, 2006). Together with other synaptic connections via the cerebral hemispheres, the cerebellum, and the visual and somatosensory systems, the vestibular nuclei coordinate compensatory ocular and motor responses during passive perturbations and self-generated movements (Gresty & Lempert, 2001; Leigh & Zee, 2006). Therefore, in response to an abrupt translational acceleration to the left, the lateral hemimacula of the left utricle is excited, which provides a low-gain compensatory horizontal eye movement to the right via the right lateral rectus muscle and the left medial rectus muscle (see Figure 4–5) (Leigh & Zee, 2006). In addition, the medial hemimacula of the right utricle is excited, causing a diminutive ocular rolling in the direction ipsiversive to the linear acceleration. This ocular ipsi-roll reflex is less robust (or non-existent) in response to brief linear accelerations secondary to the longer latency required to initiate the ocular-roll reflex (Gresty & Lempert, 2001). However, in response to a sustained linear acceleration, such as during eccentric rotational testing, both the t-VOR and the c-VOR are evident secondary to the sustained applied force on the weighted otoconia (Gresty & Lempert, 2001).

Counterrolling Macula-Ocular Reflex (c-VOR).

The c-VOR occurs in response to sustained tilting

of the head in the lateral direction (roll axis) as well as the sagittal plane (pitch axis). As the head tilts laterally, the eyes counterroll in order to maintain the horizontal meridians of the retina toward the earth horizontal plane (Tran Ba Huy & Toupet, 2001). One primary limitation to this reflex, however, is its fundamental low sensitivity or gain. As Tran Ba Huy and Toupet (2001) explain, a lateral tilting of the head by 90° yields an eye rotation of only 6°. Such a physiologic response is the equivalent to the movement of the minute hand on a clock by only 1 minute. This low-gain reflex is approximately 10% of actual head tilt (Ödkvist, 2001), and occurs with a much longer latency than the t-VOR, typically up to 300 ms (Gresty & Lempert, 2001). Provided the head tilt is static, the c-VOR is largely dependent upon the otolith maculae, specifically the utricle (Ödkvist, 2001). However, under dynamic head bobbing or sustained lateral roll conditions, such as that of a sustained jet fighter roll, the cyclotorsion of the c-VOR is under the control of the vertical SCC (Ödkvist, 2001). Thus, it is possible for the perception of tilt to be imparted from acceleration-induced canalicular activity with virtually no otolith component (Gresty & Lempert, 2001). Therefore, it is vital to understand the various stimulus conditions that contribute to a macular response in order to differentiate it from a canalicular response. It is, however, possible to provoke a c-VOR of otolithic origin from sustained eccentric linear acceleration, (to be discussed later under dynamic unilateral centrifugation testing in Chapter 8). In fact, this form of eccentric linear acceleration causes a c-VOR that is almost entirely "pure-otolithic." This is largely due to the fact that the eccentric counterroll VOR response is largely driven by the lateral centripetal linear force directed across the outwardly displaced utricular macula, rather than the more robust [dynamic] counterrolling VOR that can be produced by the vertical SCCs during dynamic head tilting or dynamic lateral rolling (Gresty & Lempert, 2001).

The anatomical connections for the c-VOR have received a greater degree of investigation than those of the t-VOR due to the advancements of eye recording techniques and better rotational testing (Leigh & Zee, 2006). As they pertain to the utricle, the c-VOR involves synaptic connections

that arise from the *medial* portion of the utricle. The medial hemimaculae has been shown to be more important for signaling head tilt, which produces a compensatory counterrolling using vertical torsional ocular muscles (Leigh & Zee, 2006) (see Figure 4–5). Therefore, in response to a static head tilt or sustained eccentric rotation to the left, the medial hemimacula of the left utricle is excited which provides a low-gain compensatory cyclotorsional eye movement to the right via the right inferior rectus and inferior oblique muscles and the left superior oblique and superior rectus muscles (Leigh & Zee, 2006).

Maculo-Spinal Reflexes

Maculo-spinal reflexes are generated by the otoliths in association with spinal reflexes in order to maintain postural stability during abrupt linear translations. During unexpected perturbations, these reflexes are generated in order to provide rapid muscular responses that counteract opposing linear forces. This maculo-spinal reflex has been described as a startle reflex. However, as Gresty and Lempert (2001) explain, "the earliest part of this startle response is purely vestibular in origin. It is very likely that this response is triggered by stimulation of the otolith apparatus, as one could tentatively suggest by the irregular units" (p. 25). Specifically, the type I striolar, non-coherent hair cells would provide the required irregular afferent response. In addition, Brandt (1999) demonstrated that these otolith-generated reflexes are critical in providing ongoing anti-gravity muscle activation. Brandt (1999) hypothesized that it is a loss of this tonic activation through the lateral vestibulospinal reflex during a crisis of Tumarkin. During such crises, patients are noted to inexplicably fall to the ground without a loss of consciousness, often describing a complete loss of postural muscle tone resulting in the inability to maintain upright stance (Brandt, 1999). Such maculo-spinal reflexes are also experienced on a daily basis by commuters who stand on a moving train. During abrupt starts and stops, maculo-spinal reflexes provide the necessary counterbalanced postural reflexes required to avoid falling. Clinically, it is this reflex that is evaluated during VEMP testing (Colebatch,

2001). Although both the saccule and the utricle are capable of producing such a reflex, the utricle is the more relevant anatomy for vestibulospinal mechanisms because most perturbations experienced in the environment occur in the horizontal rather than the vertical plane (Leigh & Zee, 2006).

Vestibulocollic Reflex (VCR)

Recently, investigation into a saccular reflex has brought new light to the examination of saccular physiology and function. Saccular function has been shown to be responsible for providing a significant contribution to the vestibulocollic reflex (VCR) (Colebatch & Halmagyi, 1992; Colebatch, Halmagyi, & Skuse 1994). Inputs from the saccule, cervical spinal cord, and cerebellum are important for mediating the cervical ocular reflex (COR), which coordinates head, neck, and eye reflexes for image stabilization. Afferent projections from the saccule course through the inferior branch of the vestibular nerve in order to innervate interneurons within the MVN and LVN (Lysakowski et al., 1998). From there, efferent fibers are sent down the descending MLF to innervate interneurons within the cervical and spinal cord via the MVST and, to a much lesser extent, the LVST. From there, synaptic connections extend to cervical anterior horn cells and both flexor and extensor cervical motor neurons within the neck (spinal accessory nuclei of CN XI) (Figure 4–6). This vestibulocollic reflex arc helps to stabilize the head on the shoulders by coordinating neck muscle contractions that resist passive movements of the head (Lysakowski et al., 1998). Stimulation of the saccule can, therefore, produce measurable responses from neck muscles known as vestibular evoked myogenic muscle potentials (VEMP). Clinically, this vestibulocollic reflex arc can provide valuable information regarding the neural integrity of the MVST, as well as saccular and inferior vestibular nerve function.

Vestibulospinal Reflex (VSR)

Vestibulospinal function is predominantly governed through the lateral vestibulospinal tract

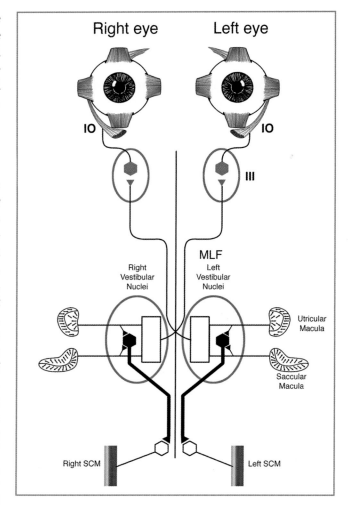

FIGURE 4–6. Vestibulospinal pathways from the maculae. Utricular neural pathways innervate the ocular motor system, whereas the saccular pathways project down the ipsilateral medial vestibulospinal tract (MVST) to innervate the anterior horn cells (AHC) of the spinal cord and the ipsilateral sternocleidomastoid muscle (SCM). Medial longitudinal fasciculus (MLF); IO (Inferior Oblique Muscle). From Vestibular-Evoked Myogenic Potentials (VEMPs) by D. L. McCaslin and G. P. Jacobson, 2016. In G. P. Jacobson and N. T. Shepard (Eds.), *Balance Function Assessment and Management*, (pp. 533–579). San Diego, CA: Plural Publishing. Reprinted with permission.

(LVST). Projections within the LVST predominantly originate from the utricle macula, as well as the vermis and fastigial nuclei, via the interneurons of the lateral vestibular nuclei. The neural input delivered through the LVST is constantly held active. This constant tonic contraction provides a dominant, and much needed, excitatory synaptic input to lower postural extensor motor neurons and muscles, which serves to hold upright posture in the presence of a continuous gravitational vector (Lysakowski et al., 1998). This excitatory pathway is known as the vestibulospinal reflex (VSR). Clinically speaking, loss of such input from a unilateral vestibular lesion significantly reduces extensor output. This creates a "weaker" side ipsilateral to the lesioned side with a tendency for patients to fall or veer to this weaker side such as that observed during the Fakuda Stepping Test.

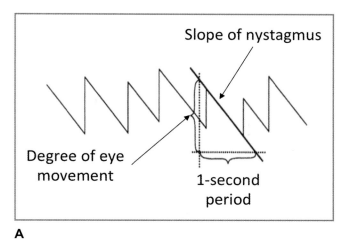

A

B

FIGURE 4–7. Right-Beating (**A**), and Left-Beating (**B**) nystagmus. Nystagmus is quantified by determining the slope of the slow-phase component, and qualified (named) according to the fast phase component. The slope of the nystagmus is determined by calculating the degree of eye movement that usually occurs over a 1-second interval. Upward on the graph is rightward eye movement and downward on the graph is leftward eye movement.

VESTIBULAR NYSTAGMUS

Nystagmus Defined

Baloh and Honubia (2001) define nystagmus as a nonvoluntary rhythmic oscillation [jerking] of the eyes. Nystagmus has an abnormal slow phase deviation of the eyes in the orbit that often has its origins from the vestibular system. The slow phase is followed by a quick "resetting" phase, which brings the eyes back to the primary position within the orbit. This fast (resetting) phase is mediated by the paramedian pontine reticular nuclei and MVN within the brainstem (Leigh & Zee, 2006). Although the slow phase component of the nystagmus is vestibular in origin, nystagmus is always named by the fast phase. That is, a right-beating vestibular nystagmus has a leftward moving vestibular slow-phase followed by a rightward fast-phase (Figure 4–7). During vestibular testing, VOR nystagmus is often induced; however, the presence of nystagmus in the absence of any head movement or clinical induction is often pathologic. Vestibular nystagmus is seldom purely unidirectional and often exhibits elements in the horizontal, vertical, and even torsional plane (Leigh & Zee, 2006). Although nystagmus can occur in any plane within the orbit, according to Ewald's first law, resulting nystagmus will always occur in the same plane as the affected canal. Horizontal nystagmus, however, is generally the most common presentation. This

is because any neural imbalance produced by the damaged vertical SCCs is usually cancelled out by the coplanar intact SCCs, leaving a dominant horizontal nystagmus (Leigh & Zee, 2006). Understanding the physiology of vestibular nystagmus is best discussed in relation to h-SCC VOR physiology. Therefore, only horizontal vestibular nystagmus will be discussed here, as it is most relevant during physiologic testing of the vestibular system.

Nystagmus from Unilateral Vestibular Lesions

As stated earlier, vestibular nystagmus can be clinically provoked, or it can occur in response to a pathologic imbalance in the vestibular system. The neurophysiology underlying pathologic nystagmus parallels that of the neural substrate of the h-VOR discussed earlier.

Central Tonic Neural Asymmetry

The physiologic symmetry of the vestibular system is ultimately determined by the tonic neural balance of the central vestibular nuclei (Baloh & Honrubia, 1996; Barin & Durrant, 2000; Curthoys & Halmagyi, 1996). Under normal physiology, an equal afferent signal is delivered to each vestibular nuclei complex, thus creating a tonic neural balance within the central vestibular system (see Figure 3–5A). A change in normal physiologic balance of the central vestibular system *at rest* dictates that an alteration, (increase or decrease), in the symmetry of the vestibular periphery sensory end organs exists. Therefore, in the state of a peripheral afferent asymmetry, a subsequent asymmetry in interneuron activity is created between the VN (Barin & Durrant, 2000) (see Figure 3–5C). Secondary to this central tonic asymmetry, an enduring spontaneous nystagmus is manifested, with concomitant vegetative symptoms of nausea and vomiting. In addition, associated or frank vertigo is often present. The vertigo is often debilitating in this stage with the patients reporting a perceptual rotation toward the non-lesioned labyrinth (Barin & Durrant, 2000). Within days or weeks, however, tonic rebalancing of the VN is possible following successful central compensation. Following complete central compensation, a tonic asymmetry no longer exists within the central VN and the spontaneous nystagmus slowly abates.

Pathoneurophysiology of Spontaneous Nystagmus

The pathophysiology of an acute spontaneous nystagmus in response to an acute unilateral vestibular insult is secondary to an asymmetrical neural tone within the central VN. In the absence of an afferent peripheral input, type I neurons within the ipsilesional VN quickly lose their input and neuronal activity. Concomitantly in the contralesional intact VN, there is a significant increase in the average *central* resting rate (Cur-

thoys & Halmagyi, 1996). This dramatic increase in resting neural activity in the contralesional VN is due to the lack of ongoing commissural inhibition from the ipsilesional VN. Unfortunately, the increase of resting activity in the contralesional VN serves to further increase their neural inhibition on the lesion side via the commissural fibers, thus silencing it even more, (if possible) (Curthoys & Halmagyi, 1996). This augmented tonic neural asymmetry within the VN is similar in physiology to that of a high velocity head acceleration toward the contralesional ear. Secondary to this asymmetry, neural stimuli are sent via the second and third-order neurons to excite the motor neuron units of the extraocular muscles causing a subsequent slow deviation of the eyes in the ipsilesional direction, (slow phase vestibular component). The slow phase deviation is followed by a quick resetting of the eyes in the contralesional direction back to their primary ocular position (fast phase component). Until central compensation is complete, a neural asymmetry will persist and an enduring spontaneous nystagmus continues. It is only when central compensation of the central VN is achieved, that tonic neural symmetry returns and the spontaneous nystagmus abates.

Nystagmus from Bilateral Peripheral Vestibular Lesions

An acute unilateral vestibular neural asymmetry will always produce a spontaneous nystagmus secondary to the tonic imbalance of the afferent system (Baloh & Honrubia, 1996; Barin & Durrant, 2000; Curthoys & Halmagyi, 1996). However, if both vestibular peripheries were affected *equally* and *simultaneously*, a neural asymmetry would fail to exist. In this case, spontaneous nystagmus would not occur because the afferent inputs between the vestibular nuclei remain balanced. In fact, in the most extreme case, where the overall sensitivity (response or gain) of the system becomes acutely *absent* in each ear, there is also a lack of spontaneous nystagmus, as the tonic afferent peripheral drive continues to remain *equal*, albeit at 0 spikes/second.

Despite the absence of any spontaneous nystagmus in cases of acute bilateral labyrinthine areflexia, the absence of a vestibular afferent neural drive is not without complication and functional impact. In the absence of any vestibular afferent input, an effective VOR cannot exist. As a consequence, a compensatory eye movement in the equal and opposite direction cannot be produced, and a resulting blurring of the visual field occurs with any head movement. In short, the VOR fails to integrate *any* head movement in order to produce an appropriate compensatory ocular response to maintain visual stability. Even in response to the smallest of head movements, fixation of a particular image momentarily slips off the retina. At this point, fixation must be redirected back onto the intended target, with a latency no shorter than 200 ms (Leigh & Zee, 2006). This is known as a corrective saccade, and can easily be identified during head impulse testing. The resulting dilemma from such a loss of bilateral peripheral vestibular input is an inability to maintain visual fixation of an intended target on the retina whenever brief head movements are introduced. The lack of visual fixation during repeated head movements, such as that during ambulation, often creates a *continuous* inability to maintain visual fixation of the environment. This creates a "shaking" or "jumping" of the visual environment, which is known as oscillopsia, and is a common indicator of bilateral peripheral vestibular damage, such as that encountered during vestibulotoxicity (Leigh & Zee, 2006).

We have discussed the consequences of symmetrical, bilateral vestibular lesions; however, what are the consequences of *asymmetrical*, vestibular lesions? In theory, labyrinthine destruction that occurs *asymmetrically* should produce a spontaneous nystagmus that beats toward the healthier ear, or at least the higher tonic neural firing rate. However, the *temporal aspects* of an asymmetrical, bilateral vestibular insult are critically important in determining the onset of any spontaneous nystagmus (and vertigo). Interestingly, there are conditions where asymmetric labyrinthine lesions could fail to produce spontaneous nystagmus and vertigo. One such clinical condition is an asymmetric decline of the peripheral afferent neural drives that specifically occur at different rates, but does so in a very chronic, and slow manner. The lack of spontaneous nystagmus and vertigo during such *slow* progression of clinical disease is due to the concomitant and ubiquitous central vestibular compensation process (Carin & Durrant, 2000; Curthoys & Halmagyi, 1996). The efficient, physiologic compensation process allows for a *continuous* rebalancing of the central neural activity that is omnipresent *during* the slow, pathologic, asymmetric change in afferent peripheral neural drive. In short, the rate of asymmetrical neural decline is equaled by the rate of central compensation. An example of such a pathologic process would be that of neurofibromatosis type II, where slow-growing bilateral vestibular schwannomas can grow and impact vestibular afferent function at significantly different rates. However, due to the slow growth patterns of the vestibular schwannomas (albeit asymmetric), acute vestibular nystagmus and vertigo are often absent, secondary to the effectiveness, and efficiency of the central compensation process. If the schwannomas were to alter their growth pattern in such a way that the afferent neural drive became acutely asymmetric, it is likely that spontaneous nystagmus (and vertigo) would ensue (depending on the residual level of remaining afferent neural drive).

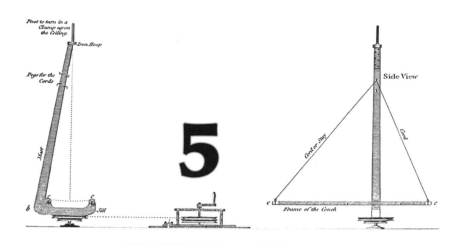

5

The Clinical Utility of Rotational Testing

INTRODUCTION TO ROTATIONAL TESTING

Now that we have a thorough understanding and foundation of the vestibular system's anatomy and physiology, we can begin to discuss the relevance and overall physiological responses generated by rotational testing. Just as the cochlea responds to a broad range of acoustic frequencies, the vestibular system equally responds to a broad range of acceleration stimuli (frequencies). Similar to the auditory system, the vestibular system's sensitivity range is significantly broader than what is needed for daily life activities. Specifically, the vestibular system's response characteristics are principally efficient and effective for a narrow range between 0.05 and 6 Hz, even though its detection sensitivity for acceleration stimuli can extend well beyond this range. Figure 5–1 illustrates this point and highlights the system's effectiveness for the narrow frequency range where natural head movements occur. Within this frequency range, the responsiveness of the vestibular system can be characterized as a linear system capable of operating with nearly perfect VOR gain and phase (Goldberg et al., 2012; Wilson & Jones, 1979). This is ideal insomuch that the operating range of the VOR is functionally matched to those activities that are most common during ambulation and particularly those active head movements that are associated with daily life activities, approximately 1 to 5 Hz.

Figure 5–1 also depicts the nonlinearity and lack of response unity (perfect gain) for frequencies that occur above and below those associated with natural head movements. For these frequencies, VOR gain and phase are significantly poorer. Unfortunately, the test stimulus that is most commonly used to clinically evaluate the vestibular system, the caloric stimulus, falls within this range and is, therefore, neither truly ideal nor representative of daily life activities. This can be seen in Figure 5–1 where the gain and phase of the vestibular system at the frequency of the caloric stimulus is quite poor. This is not to say that the caloric response fails to deliver a useful clinical result. As many clinicians who assess the vestibular system know, the caloric test offers a distinct advantage for determining laterality of vestibular pathology. However, one of the primary disadvantages of the impuissance of the caloric stimulus is that even the slightest vestibular pathology is often sufficient to deleteriously impact its ability to provoke a vestibular response. This may seem like a positive advantage of the caloric stimulus, as its

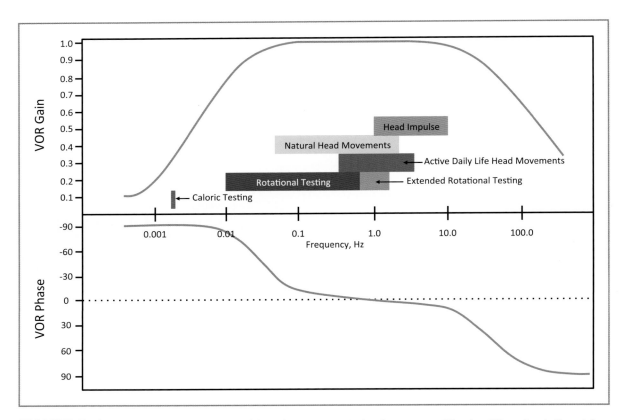

FIGURE 5–1. Distribution of tests and head movements by frequency. The traditional rotational frequency range is from 0.01 to 0.64 Hz. Extended rotational frequency range can, at times, include frequencies through 2.0 Hz. Caloric test frequency is plotted at 0.003 Hz. Head impulse testing is between 1 and 10 Hz. Response characteristics for gain and phase of the vestibular system (VOR) are superimposed on the frequency range. Note the linear response and near perfect phase of the VOR for natural and active head movements of daily life between 0.05 and 5 Hz. Adapted from Barin, 2013; Goldberg et al., 2012; Wilson & Jones, 1979.

sensitivity to identify slight vestibular pathology is good. However, a stimulus that only stimulates and reflects a very small portion of an operating (response) range is extremely limiting when characterizing the function of a system whose frequency operating range is much broader. This is even particularly more poignant for the caloric stimulus as it resides at the extreme lower end of the operating frequency range, where the majority of vestibular pathologies have their initial and greatest impact. In fact, this has always been a significant disadvantage of the caloric test, as it is analogous to confining a hearing test to 8000 Hz (where the majority of auditory pathologies have their initial and greatest impact), from which a comprehensive auditory phenotype

must be characterized (for the entire frequency range). Unfortunately, this analogy is all too true when performing vestibular assessments. Somewhere along the way since the time of Róbert Bárány, the standard clinical practice of confining vestibular assessments to caloric irrigations, and making a clinical judgment regarding the health of the entire vestibular system's frequency response, has become far too commonplace. The recent advent of the video head impulse test (vHIT) has made a concerted effort to address this problem. Video head impulse testing is a relatively new clinical assessment tool that attempts to fill the high frequency stimulus void in the comprehensive vestibular evaluation. Video head impulse testing provides a stimulus presentation range to the vestibular system, usually between 1 and 10 Hz (Barin, 2013). However, its success in extending the frequency range beyond the caloric stimulus is certainly not without merit and challenges. Although the benefits of vHIT testing have proven to be worthwhile, the consistent and accurate delivery of a quick acceleration impulse to the head remains a significant hurdle. Moreover, the stimulus frequency range is well above that stimulated during caloric irrigations, leaving a stimulus void from 0.003 to approximately 1 Hz. Rotational testing not only fills this stimulus void (see Figure 5–1), but also provides the most stable, precise, and consistent stimuli delivery mechanism available during vestibular assessment.

Principle of Rotational Testing

Rotational testing offers a repeatable, reliable, consistent, precise, and tolerable acceleration stimulus, which makes it an excellent device for investigating the physiological response of the vestibular system. Moreover, its precision for measuring detailed outcomes is unparalleled. Rotational testing evaluates the function of the VOR under highly controlled conditions. In fact, Arriaga, Chen, and Cenci (2005) indicated that the sensitivity of rotational vestibular testing was so precise that it should be the primary test of vestibular function, with videonystagmography (VNG) reserved as a complementary test.

Rotational testing is fundamentally composed of a series of back-and-forth oscillations (rotations), in addition to a series of abrupt persistent rotations that are used to stimulate the vestibular system. Rotations are delivered to a seated patient via a computer-controlled torque driven chair that can be finely tuned to apply exacting accelerations and velocities. With the head tilted downward by approximately 30°, so as to place the horizontal semicircular canal in the horizontal plane for maximal stimulation (Figure 5–2), the body and head can precisely be rotated at exacting frequencies, from as slow as 0.003 Hz (that of the caloric stimulus), to as quick as 2.0 Hz (Brey, McPherson, & Lynch, 2008b). In addition, constant

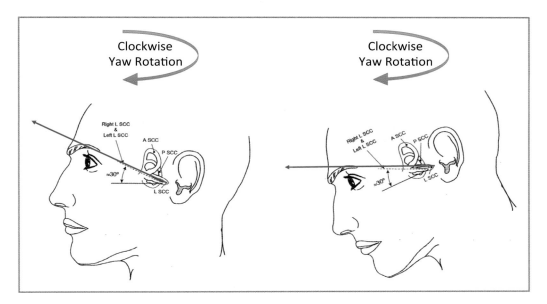

FIGURE 5–2. Rotation around the earth vertical axis is performed with the head tilted downward by 30° so as to align the horizontal semicircular canal in the optimal plane of [yaw] rotation (*red arrow*), thus maximizing excitation and inhibition in accordance with Ewald's first law. Adapted from Barin, K. & Durrant, J. (2000). Applied physiology of the vestibular system. In P. R. Lambert & R. F. Canalis (Eds.). *The Ear: Comprehensive Otology*. Philadelphia, PA: Lippincott Williams & Wilkins. Used with permission.

velocity stimuli, as fast as 400° to 600°/sec, and thrust accelerations as quick as 1000°/sec², can also be delivered (Neuro Kinetics, Inc.). Modern day rotational testing offers an array of test options for delivering precise and exacting stimulus delivery conditions.

Eye movements (VOR), in response to the varying chair accelerations, are precisely recorded through electrooculography (EOG), or via high sampling-rate videooculography (VOG) methods. Testing is generally conducted in a lightproof enclosure, or at least under vision denied conditions, so as not to allow for any visual or optokinetic contributions when measuring the VOR. Precise rotational paradigms have been well established and are applicable to a wide range of populations, from very young patients to octo- and nonagenarians. However, prior to discussing the routine (and not so routine) tests performed during rotational testing (Chapters 6, 7, and 8), this chapter discusses the equipment and patient setup, the various components of the rotational test battery, and the clinical utility and patient candidacy for rotational assessment. Furthermore, this chapter introduces the physiological response obtained during rotational testing, as well as the advantages and limitations of rotational testing, its repeatability, and overall reliability, as well as provides an introduction to the rotational stimuli.

THE ROTATIONAL CHAIR

Unlike audiometers, the options for purchasing a rotational chair are very limited. Currently, there are only a few manufacturers producing "turnkey," commercially available equipment dedicated to advanced clinical rotational testing. The two most common manufacturers in the United States are Neuro Kinetics, Inc. (NKI) and Micromedical, Inc. Figure 5–3 shows two images of the Neurotologic Test Center Suite (NOTC) produced by Neuro Kinetics, Inc. Each image comprises a lightproof enclosure and torque-driven rotational chair. The primary difference between the two images are that the NOTC on the left is a stan-

dard rotational chair, whereas the image on the right is a chair that is capable of producing angular rotations with the chair positioned slightly off vertical axis. This later testing is known as Off-Vertical-Axis-Rotation, or OVAR, and requires an upgraded torque motor that sits higher off the floor. As such, the increased rotational tilt of the chair necessitates an eight-foot diameter booth in lieu of the six-foot diameter booth used with the standard NOTC chair. Figure 5–4 shows two images of the System 2000 produced by Micromedical, Inc. Both images show the same rotational chair. The difference between the images is that because the videooculography goggles are fully enclosed, the testing can be performed without the need for a lightproof enclosure. This can offer a distinct advantage in test environments that may not be able to support a six-foot or even eight-foot diameter enclosure. Moreover, the boothless nature of this rotational chair makes it easily convertible to concomitantly perform videonystagmography testing simply by lowering the chair into a flat, or caloric position.

Rotational Chair Components

The rotational chair itself is fairly straightforward. Figure 5–5 identifies the various components to a basic lightproof booth rotational chair. Beneath all the complexities of the software and the intricacies of a finely tuned torque motor, lies a chair that rotates on the earth-vertical axis using a variety of different stimulus paradigms during which eye movement recordings are made. However, nearly all rotational chairs have certain principal components that are integral to their construction and performance. Such components often include a test enclosure, a torque driven motor, safety harnesses, head restraint devices, a computer and/or electrical console to run the chair, and a means by which eye movements can be recorded such as with videooculography goggles. Although eye movements can also be recorded via electrooculography (EOG), the use of electrode leads has almost become obsolete in routine clinical practice, as video goggles have become less expensive and offer finer detail during the collection of ocu-

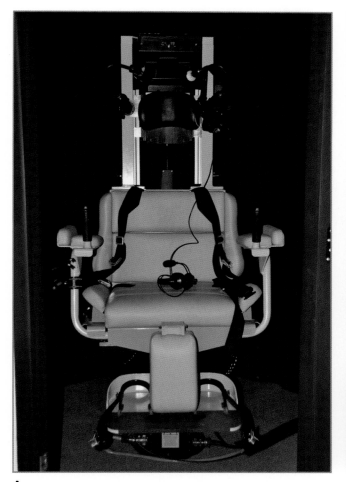
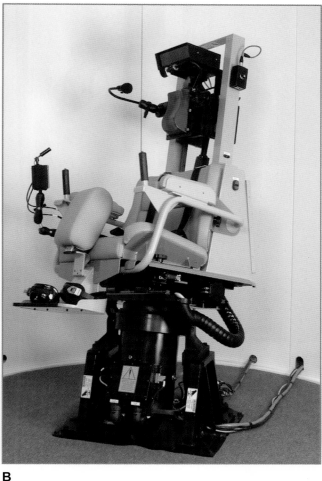

A   B

FIGURE 5–3. **A.** Earth-vertical axis rotational chair. **B.** Off-vertical axis rotation (OVAR) rotational chair shown tilted posteriolaterally by 30°. Image courtesy of Neuro Kinetics, Inc.

lar data that can be recorded, played back, and stored in secure files. Although this basic hardware is common to most rotational chairs, the individual hardware may vary slightly in design across manufacturers. Nevertheless, these components are critical to the accurate administration of rotational testing as well as the safety of the patient. Each component will now be discussed.

Rotational Test Enclosure

The most obvious component to rotational test equipment is that the chair is often housed within a lightproof enclosure (Figure 5–6). A lightproof (or

at least a vision denied) environment is required to perform rotational testing so as to ameliorate any visual cues that can augment the production of the VOR. The augmentation of the VOR by visual cues is known as visual-vestibular enhancement and is discussed in Chapter 8. Elimination of any visual cues is essential if rotational testing is to isolate the response from the vestibular system, and negate any visual contributions to the VOR.

So what are the distinct advantages of performing rotational testing within a lightproof enclosure versus a boothless test suite using a fully enclosed videooculography goggle? One advantage to performing rotational testing in a

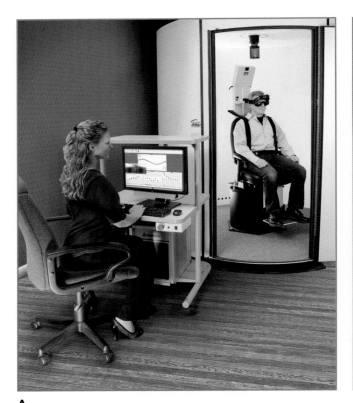

A

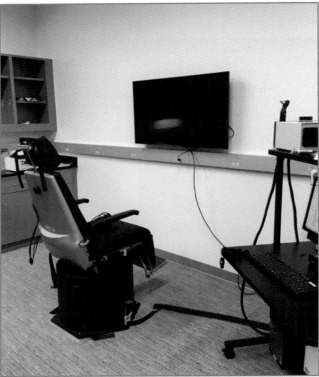

B

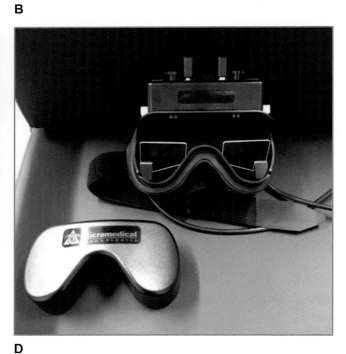

C   D

FIGURE 5–4. Images of rotational test suite (System 2000, Micromedical, Inc.). **A.** Depicts the rotational chair in a lightproof booth. Image courtesy of Micromedical, Inc. **B.** Depicts the rotational chair in a boothless setup. The LCD screen in the foreground provides the stimulus for the ocular motor stimuli, while the vision denied goggles are used during VOR applications. **C.** Depicts the video oculography goggles with the vision-denied cover in place. **D.** Depicts the same goggles with the vision-denied cover removed. Images B–D courtesy of James Madison University, Harrisonburg, VA.

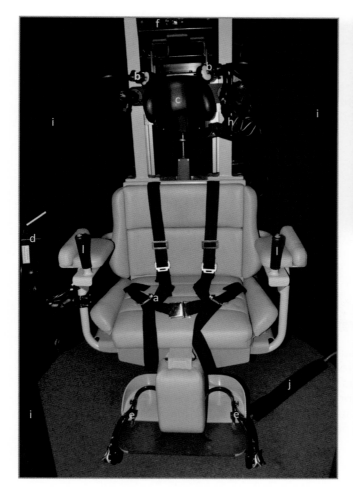

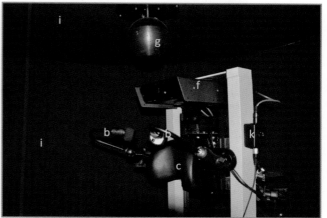

FIGURE 5–5. Earth vertical axis rotational chair with various components labeled: (a) Seatbelt restraint, (b) Articulating head restraints, (c) Headrest, (d) Infrared video camera, (e) Foot restraints, (f) Ocular motor projector,(g) Optokinetic projector, (h) Biocular cameras (hanging on head restraints), (i) Lightproof enclosure (inside walls painted black), (j) CPU/ electrical cords, (k) Talk-back patient volume dial, (l) SVV buttons and hand holds during rotations.

lightproof enclosure is that precise ocular motor testing can be conducted prior to rotational testing. Although ocular motor testing can be conducted outside of a lightproof enclosure, which is often employed during most VNG assessments, there is evidence that suggests ocular motor responses are best measured in a lightproof environment, particularly optokinetic reflex testing. Therefore, most current videooculography goggles are designed to have an "open line of sight" so the patient can effectively view the ocular motor stimuli while the videographic recordings are obtained (Figure 5–7). Use of biocular versus monocular goggles has certain advantages and disadvantages, which will be discussed a bit later. For a boothless option, ocular motor stimuli are generally presented on

an LCD screen or light bar positioned in front of the patient. A second advantage to performing rotational testing in a lightproof enclosure is the administration of certain specialty tests under a highly controlled environment. Such tests would include certain rotational tests that evaluate how the visual and vestibular system interacts together. These tests are known as visual-vestibular interaction tests, and are discussed in Chapter 8. Although boothless rotational tests can perform such tests as visual suppression testing, other tests like visual-vestibular enhancement testing, unilateral centrifugation testing, and subjective visual vertical/horizontal testing are often best performed in the absence of any competing visual stimuli.

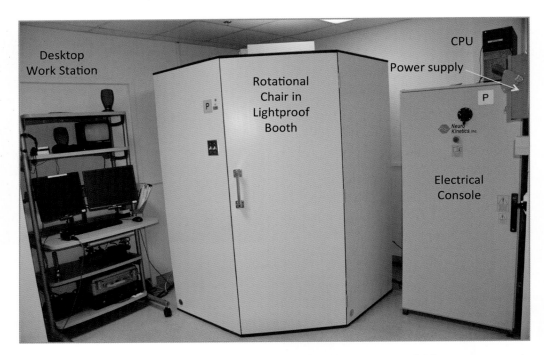

FIGURE 5–6. Rotational vestibular test suite (Neuro Kinetics, Inc.). The power supply receives "cleaned" and "stabilized" power from a remote transformer. The CPU controls the electrical console, which in turn supplies the rotational chair located in the lightproof booth with the precisely controlled stimuli for the various rotational protocols. The entire suite is managed from the workstation where the clinician monitors the stimuli, chair operation, patient safety, and data capture and analysis.

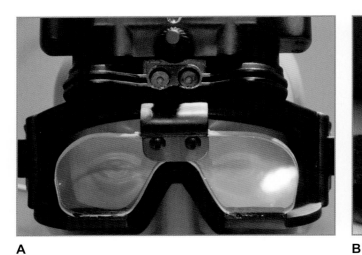

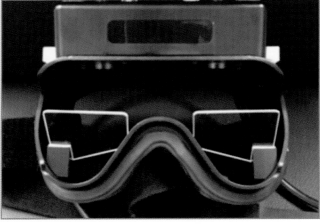

A   B

FIGURE 5–7. A. The transparency through the dichroic glass, which allows for the viewing of ocular motor signals presented directly in front of the patient. **B.** A similar transparency in another set of biocular goggles. Image courtesy of James Madison University. Both goggles have their infrared cameras mounted vertically above the dichroic glass, which allows for recording of eye movement without obstructing vision. Knobs positioned on the camera mounts allow for slight adjustments in the viewing angle of the reflective glass.

On the Horizon: Enclosed LCD Video Goggles

Currently, manufacturers are designing commercially available versions of an LCD videooculography goggle (Figure 5–8) capable of presenting a full range of ocular motor stimuli under a fully enclosed goggle. A distinct advantage of a fully enclosed videooculography goggle capable of presenting a full complement of ocular motor stimuli is its portability. This becomes a significant advantage, particularly in environments that can be outside the clinical settings, such as those of sports traumatic brain injury (TBI) "on-field" assessments, or even during military field-use immediately post concussion during combat or even non-combat related injuries.

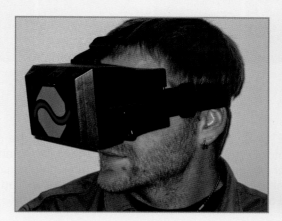 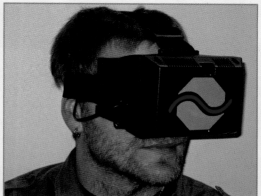

FIGURE 5–8. Images showing an LCD projection goggle known as a "3D Head Mounted Display (HMD) System." Visual field is completely enclosed using a self-contained 3D imaging LCD screen capable of projecting all ocular motor pursuit stimuli and other various visual stimuli such as three-dimensional images, reaction time stimuli, light reflex stimuli, subjective visual vertical and horizontal stimuli, vergence testing, and optokinetic stimuli able to elicit an OKN response in multiple planes. Goggles are powered and analyzed via a portable laptop making this system highly mobile in various environments, including patient rooms and frontline activities, including sports and combat situations. Images courtesy of Neuro Kinetics, Inc.

Rotational Chair Motors

All chairs sit atop a computer-controlled AC-driven torque motor (Figure 5–9). Modern torque motors (unlike their predecessors) provide an exceptionally smooth and quiet stimulus. This is essential as it helps to ameliorate, or negate, any somatosensory or auditory cues that can augment the VOR response, and sometimes provide subtle cognitive contributions, which can assist in the detection of rotation (Van Nechel, Toupet, & Bodson, 2001). Aside from being quiet and incredibly smooth, modern day torque motors are also capa-

ble of producing an incredible amount of angular momentum, specifically up to 340 foot-pounds of torque (Brey, McPherson, & Lynch, 2008a). Such a high production of torque allows for the generation and presentation of highly controlled stimuli that are capable of generating highly precise and repeatable accelerations up to $1500°/sec^2$ for a 400-pound patient. The degree of acceleration gradually increases up to $3500°/sec^2$ for lighter patients weighing 100 pounds (Brey et al., 2008a). The principle behind the torque motor is such that the same exact acceleration stimulus can be delivered to all patients independent of patient weight,

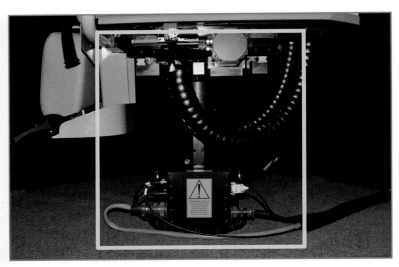

B

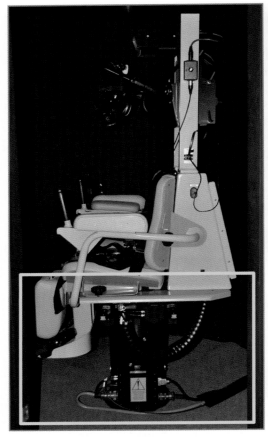

A

FIGURE 5–9. Torque motor positioned beneath the rotational chair. Motor is highlighted by the yellow rectangle (**A**) and shown in a larger scale (**B**). Electrical and programming patch cords connect to the base of the torque motor, which are supplied from the electrical console.

which is imperative if outcome measures are to be compared across patients, between clinical sites, and across repeat patient visits over extended periods of time. This was a significant advantage when rotational chairs transitioned from less reliable DC-driven torque motors to their current AC-driven torque motors in the early 1970s.

Specialized components of motors can be found on some chairs, which allow for either tilting of the chair off the vertical axis (OVAR), or displacement of the chair's center of rotation off the horizontal axis. The later is known as unilateral centrifugation (UCF) testing, and is discussed in great detail in Chapter 8. As mentioned earlier, OVAR torque driven motors are highly specialized insomuch that these motors allow for a slight tilting of the chair off the vertical axis prior to, or during, yaw rotation. With regard to UCF testing, many chairs have been designed to displace the center of rotation off to the right or

left. This is known as eccentric rotational testing. The degree of displacement can be as much as 1 meter (or greater) on some research chairs; however, many clinical test paradigms limit the displacement of the chair's center of axis no greater than 10 centimeters. These two tests, OVAR and UCF, are highly specialized tests that are used to investigate otolith (maculae) function. More will be discussed in terms of these specialized tests in Chapter 8.

Ocular Motor Projector

Above the chair is usually mounted a projection device that provides the stimuli used during ocular motor assessment (Figure 5–10). An alternative to an ocular motor projection device is the use of an LCD screen through which the various ocular motor stimuli are presented. LCD screens are often used with boothless rotational systems

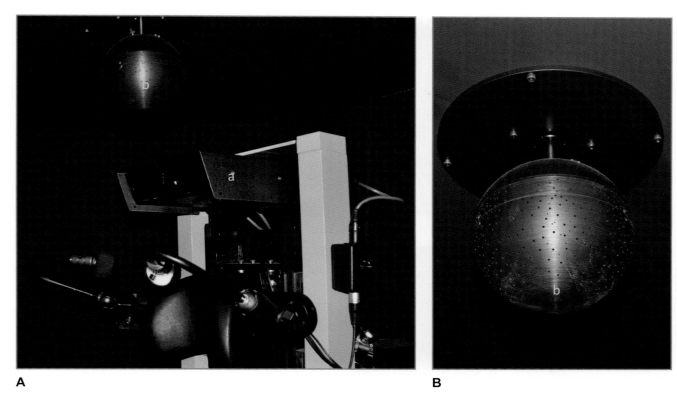

A   **B**

FIGURE 5–10. A. Ocular Motor Projector mounted above the headrest and head restraints (a). Optokinetic stimulus projector is mounted above the chair on the ceiling located directly in the center of the lightproof booth (b). In this stimulus design, the optokinetic stimulus field is a projection of random white dots similar to a star field. The optokinetic stimulus projector better visualized in **B**.

(see Figure 5–4B). It should go without saying that performing a comprehensive ocular motor assessment is absolutely essential prior to conducting any rotational assessment protocol. This is because the VOR (our measured outcome) is an "indirect" measure of vestibular function that is filtered through our ocular motor system. Any ocular motor abnormalities will invariably have a deleterious impact on the resultant nystagmus produced during rotational testing. Recall that the fast phase of vestibular nystagmus is, in fact, a saccade that is produced by essentially the same neural substrate that produces visually guided saccades (Leigh & Zee, 2006). If an abnormality is present in the production of a saccade, then there is a good chance that this abnormality will also be manifested within the VOR output, and consequently your rotational VOR results. It is imperative that such ocular motor abnormalities be identified prior to conducting any rotational testing so as not to misdiagnose a vestibular disorder in lieu of a more correct ocular motor disorder.

Patient-Clinician Talk-Back System

Every enclosed rotational chair has a two-way communication system by which the clinician and patient can communicate during testing. Boothless chair options are an exception to this setup. Figure 5–11 depicts an example of a talk-back communication system. This component of the rotational chair is critical, as most of the rotational tests performed require some form of mental tasking. Throughout this text, we will discuss the importance of tasking and its critical importance to obtaining accurate and reliable data. At times, the talk-back system can be challenging, particularly when the patient has significant hearing loss and feedback becomes a problem. For patients with little to no functional hearing (aided or

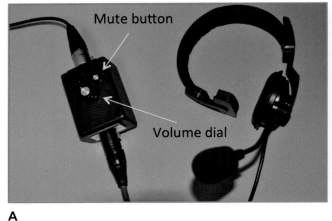

A

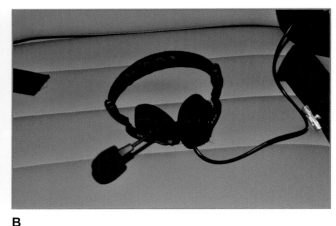

B

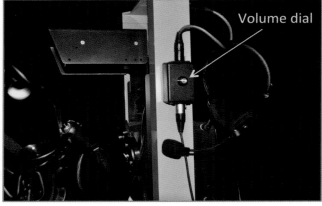

C

FIGURE 5–11. Patient talkback system. **A.** The clinician audio headset with chin microphone and volume/mute handset. **B.** The patient audio headset with chin microphone. **C.** The same headset hanging next to the volume adjustment dial mounted on the side of the rotational chair.

unaided), the talk-back system is often set aside in favor of an alternative means of tasking, such as reciting a story, recipe, or even manually signing a predetermined topic.

Infrared Patient Video Monitor

With the exception of a boothless rotational chair, each rotational chair also has an infrared video camera that is mounted to the chair and allows for *visual* monitoring of the patient during the entire test (Figure 5–12). This can be important for four reasons. First, it permits the detection of any anxiety and/or allows the clinician full observation of the patient's behavior during the test. At times, increased anxiety in a patient can be detrimental to performing rotational testing, and can often cause unwanted noisy, or spurious, data in the VOR response. The onset of anxiety may be secondary to claustrophobia experienced

from being in the lightproof enclosure, the fear of having an increase in vertiginous symptoms, or even nyctophobia (fear of the dark). Many times, patients can overcome this anxiety and will at least attempt, if not often complete, the test simply because they are comforted by the fact that you can "see" them during the entire assessment, even if they cannot see you. Second, having a video monitor can also be critically important for a select group of patients, particularly those who are deaf and use American Sign Language to communicate, or to alert the clinician to any problems they may be experiencing. The third reason for the use of a video monitor is that the clinician can monitor whether the patient has altered their position in the chair. This addresses both a safety issue as well as a standard of test-operations issue. Patient safety is the number one priority during rotational testing. Therefore, it is essential that the clinician continuously monitor the patient

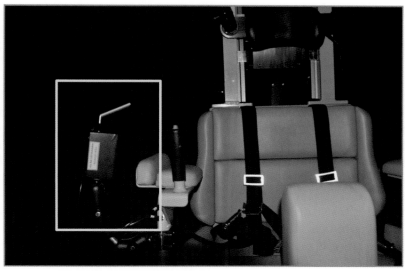

A

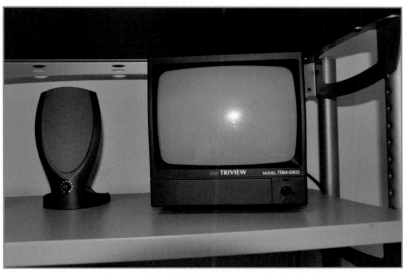

B

FIGURE 5–12. Patient visual monitoring system. **A.** The infrared camera mounted to the arm of the rotational chair (*yellow rectangle*), which provides a black and white image of the patient in the lightproof enclosure on the video screen (**B**).

to determine whether they are slipping out of position, or become agitated, confused, or disoriented. However, the concern for patients slipping in the chair should be entirely ameliorated if the patient is harnessed securely and properly in the chair. Safety of the patient is always the primary concern, particularly during higher (faster) rotational stimuli. Monitoring patient position also addresses a standard-of-testing operations issue. Confirmation that the patient's head remains in the proper test position is critical for reliable and repeatable results. Patients have a tendency to slip (slide) down in the chair during rotations, which often places them in a slouched position and can often alter the position of their head. Moreover, movement of the head during angular rotations can also incite an acute onset of severe vertigo secondary to an abrupt change in the spatial positioning of the semicircular canals relative to their pre-test orientation in space (Coriolis force). This causes an immediate response from the semicircular canals that quickly respond to the ongoing rotational stimulus. This, of course, also produces a significant change in the VOR response (your output measure) that no longer represents the intentions of the test. Rather, the new head position introduces unwanted vertical VOR responses and altered horizontal VOR responses that significantly contaminate the test data. The fourth reason a visual monitor is important in rotational testing is that it provides an alternative "recording" method by which the clinician can visualize a patient's eyes if VOG or EOG cannot be performed, such as with a baby or a toddler. Most young children will not (and often should not) perform rotational testing by themselves until they are of sufficient age to maintain an appropriate seated posture and understand their responsibility during the test. This, however, does not mean that a baby or young child cannot participate in rotational testing. In fact, they can and often do complete rotational testing. Using a slightly modified test protocol, a young child or baby can sit in a parent's lap during rotations while the clinician simply observes the child's or baby's eyes and confirms the presence of an appropriate VOR in relation to the rotational stimuli. During such testing, the video goggles are not being worn and, consequently, an objective measure of nystagmus cannot be determined. However, a binary decision regarding the presence or absence of a functional VOR can often be determined, which is sometimes all the data you need when determining the functional aspects of a child's or baby's VOR. In this sense, this "recording" method is more of a qualitative response rather than a quantitative one.

Headrest

Another basic component of the chair is the headrest (Figure 5–13). The headrest should be positioned so that it appropriately aligns the head in a slight downward 30° position (see Figure 5–2). This will properly align the horizontal semicircu-

lar canals in the horizontal (or yaw) plane and, in accordance with Ewald's first law, provide maximum stimulation of the lateral canals during upright rotation. However, slight-to-mild deviations in the orientation of the head have been shown to have minimal effects on the intensity of the VOR during rotational testing (Coats & Smith, 1967; Fetter, Hain & Zee, 1986). We discuss the effects of head position more when reviewing factors that impact rotational testing later in this chapter. Nevertheless, it is important the clinician make every attempt to standardize test procedures in order to maximize and homogenize the test results across patients.

Booth Light and Circulating Fan

Within the booth itself are usually mounted a light and a circulating fan. The fan should be strong enough to periodically refresh the air during each assessment. The light is usually red for two reasons. First, a red-light environment provides sufficient light to prepare the patient for electrooculography, if VOG is not available or appropriate, thereby significantly reducing the adaptation time needed to stabilize the corneoretinal potential (CRP). Bartley (1951) effectively showed stabilization of the CRP to the required 1 mV in a little as 5 to 10 minutes using a red-light environment, compared to 15 to 20 minutes using a white-light environment (Brey et al., 2008b). That being said, the time spent preparing your patient for EOG rotational testing can be applied to the time required to effectively dark-adapt and stabilize the CRP prior to testing. Obviously, this is less of an issue when conducting videooculography testing, which has become the standard for current rotational equipment. The second reason for the red light is that it is generally less obtrusive to a patient who needs to visually reacclimate to their surroundings prior to opening the enclosure door following completion of test procedures (rotations). The circulating fan and booth light are, otherwise, functional components of the equipment that have no effect on the VOR response, unless the light is unintentionally left on during testing. Leaving the booth light on during testing will invariably cause a suppression, (or even complete ablation), of the VOR

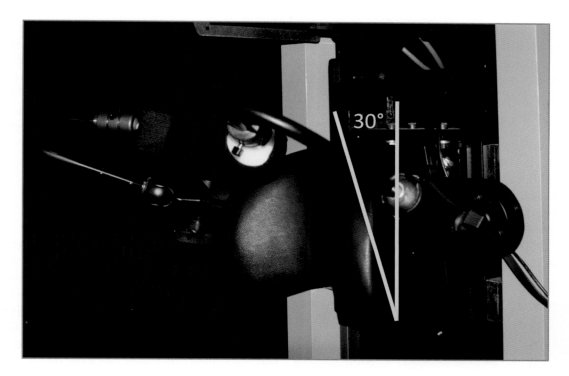

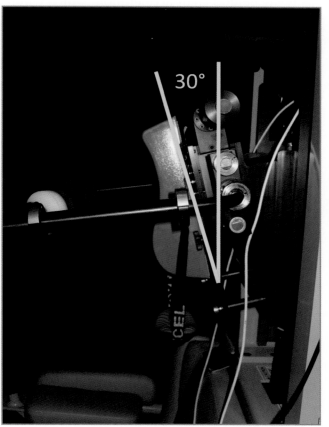

FIGURE 5–13. Rotational chair headrest. Note the slight 30° downward angle that each headrest promotes in order to align the horizontal semicircular canal in the yaw plane to maximize excitation and inhibition in accordance with Ewald's first law.

response secondary to visual fixation. In light of this, failing to turn off the light should always be considered a potential artifact when an absence of VOR response is unexpected during rotations.

Rotational Chair Safety Harness

All rotational chairs will have some form of safety restraint devices and/or harnesses. At a minimum, all chairs will have a seatbelt and many now come equipped with a four- or even a five-point harness (Figure 5–14). In addition, other safety restraint devices may be present such as knee, leg, and even foot restraints (Figure 5–15). Such restraints become increasing more important as certain tests

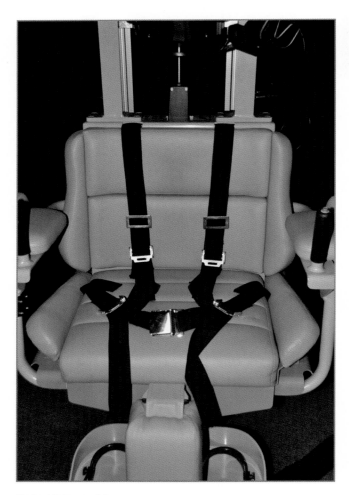

FIGURE 5–14. The rotational chair's four-point seat belt harness. Not pictured is an additional chest strap that brings the shoulder straps close together for added security and retention.

require higher acceleration and/or constant velocity stimuli. In fact, rotational stimuli greater than 200° per second can often produce a feeling of centripetal force that can give the impression or even produce a physical displacement of the body away from the chair. During these rotations, having a snuggly-fit four-point harness restraint as well as leg, knee, and foot restraints all contribute to giving the patient an enhanced degree of safety and feeling of security.

Rotational Chair Head Restraints

Another important restraint that all rotational chairs have is a head restraint device (Figure 5–16). This is one of the most critical components to rotational testing as it ensures that the angular acceleration and velocity stimuli generated by the chair's torque motor is precisely translated to the head, and subsequently to the vestibular system. Without such head restraint devices, the head would easily lag behind chair acceleration, which would produce an aberrant delay in the stimulation of the head and vestibular system relative to the chair. This would almost certainly cause a significant decrease in the sensitivity (or gain) of the vestibular system, while concomitantly producing an opposing VOR response that is not "in-time" with the applied stimulus (referred to as the "phase" of the VOR response). Without a doubt, this relationship between a poorly synchronized stimulus and vestibular response gets exponentially worse as rotational acceleration stimuli are increased (i.e., the quicker the acceleration stimulus, the greater the chance and larger the error in head-to-chair delay). As a result, a great deal of effort must be given to ensure that the head is secured tightly against the chair without sacrificing patient security, safety, and comfort. This is possibly the most (or at least one of the most) critical setup procedures prior to performing any rotational test protocol(s).

Types of Head Restraints. The most common form of head restraint is achieved through articulating arms with soft head-posts, as pictured in Figure 5–16. Such head posts are used to securely "push" and hold the head against the headrest to minimize the degree of head rotation and neck

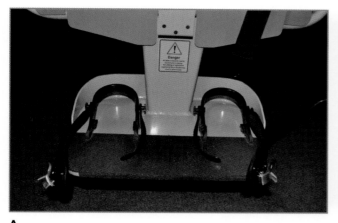

A

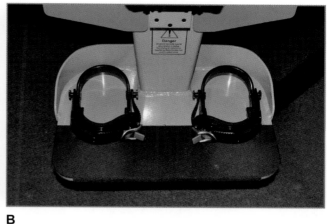

B

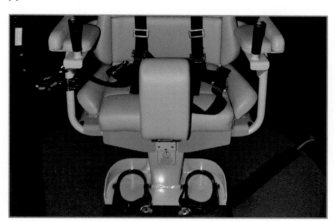

C

FIGURE 5–15. Foot restraints in both the open (**A**) and closed (**B**) positions. **C.** Depicts the center leg support / cushion, which can also be used in conjunction with a large Velcro strap that can help secure the legs around the center cushion for increased safety and support.

flexion during testing. It is important to note, however, that appropriate instructions to the patient, like asking them to refrain from moving their head and holding it as still as possible during testing, can go a long way in improving your data acquisition. Other common forms of head restraints are a head and/or chin strap (similar to a chin strap of a football helmet) (see Figure 5–16). A chin strap can help hold the head (and body) upright in the chair to prevent slouching as well as assist in keeping the head held tightly against the head restraint while still maintaining an acceptable degree of patient comfort. These additional restraints may even be applied in addition to the articulating arm soft head posts, particularly if higher rates of stimuli are applied. Always remember that a strong correlation exists between the potential for head movement and stimulus intensity, such that the greater the acceleration stimulus, the greater

the probability of inadvertent and unwanted head movement or slippage. Such unwanted head movements will always introduce noise and aberrant responses in your VOR outcome measures. Subsequently, the measured response will less accurately represent or reflect the true physiological response that was originally intended by the test stimuli. This deleterious relationship between unintended head movement and measurement artifact often exponentially worsens the quicker the acceleration stimulus. This problem often plagues test protocols such as quick head thrusts secondary to either slippage of the video goggles on the head or slippage of the head in the chair. This challenge is again discussed in Chapter 8 when reviewing how newer rotational protocols (crHIT) are attempting to apply extremely quick chair accelerations in order to thrust the head similar to that of head impulse test protocols. Less

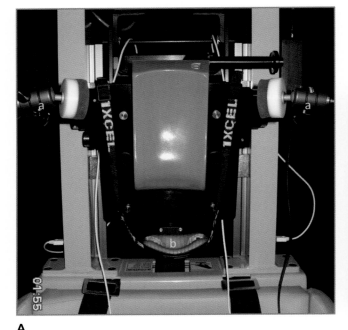

A

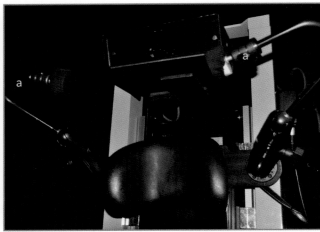

B

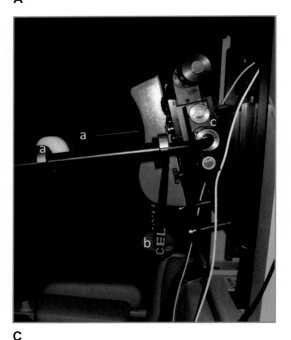

C

FIGURE 5–16. A–C. Various head restraints. Articulating arms (a) serve as head restraints. The head posts are capped with soft foam tips that can firmly be pressed against the patient's scalp for firm placement and restraint of the head against the headrest without sacrificing comfort. Optional chin strap (b) can also be used to secure the head for stability and safety. Optional self-centering head restraint (c) ensures head is positioned in the center of angular rotation. Images A & C courtesy of Neuro Kinetics, Inc.

common head restraint devices are soft moldable facemasks, self-centering head restraints (see Figure 5–16), and even bite blocks. Although these are often found only in research labs, such devices are critical if precise and reliable data are to be obtained during rotational protocols involving very high acceleration stimuli.

Computer/Software/Electrical Console

Ever since the 1960s, computer-controlled rotational chairs have permitted the control and administration of extremely precise stimuli. Moreover, the recordings of vestibular ocular reflexes through increasingly advanced eye tracking software programs have significantly enhanced the clinician's ability to track more subtle eye movements (e.g., ocular torsion), and subsequently identify more subtle pathology (e.g., internuclear ophthalmoplegia, micro-saccadic abnormalities). It goes without saying that the computer is the single most important component to the rotational test suite. It is also the one component that is constantly changing. Advances in computing software are constantly improving eye tracking recording techniques and analysis algorithms. In fact, an in-depth discussion regarding the computer and its software would be futile as the discussion would likely be outdated by the time this text was even one year old. Therefore, it is not the intent of this text to review the software for each

manufacturer. Rather, the intent of this text is to present a comprehensive understanding of the rotational chair and its diagnostic tests and physiologic results. With that being said, it is important for the reader to understand that many of the examples presented throughout this text are from personal experience and, therefore, from a single rotational system. The principles of analysis and interpretation, however, can theoretically be applied across all rotational data, regardless of the software and manufacturer.

Figure 5–17 depicts the electrical console (or the brains) behind the chair. It is a complex network of wires and switches that feed the appropriate electrical signals to the torque motor, the videooculography goggles, and/or the ocular

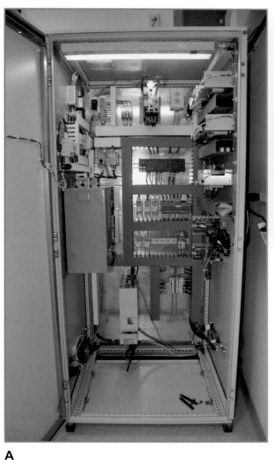
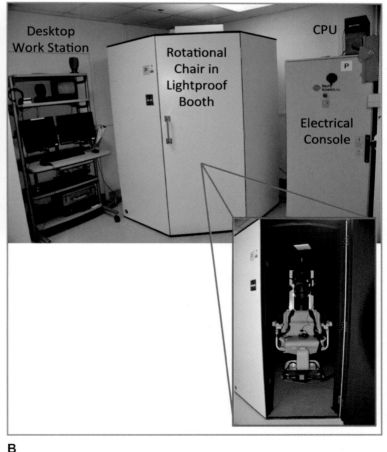

A   **B**

FIGURE 5–17. Electric console with the door open (**A**) showing the complexity of electrical engineering to control the stimulus parameters of the rotational chair (**B**). The electrical console is supplied by a ceiling mounted remote transformer (not shown) that "cleans" and "stabilizes" any fluctuations in power prior to delivering it to the console.

motor stimulus generator. Like any complex mechanical network of wires, switches, and fuses, problems can occasionally develop and it is important to establish a good working relationship with the manufacturer to ensure the unit is maintained in proper working order and any problems can be troubleshooted when the need arises.

Videooculography Goggles

The second most critical component common to all rotational chairs is the recording goggles (Figure 5–18). High-resolution goggles ensure that accurate and precise eye movements are recorded, from which a detailed analysis and video playback can be performed by the clinician. As previously alluded to, the goggles must also give the patient a clear line of sight to see visual targets

that are presented at various times throughout testing. This is accomplished through sophisticated cameras and mirrors mounted on the front of the goggles (see Figure 5–18). There are many properties of videooculography cameras that can affect their performance. We will review some of the more key components, such as their detection of infrared light, their resolution and frame rate, and various hardware components located on the goggles. However, for an excellent and comprehensive review of videooculography, and the various aspects of ocular video recording, the reader is encouraged to review "Vestibular Function Measurement Devices" by Miles and Zapala (2015).

Biocular Versus Monocular Cameras. Most rotational chairs use biocular goggles rather than monocular goggles, although both can be used

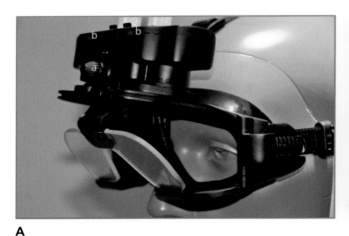

A

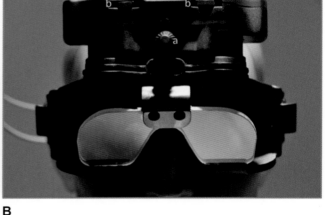

B

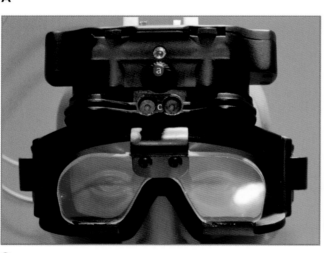

C

FIGURE 5–18. Dichroic mirrored glass. **A.** Shows the mounting angle of the dichroic glass (mirrors). **B.** Shows the reflective coating of the dichroic glass (mirrors). **C.** Shows the transparency of the mirrors, which allows for the viewing of ocular motor signals presented directly in front of the patient. A knob (a) is positioned on the camera mount, which allows for slight adjustment in the viewing angle of the dichroic lens. Smaller dials (b) allow for focusing of the cameras to each eye image. Fixation lights (c) can be presented through the goggle if the vision-denied cover was in place.

effectively. Figure 5–19 depicts both types of goggles. There may be times when there is only a single eye to record from; however, this does not preclude you from using a biocular recording and only analyzing a single eye. However, it is essential to realize that when using a biocular goggle, nearly all analysis software will report rotational *VOR* data that have been combined or averaged from both eyes. That being said, it is important to appreciate that a single-eye *VOR* recording may be more appropriate if there are significant disconjugate eye movements, or a unilateral ocular pathology prohibits biocular recording. This is particularly true if the analysis software does not permit the ability to choose between a biocular versus a monocular analysis. Keep in mind that this rule applies only to VOR assessment and not during analysis of ocular motor results, where the identification of disconjugate eye movements

is always preferred and can be critical to the differential diagnosis. Finally, there are also subtle distinctions between biocular and monocular goggles as it pertains to certain specialized tests, such as subjective visual vertical (SVV) testing. These distinctions are presented when discussing UCF testing in Chapter 8.

Use of Infrared Light. Videooculography cameras utilize infrared (IR) light to identify and capture eye movements by identifying pupil contrast from the lighter surrounding iris (Figure 5–20). The software's capability of identifying and "locking on" to the pupil allows it to track the movement of each eye over time. However, various problems can limit the software's eye-tracking algorithm. Specifically, problems with ocular tracking are most commonly the result of eye makeup. Mascara, in particular, is extremely sensitive to

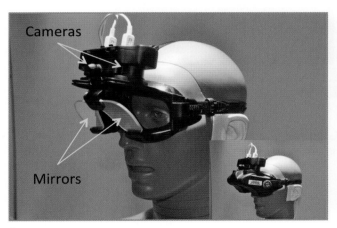

A

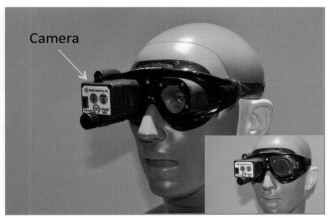

B

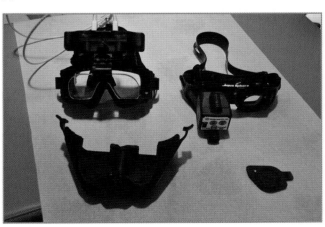

C

FIGURE 5–19. A biocular and monocular video goggle. The biocular goggle (**A**) has independent right and left infrared cameras mounted vertically above each dichroic lens that record the eye image off the mirrored glass. The monocular goggle (**B**) has a single camera mounted horizontally, which provides a direct in-line recording of the eye. The monocular camera can be mounted on either eye. Inset images depict each goggle with the "vision-denied" cover in place. **C.** Both goggles are pictured in a side-by-side comparison with their respective "vision-denied" covers placed in front of each goggle.

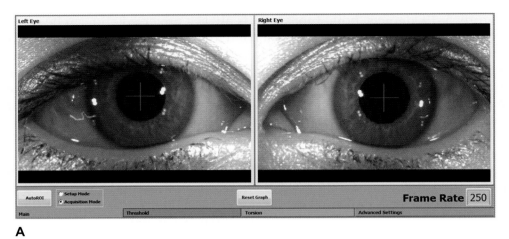

FIGURE 5–20. Videooculography (VOG) showing actual eye image (**A**) versus threshold image (**B**). Threshold detection is adjusted to maximize detection of pupil contrast from surrounding iris.

IR light and produces a reflective surface that the IR light highlights (similar to the pupil contrast). When this happens, the eye tracking software has difficulty making key distinctions between the pupil and the eye makeup (Figure 5–21). Such ocular "splatter" can cause significant problems with eye-tracking algorithms "locking on" to the intended target (pupil), which subsequently creates an extremely poor signal-to-noise ratio and a very poor (noisy) recording. Consequently, the analysis of such noisy recordings is fraught with poor signal detection and either missing or uninterpretable data. This is a similar and common problem often encountered during videonystagmography (VNG) testing. Because of this, it is often helpful to have makeup wipes available for the removal of mascara, in the event that such a situation arises. Other deterrents to accurate (i.e., "clean") eye tracking include eyeliner, ptosis, drooping eyelids, narrow eye slits, significant coloboma, cataract lens replacement surgery, and macular degeneration.

Camera Resolution and Frame Rate. Similar to the screen on your computer or television, sharper images are highly correlated to higher image resolutions. This translates to a greater number of available pixels, which means a greater degree of available visual information and, subsequently, a higher degree of ocular detail (data) acquired during eye movement recordings. Furthermore, the camera's frame rate (i.e., the number of frames

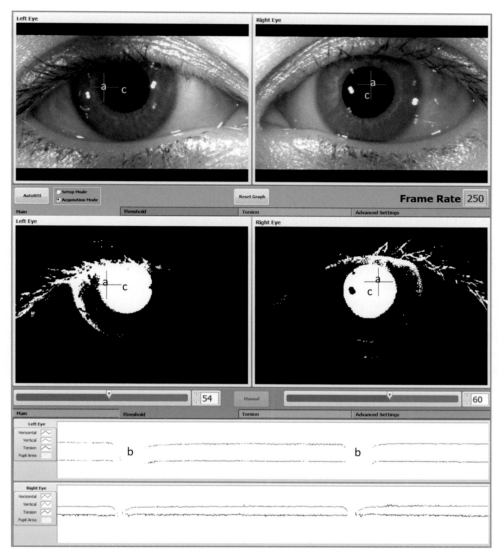

FIGURE 5–21. Videooculography (VOG) images showing oversaturation of the pupil threshold detection due to mascara. This example demonstrates a slight-to-mild impact, which can often be corrected by adjusting the threshold detection parameters. However, at times, such corrections are more difficult to resolve and can easily obscure pupil detection, which is depicted by the offsetting of the cross-hairs (a) from the actual center of the eyes (c). Such offsetting can significantly impact the reliability of your data acquisition. Excessive threshold saturation most often occurs as a result of an inappropriately calibrated threshold detection setting or continuing to test with irreconcilable noise (such as excessive mascara). As a result, consistent VOG capture is either lost (b) or collected as noise, significantly impacting the signal-to-noise ratio.

or "images" the camera is able to capture per second) also correlates to the amount of detail (data) that can be captured during each second of recording time. The higher the frame rate, the greater amount of acquired data. This becomes important during quick eye movements, particularly for some eye movements like saccades, which can be as fast as 900° per second. Keep in mind that the fast phase produced during vestibular nystagmus is physiologically identical to that of a saccade. In light of this, higher frame rates allow for a greater amount of data collection and a greater likelihood of capturing subtle abnormalities associated with extremely transient or quick eye movements (e.g., microsaccades).

Traditional analog cameras have a frame rate of 60 Hz, however, purely digital cameras have a much higher frame rate of 100 Hz, or even as high as 250 Hz. Such frame rates can significantly increase the degree of ocular movement (data) captured. This can be extremely beneficial, particularly for some of the more subtle eye movements, such as torsional nystagmus, as well as even some of the more highly detailed and rapid eye movements, such as micro corrective saccades or ocular flutter. However, it is important to recognize that frame rates can sometimes unknowingly decrease when concurrent or added demands are placed on the software running the eye-tracking algorithms. Such demands may include the addition of pupilometry, torsional tracking, and even increasing the ocular region of recording interest. In general, the less number of the lines the eye-tracking algorithm needs to scan from the image (i.e., the eye), the higher the recording frame rate. Thus, if you increase the region of interest (ROI) of the eye being recorded, (i.e., expanding the recording region to include a larger portion around the eye), the frame rate is going to decrease below the maximum allowable limit the camera is optimally designed to record, (such as dropping from 250 to 200 Hz or lower). Figure 5–22 illustrates a few frame rate examples relative to different recording regions of interest. In light of this, the clinician needs to be cognizant that there is often a compromise or tradeoff that occurs between the desired recording image size, other recording features (e.g., pupilometry), and frame rate. As a clinician, you need to decide which features are important.

Miscellaneous Components of the Video Goggles. There are certain components of the goggles that will require regular attention and routine maintenance. First, prior to making any ocular recordings (whether ocular motor assessment or VOR testing), it is important to properly focus the IR camera image for each eye. This will ensure accurate measurement of even the most subtle of eye movements (e.g., torsional). Because each patient's facial dimensions will vary, the focal length between the eye and the camera will similarly vary from one patient to another. Therefore, it is important to refocus each camera prior to testing each patient. Furthermore, because IR light has a different focal length than visible light, if you focus the cameras in a well-lit room and then proceed to test the patient in a light proof enclosure, do not be surprised if the camera seems out of focus. This being said, it is often better to focus each camera with minimal lighting, such as with the booth's red light, or in a dimly lit room. Note that this is different from the adaptation of the CRP, which requires 20 minutes.

Second, it is important to maintain care of the goggle's face mask and headband, as maintaining a light proof seal against the face is critical to testing, particularly if you are not using a light proof enclosure. Cleaning with an alcohol-based solution should be avoided, as alcohol can dry out the rubber mask and head strap (if made from rubber) and can cause premature cracking.

Finally, inspection of the IR reflective dichroic mirrors (lens) that are fitted directly in front of the eyes should be performed prior to each patient test (see Figure 5–18). It is important to look for any debris, smudges or even cracks that may prevent the eye-tracking algorithm from accurately following eye movement. Use a soft lens cloth to wipe clean and avoid any harsh cleaner (e.g., window cleaner), as this can damage the IR reflective coating.

TEST PREPARATION AND PATIENT SETUP

Now that we are familiar with the principle hardware components of the chair, it is important to discuss key elements that are critical to preparing the patient for rotational testing. These include pretest procedures such as dizziness questionnaires, patient instructions, calibration, and a pre-rotational ocular motor assessment.

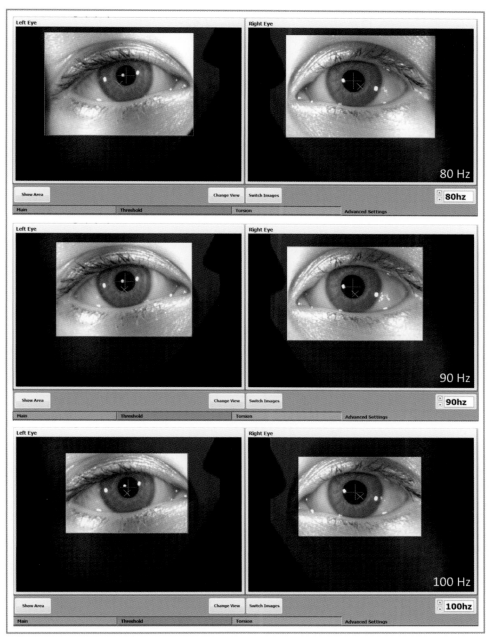

A

FIGURE 5–22. Videooculography (VOG) sampling rate as a function of Region of (Recording) Interest (ROI). **A.** From a 100 Hz VOG goggle. *continues*

Preappointment Fundamentals

When scheduling patients for a rotational assessment, there are two things that are helpful to address prior to the patient arriving for their appointment. The first is to give them any pretest instructions. Pretest instructions would include avoidance of any mascara that could obscure ocular tracking, or the use of alcohol 48 to 72 hours prior to their appointment. Pretest instructions

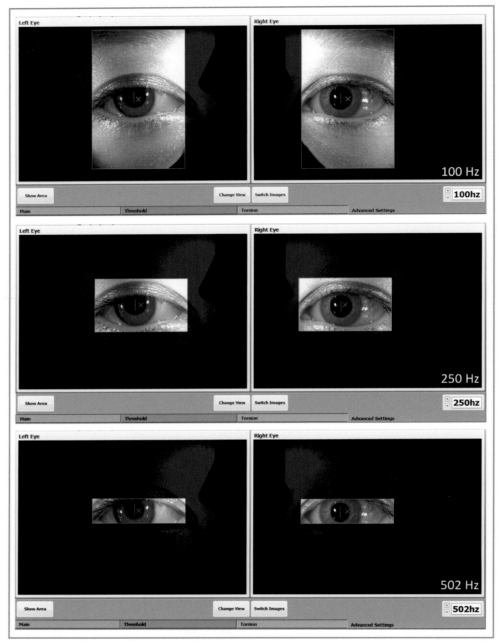

B

FIGURE 5–22. *continued* **B.** From a 250 Hz VOG goggle. As the ROI decreases (smaller), the VOG sampling rate increases (indicated on the lower right corner for each image).

would also include avoidance of any medications that could potentially alter the VOR response (usually suppression of the response), or produce any aberrant findings that would suggest a central pathology. A list of drug classifications and the respective potential abnormality associated with each can be found in Table 5–1. Termination of any medication should be done in conjunction

Table 5–1. Vestibular Assessment Abnormalities Associated With Various Drug Classifications

Drug Classification	Abnormality
Alcohol (ethanol)	Vestibular dysfunction: positional nystagmus; Brainstem-cerebellar dysfunction pattern

Aminoglycoside Antibiotics
  Streptomycin
  Gentamicin
	Vestibular dysfunction: chronic and irreversible vestibular hypofunction, can cause total loss of labyrinthine response

Anticonvulsants
  Dilantin (phenytoin)
  Tegretol (carbamazepine)
	Brainstem-cerebellar dysfunction: vertical or oblique up-beating nystagmus; saccadic intrusions (i.e., cogwheeling) in pursuit pattern

Antidepressants
  Tricyclic (Elavil, Pamelor)
  Others (Prozac, etc.)
  Lithium
	Central sedation pattern; static positional nystagmus; Internuclear ophthalmoplegia; slow peak saccade velocity; opsoclonus; partial or total gaze paresis. Brainstem-cerebellar dysfunction pattern

Chemotherapeutic Agents Cisplatin	Vestibular dysfunction: chronic and irreversible vestibular hypofunction, can cause total loss of labyrinthine response

Diuretics
  Lasix
  Ethacrynic Acid
	Vestibular dysfunction: temporary labyrinthine hypofunction

Antipsychotic Haldol	Opsoclonus

Industrial Solvents
  Xylene, Toluene
  Trichloroethylene, Styrene
	Brainstem-cerebellar dysfunction pattern;
	Vestibular dysfunction; central positional nystagmus; exaggerated VOR; impaired VOR fixation suppression

Marijuana	Brainstem-cerebellar dysfunction pattern
Methadone	Brainstem-cerebellar dysfunction pattern; saccadic undershoot
Opiates	Brainstem-cerebellar dysfunction pattern; downbeat vertical nystagmus
Quinine	Vestibular dysfunction: positional nystagmus
Salicilates (aspirin)	Vestibular dysfunction: transient labyrinthine hypofunction

Stimulants
  Amphetamine
  Cocaine
  Ritalin (methylphenidate)
	Impaired gaze convergence
	Shortened saccade reaction time
	"Rippled" saccade waves with decreased amplitude. Saccadic abnormalities

Sedatives Barbiturates	Brainstem-cerebellar dysfunction pattern Central positional nystagmus
Tobacco, Nicotine	Upbeat nystagmus; square-wave jerks

continues

Table 1–1. *continued*

Drug Classification	Abnormality
Tranquilizers	Central sedation pattern
Benzodiazepines (Valium, Ativan, Xanax)	Brainstem-cerebellar dysfunction pattern
	Downbeat nystagmus, impaired OKN response
Vestibular Suppressants	Central sedation pattern
Meclizine, Scopolamine, Phenergan, Benadryl	Reduced peak velocity; optokinetic nystagmus;
	Decreased slow component velocity (VOR) in caloric and rotational chair testing

Source: Adapted from Cass & Furman, 1993.

with the patient's primary medical provider, as cessation of certain medications may not be possible or medically advisable.

A second preappointment fundamental is to have the patient fill out a dizziness questionnaire. There are many questionnaires to choose from, such as the Dizziness Handicap Inventory (Jacobson & Newman, 1990). Questionnaire(s) can be sent to your patient prior to their appointment, which can facilitate the use of their time during their actual vestibular assessment. Included with the questionnaire could be a brief letter or brochure that briefly discusses the tests the patient with be receiving, but being careful to do so in a nonthreatening way. It is sometimes helpful to include images of the rotational chair, as it can be somewhat threatening for some patients when viewing it for the first time.

Patient Setup

When the patient arrives, it is important to familiarize the patient with the chair. Making them feel comfortable and safe is the priority. This will help to reduce any anxiety, which could deleteriously impact your ocular data. When placing the patient in the rotational chair, the safety restraints and harnesses should be fit tightly against the patient without sacrificing comfort. A firm contact between the goggles and the face is also critical, as any slippage of the goggle during testing can create spurious (often reduced) eye movement data. In addition, the head restraint posts and head/chin straps should be tightened firmly against the head to hold it securely against the headrest and

prevent any movement of the head in either the vertical or horizontal direction. This is the most critical element to securing your patient in the rotational chair, as the degree of head movement will be inferred directly from the degree of chair movement. Any difference between the two will decrease the signal-to-noise ratio and reduce the reliability and accuracy of your results, which can often be subtle in nature.

Instructions to the patient should be straightforward and simple. Placing the two-way talkback communication headphones on your patient will further alleviate any patient anxiety, and provide an excellent way to reduce any test anxiety, further instruct the patient throughout the testing protocols, and provide any necessary mental tasking during certain portions of the test. Communication with your patient is imperative, as good feedback is essential in recording quality eye movements. Periodic reminders to maintain an "eyes open" posture in the dark are absolutely critical to obtaining quality recordings. There is a simple relationship here; good quality and clean recordings will always produce the best possible analyses from your data. Conversely, poor ocular recordings secondary to noisy and insufficient eye tracking, excessive blink artifact, and/or a complete loss of data due to drooping (sleepy) eyelids cannot be recovered or improved, even with the best post hoc analysis filters. Without a doubt, obtaining the "cleanest" eye movement tracking with video goggles is the most critical goal when performing any vestibular assessment. Simply put, analyzing noisy data is no fun. Moreover, analyzing missing data is impossible. *The most important responsibility during the assessment is to constantly maintain good eye tracking data at all times.* This often means online monitoring of the pupil tracking software to ensure good tracking of the eyes rather than focusing one's visual inspection of the recorded eye movement data (Figure 5–23). Periodic adjustment of the IR threshold for pupil, detection may be required throughout testing, as ocular position in the orbit, combating eye detection "jitter" between pupil and makeup contrast, and even very lightly colored pupils, can often cause transient problems with the IR software "locking on" the pupil with good reliability. I have often found poor pupil tracking to be one of the primary shortcomings when performing rotational tests, particularly when conducting rotational testing for the first time. For various reasons, visual attention by the clinician (online visual inspection of the real-time data) is usually directed to the recorded eye tracings (i.e., the ensuing VOR response data) rather than the VOG data and "real-time" eye-tracking data (see Figure 5–23). This is similar to directing one's visual attention to the cumulative-averaged response of an auditory brainstem response (ABR) rather than inspecting or monitoring the online EEG data for noise. The primary difference between ABR recordings and VOG recordings, however, is that once the moment of eye-tracking data has passed, and a portion of the VOG data is lost (due to a loss of eye tracking or eye closure), there is no going back or extending the recording time to collect more eye tracking data (i.e., similar to extending the ABR runtime to collect more ABR sweep data). This is largely because rotational protocols have a predetermined time domain for data collection. There is no "extension" of the immediate test rotation past the predetermined number of chair rotations if data are lost. The analysis is either performed with missing data (never easy) or the specific rotation must be repeated, which can significantly extend the overall test session time (not to mention potential patient discomfort and/or fatigue).

Calibration Test

Prior to performing any test that involves the presentation and recording of stimuli (i.e., eye movements in our case), it is vital to validate the degree (i.e., size) of eye movements before performing any vestibular test protocols. For vestibular testing, this often means validating the size and direction of eye movements relative to the size and direction of known target movements. This *validation* is known as calibration and should always be the first test performed before any test protocols are administered. Although it is understandable that we all may not be experts on reciting the exact calibration standards for vestibular testing, it is important that we all have a thorough appreciation for *why* we calibrate and *how* an inaccurate calibration can negatively impact your test results.

Calibration of the VOG response involves the precise measurement of the change in pupil position within a video image against a known target visual stimulus. Specifically, calibration measures the change in number of pixels the eye image travels as it moves from one position on the video screen to another in relation to a known change in stimulus (target) position. For example, if the eye were to move 200 pixels in relation to a 30° visual stimulus, then the calibration for eye movement would be 200 (pixels) divided by 30 (degrees), or 6.67 pixels for every degree of eye movement. Once calibration has been performed in both the horizontal and vertical directions, the computer software uses this pixel per degree of eye movement to calculate the degree of eye displacement (i.e., degree of nystagmus) in relation to any eye displacement tracked by the video goggles during the assessment. In doing so, the degree of eye movement can be determined for any eye deflection, even torsional eye movements.

It is important that calibration be performed for each patient, as small differences in facial features can produce small to moderate changes in the depth between the goggle lens and the pupil, which can create large differences in the pixel per degree calculation. This can create significant differences in how the algorithm determines the degree of nystagmus from one patient to another. Although the *direction of movement* will be the same for every patient, (positive sloping eye changes for left-beating nystagmus and negative sloping eye changes for right-beating nystagmus), the specific *degree of nystagmus* will not be valid unless patient-specific calibration is performed. The same principle applies if the video goggles

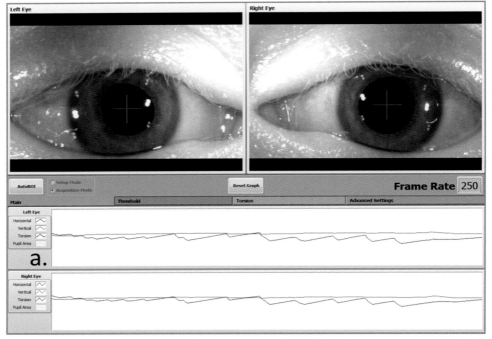

A

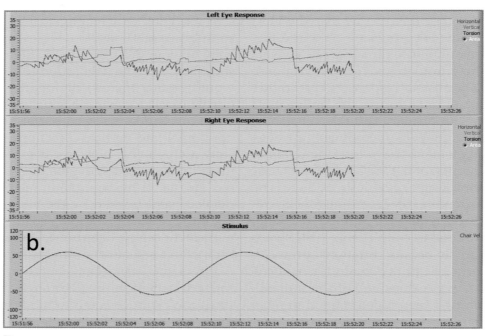

B

FIGURE 5–23. Examiner screen views offer one viewing image showing real-time data acquisition (**A**) similar to that of an EEG response during acquisition of an Auditory Brainstem Response. Horizontal (*blue*) and vertical (*red*) data for each eye are captured in real-time and traced in the graphs (a). Quality eye tracking is essential for the acquisition of high value data and should constantly be monitored for any eye tracking problems, including pupil detection noise (e.g., excessive mascara), loss of eye tracking (disappearance of red and blue crosshairs), excessive blink artifact, eye lash obstruction, ptosis, eye closure, and any significant gaze deviation from primary center. Data for each eye response are then recorded directly from the acquisition screen and stored for analysis (**B**). Stimulus feedback is provided for monitoring of chair velocity (b)

are moved on the patient's head midway during an assessment. Such changes may be minimal, but even small changes can produce surprisingly large changes in the number of pixels per degree. The same is true for using a default calibration, which can introduce measurement errors of up to 25% from the actual value (Miles & Zapala, 2015). Although the use of a default calibration is unavoidable at times (e.g., pediatrics), it is vital to realize that any eye movements recorded during a vestibular assessment (ocular motor movements, VOR, or vestibular nystagmus) and subsequently analyzed using a default calibration can only be interpreted qualitatively, not quantitatively.

Ocular Motor Testing

Following calibration, and prior to conducting any VOR rotational assessment, it is vital to have each patient perform a complete ocular motor assessment. Because the VOR is measured through the ocular motor system, it is critical to identify any potential deficits secondary to central or ocular motor lesion(s). Such deficits will invariably manifest themselves in any VOR recordings during rotational assessments. Therefore, it is important to identify any ocular motor abnormalities prior to conducting any rotational test in order to avoid inappropriately assigning an abnormal rotational test result as a vestibular lesion (when in actuality, the abnormal result is secondary to an ocular motor palsy/paresis, or central visual disorder).

Ocular motor assessment is best conducted in a [rotational] lightproof enclosure. In fact, this test environment is ideal for ocular motor assessment as the target stimulus is the only stimulus within the retinal field of vision. The absence of any visual markers within the field of vision is critical for some tests like optokinetic testing, as these markers can provide subtle cues that can erroneously inflate eye-to-target velocity (Leigh & Zee, 2006). Moreover, optokinetic testing performed in the presence of any stationary visual cues within the retinal field often fails to recruit neural pathways specific to optokinetic reflex pathways (i.e., the Accessory Optic System [AOS] and the Nucleus of the Optic Tract [NOT]) (Leigh & Zee, 2006). It is beyond the scope of this chapter to discuss how to perform the various ocular motor tests or the various abnormalities associated with ocular motor testing, but the reader is encouraged to follow up with McCaslin (2015), as well as Jacobson and Shepard (2016), and Leigh and Zee (2006, 2015) for comprehensive discussions on this topic.

ROTATIONAL TEST PROTOCOLS

Now that we have a better understanding of the various aspects involved with preparing the patient for rotational assessment, let us turn to a brief overview of the various test protocols associated with rotational testing. There are two principal test protocols that are essential to a basic or routine clinical rotational vestibular assessment; sinusoidal harmonic acceleration (SHA) testing and velocity step testing (VST), which is also commonly referred to as trapezoidal step testing, or simply step testing. These two tests comprise the fundamental rotational assessment and, when performed in their entirety, take approximately 30 to 45 minutes to complete. That being said, when these two test protocols are combined with a standard calibration assessment and a comprehensive ocular motor assessment, the basic rotational assessment will take approximately 45 to 60 minutes. Additional rotational tests are available but may not be routinely performed during a standard clinical assessment. Such rotational tests include fixation suppression, visual-vestibular enhancement, subjective visual vertical, subjective visual horizontal, unilateral centrifugation (UCF), off vertical axis rotation (OVAR), and chair head impulse testing (crHIT).

When performing rotational testing, the primary test most often performed is SHA testing. Sinusoidal acceleration testing provides critical data regarding the responsiveness of the vestibular system across a much broader frequency range than the much more common VOR test performed during videonystagmography (VNG) testing; that is caloric testing (see Figure 5–1). In particular, SHA testing provides valuable insight into the responsiveness of the vestibular system for frequencies that are closer to those experienced during daily life activities (see Figure 5–1). This is essential when considering the role of rotational testing in a comprehensive vestibular assessment. Initially, vestibular lesions often impact the effectiveness of the vestibular system for detecting and transducing *low* frequency accelerations. Because of this, a bilateral vestibular lesion will often yield absent caloric responses even though residual (and even normal) vestibular reactivity can objectively be measured for higher frequency stimuli, such as those elicited during SHA testing. Sinusoidal harmonic acceleration testing is discussed in detail in Chapter 6.

Velocity step testing is often included in a routine rotational assessment, as it complements the SHA data and can also assist in the lateralization of peripheral vestibulopathies. Velocity step testing is the oldest of all rotational tests, initially introduced to the vestibular clinic by Róbert Bárány (Chapter 1). It consists of a quick acceleration of the chair to a sustained constant velocity rotation before an equally quick deceleration brings the chair back to a full stop. Depending on the intensity of the acceleration stimulus, the velocity step test can either give unique insight into the central functioning of the vestibular system or can offer valuable insight into lateralizing a peripheral vestibular lesion. Velocity step testing is discussed in detail in Chapter 7.

Collectively, SHA and velocity step testing are often performed together. Jointly, their data can provide invaluable diagnostic insight into peripheral and central vestibular function that no other test can equally deliver. However, SHA and velocity step testing are not without their shortcomings. Each test has its own advantages and limitations, but these are examined independently when discussing each test in Chapters 6 and 7, respectively. The remaining additional tests that can be performed (VOR suppression, visual-vestibular enhancement, etc.) offer additional unique insights into vestibular physiology and should be performed when clinical needs indicate their use. Table 5–2 provides a quick summary of the various rotational tests. The use and clinical indications for these ancillary and specialized tests are discussed in Chapter 8. The determination for the use of these tests lies heavily in the judgment of the clinician. In 2008, Jacobson and colleagues

Table 5–2. Summary of the Various Rotational Tests

Test	Site of Lesion	Response Parameters
Calibration		
Ocular Motor	Central	Test dependent (see Leigh & Zee, 2012 for an excellent review)
Sinusoidal Harmonic Acceleration (SHA)	Peripheral & Central	VOR Gain, VOR Phase, VOR Symmetry, Spectral Purity
Velocity (Trapezoidal) Step (VST)	Peripheral & Central	VOR Time Decay Constant (low velocity), Peak VOR Response Symmetry (high velocity)
VOR Suppression	Central	VOR Gain
Visual-Vestibular Enhancement	Central	VOR Gain
Unilateral Centrifugation	Peripheral	Subjective Visual Vertical (SVV), Ocular Counterroll (OCR; or cVOR)
Off-Vertical Axis Rotation (OVAR)	Peripheral & Central	VOR Gain, VOR Phase, VOR Symmetry

wrote that the "clinician's end goal is to be 'one-step ahead' during the assessment, and that the hypothesis generating process should continue as each bit of new information is acquired through quantitative testing." This is true on a smaller scale during rotational assessment. The administration of certain tests, such as high frequency VOR suppression testing, can be (and should be) supplemented to the "standard" rotational battery of SHA and VST when results indicate the need for further exploration of an abnormal finding. Although we will not discuss the clinical indications for high frequency VOR suppression testing, or visual-vestibular enhancement testing until Chapter 8, the addition of those tests is indicated when central (cerebellar) lesions are suspected, or when results suggest a problem with effective cen-

tral compensation mechanisms. Table 5–3 details the clinical test protocols that should be performed during a standard or routine rotational assessment, as well as the typical stimuli that should be conducted for each test. In addition, various specialized rotational test protocols are listed, which should be performed (or recommended) when clinically indicated.

CLINICAL INDICATIONS FOR ROTATIONAL TESTING

Some of the most common questions asked about rotational testing include, "What are the clinical indications for performing the test?" "How does

Table 5–3. Standard Rotational Clinical Test Battery

Test	Protocol	Stimuli Parameters
Calibration	10° gaze right, left, up, and down.	Smooth pursuit between gaze positions or saccades.
Ocular Motor	Routinely performed	Saccades, smooth pursuit, gaze, optokinetic pursuit, spontaneous testing
Sinusoidal Harmonic Acceleration (SHA) (Chapter 6)	Routinely performed	0.01, 0.02, 0.04, 0.08, 0.16, 0.32, 0.64 Hz* (higher frequencies optional)
Velocity (Trapezoidal) Step (VST) (Chapter 7)	Routinely performed	Low (60°) Velocity Step Testing High (240°) Velocity Step Testing
VOR Suppression (Chapter 8)	Routinely performed	0.08, 0.16, 0.32, 0.64 Hz (no higher than 1.0 Hz)
Visual-Vestibular Enhancement (Chapter 8)	Perform when clinically indicated (central/cerebellar/migraine)	0.08, 0.16, 0.32, 0.64 Hz (no higher than 1.0 Hz)
Unilateral Centrifugation (Chapter 8)	Perform when clinically indicated (otolith)	SVV or SVH during static, On-Center Rotation, UCF-R, and UCF-L eccentric rotations; Generally high velocity 300°/sec.
Off-Vertical Axis Rotation (OVAR) (Chapter 8)	Perform when clinically indicated (otolith)[†]	VOR Gain, VOR Phase, VOR Symmetry

*Minimum of two cycles performed for 0.01 to 0.02 Hz, four cycles for 0.04 to 0.08 Hz, and eight to10 cycles for 0.16 to 0.64 Hz. [†]Currently restricted by the FDA to research applications only.

the clinician triage which patients are expected to gain the most from rotational testing?" And "what criteria constitute an appropriate referral for rotational testing?" We began this chapter by highlighting a comment made by Arriaga and colleagues (2005), that the sensitivity of rotational testing is so precise that it should be the primary test of vestibular function. The evidence for this clinical position comes from a number of factors. First, the test's ability to evaluate the vestibular response over a broad frequency range is unmatched by any other vestibular test. Second, the frequency range rotational testing evaluates is more relevant to those that occur during daily life activities. Third, the precise delivery of the rotational stimuli is not only extremely repeatable and highly accurate, but also very tolerable for most patients. Fourth, the ability to expand investigation of the vestibular system to include central function is essentially exclusive to rotational testing. Fifth, the rotational test's ability to investigate uncompensated vestibular lesions in patients with chronic dizziness is unparalleled within the comprehensive vestibular test battery. Finally, the rotational stimulus is a natural physiologic stimulus (i.e., movement), versus a non-physiologic stimulus (i.e., the caloric stimulus). Shepard and Telian (1996) emphasize the importance of this final point through an analysis of 90 patients diagnosed with Friedrich's ataxia, or olivopontocerebellar atrophy. In their analysis, they identified 5% of patients who demonstrated consistent reductions in rotational chair responses, while concomitantly exhibiting normal caloric responses. Although they acknowledged the fact that cerebellar pathology has been known to cause mid-to-high frequency vestibular abnormalities (thus sparing any reduction in the caloric response), they offered an alternative reason that the disparity between the observed rotational and caloric responses might be due to the fundamental differences between the stimuli (physiologic versus non-physiologic).

Given these six reasons for supporting rotational testing as the primary vestibular test, would it not then seem reasonable to suggest that nearly *every* vestibular or balance-disordered patient is a potential candidate for rotational assessment? The statements above would certainly support this notion. Simply stated, there is sufficient evidence to suggest that rotational testing should be the primary test of vestibular function, largely because it is capable of evaluating both peripheral and central function across a broad frequency range, all while using a natural stimulus that is both tolerable and precise. Then why is it not the primary test of vestibular function? It is clear that the clinical indications for performing the test for most (if not all) vestibular patients are demonstrable. However, despite the unambiguousness of these clinical indicators, rotational testing has failed to establish itself as the gold standard for vestibular assessment; that honor likely goes to the caloric test and videonystagmography.

Several factors have likely limited the elevation of rotational testing as the primary test of vestibular assessment. One of the more salient factors limiting widespread use of rotational testing is likely its reduced accessibility. The reason for this is probably a complex interaction between cost, reimbursement, demand, and space. One traditional argument is that rotational assessment fails to effectively lateralize peripheral vestibular pathology (which many consider to be the most pertinent aspect of any vestibular test). Indeed, lateralization of vestibular pathology is important; however, the fact that rotational testing fails to lateralize peripheral pathology is debatable, as we will see when discussing high velocity step testing in Chapter 7. Accessibility to rotational chairs remains one of the most significant hurdles in advancing the widespread use of rotational testing for every vestibular patient. However, as technology increases and further clinical advances are made regarding the diagnostic power of rotational testing, perhaps the availability of rotational test suites will concomitantly expand. Although the current limitations for the accessibility of rotational testing may restrict the feasibility of completing such testing, it does not change the fact that the clinical indicators used to identify potential patients for undergoing rotational testing remain the same. Whenever possible, rotational vestibular testing should be performed as part of a routine vestibular assessment, or recommended for any patient meeting the indicators alluded to above. In particular, rotational testing should be given a high priority to patients for whom caloric irrigations suggest a bilateral peripheral pathology or for patients that present with a clinical history suggesting chronic uncompensated dizziness.

Considerations for Confining a Vestibular Assessment *Only* to Rotational Testing

With regard to confining a vestibular assessment *only* to rotational testing, there is some evidence to suggest that, when rotational results are *completely* within normal limits, it is unlikely that the results from other *VOR* tests (i.e., caloric testing) will reveal any gross abnormalities (Jacobson, McCaslin, Grantham & Shepard, 2016; Kaplan et al., 2001). In fact, it is unlikely that even a "slight-to-mild" peripheral vestibulopathy would occur without manifesting even the most subtle rotational abnormality, (such as a slight prolonged low-frequency VOR phase lead; although writing this is like placing the cart before the horse as we have yet to discuss SHA testing). Previous studies have investigated associations and correlations across various vestibular test results within the same individuals. Jacobson and colleagues (2016) conducted a within-subject data analysis involving multiple vestibular tests. In this report, they reported a high correlation between caloric test results and rotational SHA gain at the lowest frequency of 0.01 Hz. Although we have yet to discuss the various parameters associated with SHA testing, this finding suggests that patients are likely to exhibit similar labyrinthine responses (VOR gain) on caloric testing and low frequency rotational testing. These data would suggest that those patients who are normal on one measure are likely to be normal on the other measure. Conversely, those patients who exhibit reduced labyrinthine responses (VOR gain) during low frequency rotation are also likely to exhibit reduced caloric responses.

These data would certainly argue that, while certain tests results should often agree, they fail to explain why the same tests don't *always* agree. That is, it is possible for a vestibular pathology to elude identification by caloric testing but not rotational testing (and vice versa). In fact, it would be shortsighted to truly believe that the diagnostic sensitivity of rotational testing is absolute. Shepard

and Telian (1996) reported that during a review of 2266 patients, there was a subset of patients who, due to reasons other than vestibular dysfunction, exhibited mildly reduced caloric responses with completely normal rotational results. Moreover, they also reported a lower sensitivity for identifying peripheral vestibular involvement in a group of patients with Ménière's disease, labyrinthitis, or vestibular neuritis, using rotational testing (66%) than by electronystagmography (ENG) testing (90%). One reason for the disagreement between ENG results and rotational results could be the presence of a borderline or "slight" unilateral caloric paresis. Such borderline vestibular pathologies may elude identification by rotational testing because the normal reference ranges (and associated variances) used to categorize normal versus abnormal patients are not only large, but may [inadvertently] include data from "healthy" individuals that actually have subclinical vestibular pathology (Kerber, Ishiyama, & Baloh, 2006). In addition, most vestibular normal reference ranges are generally not segregated by unique age ranges, but rather encompass a single, more generalized age range inclusive of a broad sampling that can span multiple decades up until 50 or 60 years of age. Such large reference ranges can potentially lead to difficulty in effectively identifying or segregating abnormal vestibular responses from one test (i.e., rotational testing) and having them correlate with another test (i.e., caloric testing). Finally, Shepard and Telian (1996) argued that when tests of VOR function fail to agree, such as rotational and caloric tests, technical error in the administration of either test should always be considered as a possible reason for the disparity. In such an event, readministration of one, if not both tests, should be considered.

Conclusions Supporting a Comprehensive Vestibular Assessment

There is currently no single clinical vestibular test that is capable of eliciting a response from *every* labyrinthine end organ. As such, it is extremely rare that a single vestibular test will ever be successful at revealing the complete vestibular phenotype for any patient, not even a complete rotational assessment. In the study cited above from Shepard and Telian (1996), where the sensitivity for the identification of vestibular dysfunction differed by approximately 20% between rotational and caloric testing, these authors went on to report an increase in the sensitivity to 100% for identification of vestibular dysfunction when considering results from *both* assessments. Overall, this is true for most vestibular assessments, as the sensitivity for the identification of vestibular pathology always increases with a more comprehensive test battery. Therefore, it stands to reason that a comprehensive vestibular assessment should always be considered for every patient. If a comprehensive assessment is not possible, the vestibular clinician should effectively prioritize which tests are going to be the most successful at identifying a suspected vestibular pathology. All things considered, rotational testing is often an excellent initial assessment choice for the many reasons discussed above.

Specific Patient Populations Ideal for Rotational Assessment

We have just discussed the various clinical indicators for when to perform rotational testing. However, there are a number of specific patient populations for whom rotational testing should be considered an absolute necessity. The first clinical population for whom rotational testing is a necessity is when caloric irrigations reveal bilateral vestibular areflexia. Rotational assessment is required is this situation in order to investigate whether there is a true and complete absence of vestibular reactivity. As previously mentioned, nearly all vestibular lesions first impact the lower stimulus frequencies (i.e., the caloric stimulus). This is analogous to the manner in which hearing loss nearly always impacts the higher frequencies first. Similar to the preservation of low-to-mid frequency hearing sensitivity in presbycusis, there is often preservation of residual vestibular function for higher frequency stimuli in the presence of vestibular pathology. Such residual vestibular function for higher frequencies can effectively and objectively be quantified through rotational assessment. This is critical as the presence of residual vestibular function is essential if physical therapy and vestibular *rehabilitation* efforts are to

be successful. Alternatively, if vestibular areflexia is determined for the entire frequency range, this also becomes critical information as vestibular *substitution* therapy is then recommended. Use of rotational testing can also confirm the validity of the bilateral absence of the caloric response. That is, if the caloric response is truly absent, then an abnormal VOR response is highly predicted at the lower end of the rotational test frequencies (Jacobson, McCaslin, Grantham, & Shepard, 2016). However, if the VOR response during rotational assessment is entirely within the normal limits for the lowest test frequencies, then a technical error in the delivery or recording of your caloric response should be considered as a possible contributing factor to the finding of bilateral caloric areflexia.

The second clinical population for whom rotational testing is necessary is when questioning the status of vestibular compensation. For case histories where persistent dizziness, vertigo, or imbalance is reported, a differential diagnosis should include an uncompensated vestibular lesion. Although most peripheral vestibular lesions effectively compensate statically within one to two weeks, and dynamically within a few months, there may be select cases where compensation is incomplete or slow to respond. In such cases, rotational assessment is one of the only clinical tools that can effectively investigate this concern. The use of SHA and velocity step testing can often highlight problems with the compensation process. Moreover, the use of rotational testing (due to its precisely controlled stimulus) makes it an excellent tool for monitoring central compensation progress over time, which is the next clinical population for whom rotation testing is highly recommended.

As mentioned, the third clinical population that would highly benefit from rotational testing are those patients who require monitoring for vestibular degenerative diseases, toxicity, pre- and postoperative status, compensation status, or rehabilitation progress. One of the greatest strengths of rotational testing is its ability to continuously deliver a precise stimulus over repeated clinical visits. Because of this, rotational testing offers a tremendous advantage when monitoring vestibular physiology over an extended period of time, even years. Although there is some variability in how various clinicians may interpret the results (more to be discussed on test-retest variability later in this chapter), or even some variability with how the test is administered (differences in mental tasking procedures), the stimulus delivery will remain exactly the same over time, provided the chair is regularly maintained and calibrated. This is a significant advantage over other assessment tools such as caloric irrigations, which have a number of inherent factors that contribute to a much higher rate of variability (McCaslin, 2012). This is a distinct advantage when monitoring vestibular function during administration of potentially vestibulotoxic medications, whether for medical treatment or labyrinthine ablation. Moreover, the monitoring of vestibular function to show compensation, rehabilitation, or disease progression can be critical to the effective management of your patient.

A fourth clinical population for whom rotational testing is often a necessity is pediatric patients. The noxious nature of the caloric test, concomitant to the wearing of vision-denied video goggles, often precludes the successful administration of caloric testing to young patients. Testing VOR function in very young patients is often limited to a binary "yes/no" decision when determining the presence or absence of a vestibular response. In these cases, it is sometimes best to simply identify the presence or absence of a VOR response during chair rotations while the young patient is seated on a parent or caregiver's lap. If the child can tolerate the video goggles, this is even better. However, very young patients often have a low tolerance for tight-fitting goggles, or many goggles are not designed for very young pediatric faces. Therefore, it is often best to simply observe the child's eyes to determine the presence of a nystagmus response that beats appropriately to the rotations of the chair. This can effectively be accomplished while the patient is seated on a parent or caregiver's lap with the video monitoring system focused on the child's face and the parent securely holding the child's face in the straightforward position (thus maximizing the orientation of the hSCC). In this way, it is possible to confirm the presence or absence of a VOR, even in an infant. Although laterality of a vestibular lesion or general vestibular weakness cannot be determined from simple VOR observation, this approach can be effective when determining complete absence of vestibular reactivity for a patient who is late to walk or has a congenital malformation, such as bilateral enlarged vestibular aqueduct (EVA), or Mondini malformation.

ADVANTAGES AND LIMITATIONS TO ROTATIONAL TESTING

At this time is may be beneficial to present the advantages and limitations of rotational testing as there is significant overlap with the four clinical populations just discussed. As such, some of the points may be highlighted again as many of the above-mentioned indications for clinical use, are also distinct advantages to performing rotational testing. Table 5–4 summarizes the advantages and limitations to rotational assessments.

Advantages of Rotational Vestibular Testing

Rotational testing offers some distinct advantages for assessing the vestibular system. There are eight primary advantages for performing rotational testing. First and most important, rotational testing provides exacting stimuli that are precisely controlled. Second, because the stimulus is precisely controlled, the recorded response exhibits an extremely high degree of repeatability (Brey et al, 2008b; Furman et al., 1994; 2000; Maes et al., 2008). This advantage alone, allows rotational testing to effectively monitor vestibular physiology during recovery or deterioration from vestibular disease or toxicity. Third, rotational stimuli are far less noxious than other stimuli (i.e., the caloric stimulus). Although slower rotational stimuli can produce slight vegetative symptoms of nausea and vertigo, the degree of subjective vertigo present during most rotations is often minimal, making rotational testing more tolerable for patients. Fourth, rotational testing allows for the assessment of pediatric patients when caloric irrigations are often contraindicated (Cumberworth, Patel, Rogers, & Kenyon, 2006; Cyr, 1991; Fife et al., 2000; Phillips & Backous, 2002). Although precise objective measures may not always be obtained due to the inability of fitting infrared

Table 5–4. Advantages and Limitations of Rotational Assessments

Advantages	Limitations
Precisely controlled stimuli	Difficult (but not impossible) to lateralize unilateral vestibular lesions; particular mild paresis
High degree of stimulus and response repeatability (when tasking is consistent)	
Tolerable stimulus / less noxious than caloric stimuli	Equipment cost
Pediatric friendly	Directly stimulates only a portion of the peripheral vestibular system (horizontal semicircular canal), however, the response reflects both peripheral and central contributions)
Broad, more natural stimulus frequency range	
Able to measure central contributions to the VOR (Phase, Time Decay Constants)	
Able to confirm / evaluate bilateral vestibular loss	Response can be complex and not always straightforward to interpret
Monitor/examine central compensation process	

goggles to a child, or even, an infant's head, the observation (or lack thereof) can provide a binary decision of an intact VOR while the child is seated on a parent's lap (Cyr, 1991). Fifth, rotational stimuli assess the vestibular system at frequencies that approach those encountered during normal daily life activities and are, therefore, a more functional measure (see Figure 5–1) (White, 2007). Sixth, rotational testing allows for the precise calculation of the timing relationship (or phase) of the VOR to head movement. This is an important parameter of the VOR as it is a representation of the velocity storage of the system and indirectly reflects central vestibular function (Shepard & Telian, 1996). Seventh, rotational testing provides a measure of investigating bilateral vestibular lesions (Shepard & Telian, 1996). It is well documented that a bilateral absence of any VOR in response to caloric irrigations does not necessarily mean a complete absence of vestibular function. Often, vestibular decrement will first appear for lower frequencies prior to higher frequency involvement (opposite that of cochlear dysfunction) (Brey, McPherson, & Lynch, 2008a). In light of this, caloric testing may not provide an adequate stimulus needed to produce or confirm a vestibular response. Finally,

rotational testing allows for the determination of the progress of central compensation following vestibular insult or vestibular rehabilitation (Paige, 1989; Shepard & Telian, 1996). This is often documented by a recovery in the sensitivity (gain) of the VOR response back to normal levels. However, other subtle abnormalities frequently remain, even following effective compensation, such as a permanent deficit in the timing (or phase) of the VOR (Shepard & Telian, 1996). More will be discussed on this in Chapter 6 when examining the sinusoidal acceleration test.

Limitations of Rotational Vestibular Testing

The primary limitations of rotational testing are few; however, they are significant. First and most relevant is that the laterality of a vestibular lesion cannot always be determined from rotational testing (Baloh, Sills, & Honrubia, 1979). Because both vestibular labyrinths are rotated simultaneously within the head, both excitatory and inhibitory responses are simultaneously generated (Brey et al., 2008a; Shepard & Telian, 1996; Shepard et al., 2016).

Therefore, determining an independent response from a single labyrinth (h-SCC) is challenging. Simply stated, a reduction in VOR sensitivity may be secondary to a lack of inhibition from the trailing ear or a lack of excitation from the leading ear. Although this limitation can be addressed through high velocity step testing (Chapter 7), the lack of lateralizing peripheral vestibulopathies is duly noted. This is probably the most significant weakness of rotational testing, and often the first and foremost criticism cited from clinicians. However, with the advancement of new tests like chair head impulse testing (crHIT), this limitation may only be a transient hurdle.

A second limitation is that rotational equipment is extremely expensive and sizable, which does not make purchasing the equipment very feasible for most clinicians or facilities. At the time of this publishing, the approximate cost of a *basic* rotational system is $110,000 for a chair and lightproof booth, and $70,000 for a boothless version. The primary cost of the chair is due to the highly specialized torque motor. Other features can be added onto the purchase (e.g., off-vertical axis motors, higher frame-rate goggles, specialized analysis research software, etc.), which can quickly inflate the cost of a rotational system above $250,000. Although boothless chairs and virtual LED goggles assist in alleviating some of the cost and space considerations, vestibular equipment is, in general, expensive. The comprehensive vestibular lab is generally associated with a well-funded research university, a well-funded clinical site, or a government facility. In addition, a comprehensive vestibular lab is often only present in more urban or metropolitan areas. Because of these issues, such well-equipped comprehensive vestibular labs are few when considering the comprehensive clinic per capita ratio. Unfortunately, rotational chairs are some of the higher priced pieces of vestibular equipment in the lab, and consequently often the first piece of vestibular test equipment eliminated from the budget when considering all the vestibular tests currently available.

A third limitation is that standard rotational testing directly stimulates only a portion of the peripheral system, specifically the horizontal semicircular canal and the superior vestibular nerve branch. Consequently, the vertical semicir-

> ## Can rotational testing be used to evaluate function from a sensory end organ other than the horizontal semicircular canal?
>
> It is important to note that it is possible to use rotational testing to evaluate vestibular sensory end organs other than the horizontal semicircular canals. Although the use of rotational testing still remains quite limited for evaluating the VOR response from the vertical canals, it is possible to utilize rotational testing to evaluate the ocular counter-roll VOR response from each utricle, as well as a collective response from both maculae. Although not part of the standard or routine rotational test battery, such investigation into the function of each utricle during unilateral centrifugation testing and, collectively, from both the saccule and the utricle during off-vertical axis rotational testing is possible. However, these tests are highly specialized and are rarely performed as part of a routine clinical assessment. These tests are discussed in Chapter 8.

cular canals and the maculae fail to contribute to the observed VOR response and are not directly evaluated.

The limited anatomical contributions to the observed VOR response during rotational testing create challenges when using the output to adequately reflect the physiology from the remaining peripheral sensory end organs of the vestibular system (i.e., the vertical semicircular canals and the maculae). This challenge is similar to making assumptions of the physiological response of the entire vestibular periphery (all five sensory end organs) based solely on the caloric test. Although rotational testing does offer valuable and unique insight into central functioning of the neural integrator and velocity storage, the results generated must be interpreted as representing only a portion of the peripheral system contributing to the overall response.

One final limitation to rotational testing is that analyses of the response can be complex, and often requires a great deal of experience and training to fully interpret the array of results that are generated from all the various tests. Given the paucity of rotational equipment available, this is a problem that may be inherent to the lack of exposure and/or training that can effectively be given to students and clinicians. Moreover, the shortage of rotational chairs in standard vestibular clinics has likely created a void in the dissemination of research and clinical findings that has circuitously and intrinsically contributed to a blunting of its clinical demand. In addition, there is also a secondary obstacle that has almost certainly led to the shortage of rotational testing in more general routine clinical practice. This obstacle is the cost to benefit ratio of the equipment versus re-imbursement. It would be a severe omission not to recognize that the lower insurance reimbursement for rotational testing, when compared to the equipment cost, has likely contributed to the scarcity of rotational test equipment available in most clinics or health care centers performing only routine vestibular testing (i.e., videonystagmography).

FACTORS IMPACTING ROTATIONAL DATA

There are a number of factors that can deleteriously impact the recording of the VOR response during rotational testing. Deterioration of the signal-to-noise ratio in the response is most often due to the introduction of excessive physiologic artifact into the signal (such as ocular noise). Keep in mind that any introduction of physiologic artifact is unwanted, but it is particularly detrimental to the signal during *low-frequency* rotations because the power of the physiological response to low frequency stimuli is inherently low. Therefore, during such low-frequency rotations, the inherently weak recorded response (VOR) can more easily be corrupted or obscured by even a minimal amount of noise or inadvertent suppression introduced into the signal. This can often be a problem because the test time required to complete low frequency rotations is often long and a subsequent decrease in mental tasking is more probable. This point is highlighted again when discussing low frequency stimulation during SHA testing in Chapter 6.

Physiological artifact can be introduced by a number of factors, such as ocular noise, ocular position, head position, mental tasking, and medications. Each of these will now briefly be reviewed.

Ocular Noise and Ocular Position

One of the most common (if not the most common) factors negatively impacting the signal to noise ratio of the VOR response is ocular noise and ocular position. Specifically, excessive ocular blink, ocular jitter, and excessive saccadic jerks, and even ocular position within the orbit can all have a significant impact on reducing the signal to noise ratio (Leigh & Zee, 2006). Regarding ocular position within the orbit, Fetter and colleagues (1986) reported that the gain of the VOR during yaw rotations was attenuated by the cosine of the angle between the visual axis and the plane of head rotation. In other words, they concluded that the VOR response was maximally elicited when both the head and the eyes were oriented in the lateral plane (equal to that of yaw rotation), or when the eyes were deviated in the opposite direction, but equal to the pitch of the head either up or down. In either of these eye-to-head orientations, the VOR was maximized secondary to the line of sight was always in the plane of yaw rotation. Minor and Goldberg (1990) also reported that maximal VOR responses were obtained (in squirrel monkeys) when the head is placed in the position equal to the average muscle plane of the lateral and medial rectus muscles. Finally, Goebel, Stroud, Levine, and Muntz (1983) reported a significant inhibition of vestibular induced nystagmus simply by having the eyes deviate superiorly within the orbit, an occurrence known as Bell's phenomenon.

Head Position

Alternatively, head position has been shown to have only minimal (if not negligible) effect on the VOR response. Coates and Smith (1967) were some of the first to show that altered head positions from the traditional 30° pitch-upward plane during caloric irrigations have minimal effects in the overall VOR response. With respect to angular stimulation, Fetter and colleagues (1986) reported no significant change in VOR response intensity during yaw rotations with the head positioned at 0°, +30°, and −30° respect to earth horizontal. Although Van der Stappen, Wuyts, and Van de Heyning (1999) did report a significant difference in VOR gain between the head upright position (oriented to the yaw plane) and a downward pitch of the head by 30°, the mean difference was quite small (0.578 ± 0.029, *SD* 0.15; 0.547 ± 0.025, *SD* 0.15, respectively) and would likely only have minimal effects on altering the classification of normal versus abnormal gain. These mixed findings suggest that head position could be a potential variable to the VOR response, particularly because it could impact ocular position. Subsequently, the position of the head in relation to angular rotations should be considered a possible source of variability, and therefore, monitored during testing.

Finally, with regard to head position, changing head position *during* a test (such as introducing sudden pitch-oriented head changes as in the "yes/no" nodding plane) can introduce significant artifact and spurious ocular responses that no longer represent data solely from the horizontal canals (coriolis effect). When such pitch-oriented head changes are produced during rotations, additional data from the vertical canals will likely introduce novel vertical canal VOR data in the output response, thus seriously confounding the test results. Every attempt should be made to prevent such head changes *during* rotations in order to ensure good quality data (not to mention prevention of a sudden onset of significant vertigo likely to be reported by the patient in response to such acute stimulation of the vertical canals).

Mental Tasking

Mental state is also critically important when performing rotational testing. Specifically, poor mental tasking can produce inaccurate sensitivity (VOR gain) data. It has been well reported that insufficient mental tasking can significantly reduce vestibular ocular reflex gain (Formby et al., 1992). This is often secondary to an inadvertent absence of tasking or even an inappropriate type of task-

ing. Tasking procedures that are too simple have been shown to cause a decrease in VOR gain due to mental "wandering" (Formby et al., 1992). Conversely, tasking that is too difficult can also lower VOR gain due to ocular tension or even increased anxiety (Leigh & Zee, 2006).

There are six factors that should be considered when ensuring that a mental agility task is effective in maximizing the VOR response (Formby et al., 1992). These factors are summarized in Table 5–5. First, the task must be at a level that is appropriate for the individual. It goes without saying that this level will certainly be different when assessing patients of different age ranges, particularly younger children. Second, the mental task should maintain a consistent level of concentration. This will prevent periods of recording where even transient episodes of suppression can impact VOR gain. This becomes increasingly important during critical periods of data capture that often occur during intervals of abrupt angular accelerations, or during higher frequency rotations where the periods of nystagmus production are extremely brief (e.g., high velocity step testing, or high frequency SHA testing). Third, the task should require little if any practice by the patient. That is, the task should not be so difficult that the patient feels as though they are performing it incorrectly and need time to improve their performance. In such cases, patients may either put minimal mental effort into attempting the task, or, the degree of mental tasking (con-

Table 5–5. Factors Impacting Adequate Mental Tasking

1. Task should be at the appropriate level to the patient
2. Task should maintain a constant and consistent level of mental tasking
3. Task should require minimal practice
4. Task should have minimum interaction with the clinician
5. Patient's role should require *active* thinking
6. Type of task may change within a single test session

Source: Adapted from Formby et al., 1992.

sistency of tasking) may be significantly different from the start to the completion of testing. Fourth, the task should require as little interaction with the clinician as possible. Inconsistent dialogue and periods in the interruption of thought often prevent the subject from achieving a consistent level of mental provocation. The more time the clinician spends in discourse with the patient, the greater the opportunity the patient has to suppress the VOR response. In turn, this only creates additional opportunities for periods of reduced VOR gain, which can be catastrophic to VOR gain if those periods occur at highly critical stimulus intervals (e.g., immediately post velocity step stimuli). Fifth, the patient's role should be as active as possible. Avoid tasks that involve the patient in a passive role such as recalling a story. Tasks involving the retelling of personal stories tend to place the patient in a passive role that places little demand on active thinking. Finally, the sixth factor to consider when selecting an appropriate and effective mental tasking procedure is to select one that is motivating for the patient. Above all, the best mental tasking procedure involves one that is appropriate to the patient's abilities and interests, as well as one that motivates the patient to perform at a consistent level in order to elicit a VOR response that remains constant throughout the test.

When considering the various types of mental tasking, Formby and colleagues (1992) reported that the best mental tasks were those that required the patient to name or list items pertaining to certain categories (cities, names, body parts, colors, etc.). They reported the lowest mental tasking procedures were those associated with backward counting exercises and reflexive quizzing. They concluded that the ideal alerting tasks should be simple exercises that are characterized by low uncertainty (i.e., categorical naming). Reflexive quizzing tasks (i.e., naming siblings, house address, etc.) often require minimal thought with simple, known answers. Such tasks often fail to generate "active" thinking. Finally, Formby and colleagues (1992) stressed that the selection of the appropriate mental task may rapidly change throughout testing, as both the clinician and the patient merge in their thought process to find a task or topic category, that best suits the motivation and interest of each patient.

Medications

Finally, the presence of contraindicated medications, such as central suppressants and/or stimulants can deleteriously impact the VOR output. This is particularly true of the elderly population where pharmacodynamics and pharmacokinetics can significantly alter the sensitivity, absorption rate, or elimination rate of drugs from organs or cells within the body (Shoair, Nyandege, & Slattum, 2011). If possible, such medications should be temporarily suspended prior to rotational testing (in conjunction with the patient's medical providers), similar to that employed during VNG test protocols.

TEST-RETEST RELIABILITY OF ROTATIONAL VESTIBULAR TESTING

Adequate test-retest reliability is essential for any clinical measure. Ensuring the reliability of a test measure is vital if comparisons are to be made from one trial to another, and even more critical when determining if intersubject differences are not obscured by intrasubject differences (Jenkins & Goldberg, 1988). Maes and colleagues (2008) investigated the test-retest reliability of rotational testing. In their report, they concluded that the various parameters of rotational testing (VOR gain, phase, and symmetry) are highly reliable for SHA and velocity step testing. They further indicated that VOR phase is the most stable response parameter, with VOR gain displaying the greatest variance. However, despite this variance, Maes and colleagues (2008) were careful to note that both parameters were within statistical tolerance for all frequencies. The authors highlighted the importance of this finding because the VOR gain parameter can be influenced by many subject variables, which can negatively impact measures of VOR phase and symmetry. Although this concept is covered in Chapter 6, it is important to realize that certain parameters of the VOR response (phase and symmetry) are highly dependent on the gain (sensitivity) of the VOR, as both parameters are measured from the VOR gain response. Hence, if the sensitivity of the VOR response is poor, the validity of phase and symmetry may also be questionable.

Test-retest reliability is critical, as results must also be reliable from one facility to another. Furman and colleagues (1994, 2000) investigated the variability of rotational chair analyses from different facilities using data analysis programs with the same patient's raw data. Surprisingly, they demonstrated significant variability among laboratories for both VOR gain and phase parameters when various software programs analyzed the raw data files. However, when clinician intervention and judgment were permitted during analysis, the variability was significantly reduced. The authors concluded three things from this study. First, this interlaboratory variability would negatively impact the value of monitoring vestibular function, particularly if testing was performed at different locations. Second, a reduction in the diagnostic power of rotational testing and the possibility of assigning an inappropriate diagnosis may exist if individual analysis algorithms are not robust. Finally, the authors concluded that such variability would compromise comparisons with published data, including use of published normative data and subsequent patient outcomes. Furman and colleagues questioned the uncertain effect of using "actual" raw data with "real" patient artifact. They speculated whether the significant variability occurred as a result of how the different analysis methods filtered out patient artifact. As a result of this concern, Furman and colleagues (2000) repeated the same study design but used simulated data to control for the amount and type of artificially introduced "physiologic" artifact. They demonstrated a significant effect of signal-to-noise ratio during the data analysis. Specifically, they showed that a higher signal-to-noise ratio (lower "physiologic" artifact) generated a significant improvement in data analysis and reduced variability across facilities. Conversely, they concluded that data with higher artifact may be unsuitable for analysis and subsequent comparison across facilities and published reports should be interpreted with caution. Finally, Furman and colleagues (2000) replicated their earlier findings that an improvement in accuracy and a subsequent decrease in inter-laboratory variability occur when operator intervention is permitted.

The most pertinent conclusions from both of these studies is the fact that expert clinical intervention in the clinical analysis of the data was significant in reducing the discrepancies and statistical significance with disparate data analyses across the various clinical sites. In short, clinical experience matters. There is a significant difference between what I refer to as *clinician* analysis versus *algorithm* analysis. As experienced clinicians, we are trained to scrutinize, appropriately filter, and analyze data when the signal-to-noise ratio is poor. Perhaps the most relevant and important concept presented throughout this entire text is this; that clinical experience and knowledge provided by the vestibular clinician is the most instrumental and influential component in vestibular assessment. Without a doubt, the knowledge and experience of the clinician is paramount to providing quality vestibular assessments and accurate vestibular diagnoses.

TWO FUNDAMENTAL CONCEPTS OF ROTATIONAL TESTING

Prior to examining the specific tests conducted during rotational assessment, it is important to understand a few basic concepts that are integral to the administration and understanding of the rotational stimulus and the response. These concepts refer to the input stimuli and the output response that occur during rotational testing. Specifically, regarding the input stimuli, it is important to understand the difference between acceleration and velocity. In addition, with regard to the output, it is important to understand the basic outcome measure of any rotational test is inherently an ocular response. Let's first briefly discuss the various elements related to the input and output parameters associated with rotational assessment before examining the specifics of each test.

Differences Between Acceleration and Velocity

Prior to discussing the various tests and rotational protocols associated with rotational testing, it is a good idea to become acquainted with the difference between velocity and acceleration, as these two terms will often be referenced during rotational testing. Velocity refers to the rate at which an object changes its position in space, whereas acceleration is defined as the rate at which an object changes its velocity. Simply stated, velocity is how fast an object is moving, and in what direction (you cannot have velocity without indicating its direction), whereas acceleration is how quickly the object achieves its target velocity. Just because an object is moving fast does not mean that it has, or that it is, accelerating. Conversely, an object experiencing constant changing velocity is always undergoing some form of acceleration (or deceleration).

The distinction between acceleration and velocity is important because every single vestibular receptor in the labyrinth (i.e., the cupulae and maculae) responds to acceleration, not velocity. Within the literature, you may find seemingly contradictory statements indicating how the vestibular system behaves as a "velocity-matching" or an "acceleration-matching" system. However, such statements describe the behavior or *output* of the vestibular system (eye movements), not the input. Indeed, for mid-frequency stimuli (0.25 to 25 Hz), which include the frequency range where natural head movements occur (1 to 5 Hz), the output (as measured by velocity of eye movement), does, in fact, more closely match head velocity. For this reason, the vestibular system's mid-frequency response is often referred to as an angular-*velocity* transducer. Conversely, when examining eye movement (velocity) data during very low frequency angular stimuli (at or below 0.25 Hz), the eye velocity data less resembles head velocity and more closely resembles head acceleration. For this reason, the vestibular system's low frequency response is often referred to as an angular-*acceleration* transducer.

Let's explore this concept further. The fundamental explanation for the difference between low-to-mid frequency response characteristics is that these statements are meant to describe the *output* or behavior of the vestibular response (eye movement) with respect to the input (acceleration). That is, these statements characterize the manner in which the vestibular system integrates and transduces different rates of acceleration stimuli. This can be visualized in Figure 5–1 where the eye velocity response to mid-fre-

quency stimuli more closely parallels head velocity with a gain of 1.0 and a phase of 0°. That is, eye-measured velocity precisely parallels head velocity (gain of 1.0), only in the opposite direction without any temporal slip or phase shift (0° phase). Conversely, low-frequency stimuli produce an eye movement velocity response that more closely parallels head acceleration. Simply put, the output of the vestibular system behavior, or its response characteristics, largely depends on the rate of acceleration. This one single concept will continue to resurface during our discussion of the various response parameters obtained during rotational assessment. Irrespective of whether the eye velocity output resembles head acceleration or head velocity, it is critical to remember that every labyrinthine sensory end organ responds to acceleration and *only* acceleration. For the remainder of this text, we will continue to review and reference the unique relationship between acceleration and velocity. However, for a greater discussion of this topic, the reader is strongly encouraged to review Goldberg, Wilson, and colleague's (2012) discussion on vestibular physiology.

VOR Response During Rotational Testing

If the vestibular system is functioning properly, the VOR will generate an equal and opposite eye movement that is relative to the rate of acceleration and direction of chair rotation. In its most basic form, modern rotational testing captures video-graphic recordings of the VOR during whole body rotations via infrared video cameras, and plots the ocular response (VOR) in relation to the chair's oscillations or rotations. Computer algorithms analyze the resulting VOR response and, specifically, the vestibular portion of the nystagmus (i.e., the slow-phase) is quantified. It is safe to assume that in a normal healthy functioning vestibular system, the VOR will always be in the opposite direction. However, as we have already discovered, the intensity of the vestibular response (i.e., the slow-phase nystagmus compent) will vary depending on the frequency of chair rotation (i.e., the rate of acceleration), with much lower vestibular sensitivity (gain) appreciated for lower frequency stimuli. Given this, we now know that its ability to *truly equal* head velocity is, therefore, acceleration dependent. The reasons for this are discussed at length in Chapters 6 and 7.

In summary, a healthy VOR response will always be opposite that of chair acceleration, but not always equal in response intensity, as the vestibular system's physiologic-efficiency is consider-ably poorer for low frequency rotational (angular) stimuli. Overall, rotational testing essentially measures the efficiency of the VOR in response to various rotational frequencies (angular accelerations). Now, let us consider the various vestibular responses that occur in response to different types of chair rotations, namely, sinusoidal accelerations and velocity step stimuli.

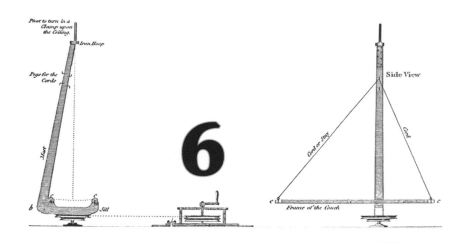

6

Sinusoidal Harmonic Acceleration (SHA) Testing

Rotations of an upright head and body about a fixed earth vertical centric axis are the simplest and most fundamental stimuli provided during rotational vestibular testing (Figure 6–1). This form of rotational stimulation efficiently produces a horizontal vestibular ocular reflex (VOR) and a subsequent peak eye velocity that approximates a given rotational velocity (Brey, McPherson, & Lynch, 2008a; Goulson, McPherson, & Shepard, 2016). In general, as the velocity of chair rotation increases, so does the peak eye velocity of the responding VOR. By comparing the velocity of the responding VOR against a known velocity of chair rotations (for a variety of stimulus frequencies), the reactivity of the vestibular system can be inferred across a broad frequency range. Examining the responsiveness of the vestibular system across a broad frequency range provides a more comprehensive evaluation of vestibular integrity, particularly in the presence of a bilateral absent caloric response. Similar to an audiometric assessment, which identifies normal to near normal low frequency hearing with a concomitant profound high frequency hearing loss, the ves-

tibular system is also subject to frequency dependent damage. Assuming an absence of vestibular response based on an absence of caloric response would be similar to concluding complete anacusis based on a single absent audiometric threshold at 8000 Hz.

When a vertically upright individual is rotated (or oscillated) back and forth in the horizontal (or yaw) plane, the responsiveness of the vestibular system to such rotations can be determined across a known frequency range of stimuli. Rotational stimuli are most commonly presented as sinusoids, with the chair first accelerating in one direction until a peak target velocity is achieved (usually $50°$/sec or more commonly $60°$/second), after which the chair slows and reverses to the same peak velocity in the opposite direction. This periodic motion, whereby the chair (head) oscillates about a centric position, is known as sinusoidal acceleration testing. Provided the rotational frequencies being administered are simple harmonics of one another, this form of stimulation is known as sinusoidal harmonic acceleration testing, or SHA testing (Stockwell & Bojrab, 1997a). For a visual introduction into the various SHA rotational stimuli (or harmonic frequencies), the reader is encouraged to review the companion website for an example of each rotational SHA frequency.

153

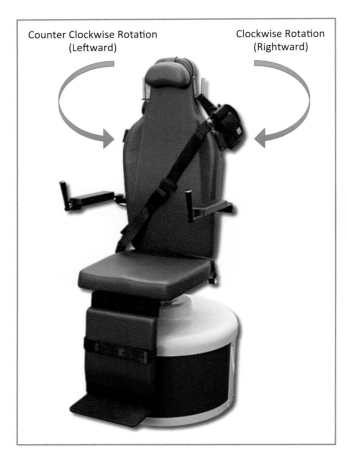

FIGURE 6–1. Rotational chair showing direction of clockwise (rightward) and counterclockwise (leftward). Image courtesy of Micromedical, Inc.

Although rotational testing can be composed of a variety of rotational frequencies, it is not required that SHA testing be administered in octave or harmonic intervals. Certain test paradigms may often omit certain frequencies to conserve clinical test time, whereas other rotational paradigms can also be administered whereby a series of oscillation frequencies can be combined and presented simultaneously. This later rotational paradigm is known as *sum of sines* and is rarely (if ever) performed in the clinical assessment of vestibular function. The primary reason for the infrequency by which a sum of sines rotational paradigm is used is due to the significant loss of energy (physiologic response) that occurs secondary to a significant spread of VOR response over multiple frequencies of simultaneous stimulation (Wall, 1990). Although the single-frequency

oscillation paradigm employed during the more common type of SHA testing takes considerably longer than the sum of sines paradigm, having all the response energy concentrated at a single frequency of rotation is quite adventitious when analyzing response parameters, particularly those produced from weak vestibular physiology (either by a low-frequency stimulus or pathology) (Wall, 1990).

SINUSOIDAL HARMONIC ACCELERATION (SHA) STIMULUS

Chair rotations, or oscillations, are most often delivered in the yaw, or horizontal, plane in both the clockwise and counterclockwise directions.

Chair rotations are defined by the frequency of rotation, or simply, how many back-and-forth oscillations are delivered within a given time period (usually one second). Rotational frequencies are expressed in hertz (Hz). The frequencies

Determining the Difference Between Clockwise and Counterclockwise Rotations

For those just becoming acquainted with visualizing the direction of rotation, the clockwise or counterclockwise vector is best described from a vantage point above the rotational chair (Figure 6–2).

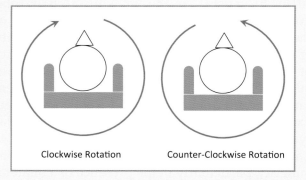

Clockwise Rotation   Counter-Clockwise Rotation

FIGURE 6–2. Rotational chair showing direction of clockwise (rightward) and counterclockwise (leftward) rotation as viewed from above.

most commonly administered are harmonic or octave frequencies between 0.01 and 0.64 Hz (that is; 0.01, 0.02, 0.04, 0.08, 0.16, 0.32, and 0.64 Hz). Additional frequencies can be administered, which include 1.28 Hz and even 2.0 Hz (or higher). However, stimulus frequencies above 1 Hz can be progressively problematic for many reasons. Most notably, the resulting VOR eye data become increasingly difficult to accurately capture, as the precise acceleration of the chair is not exactly translated to the head due to dermal slip against the skull for most standard head restraint devices. As a result of the slight dermal slip, head acceleration lags slightly behind chair acceleration and produces an inadvertent delay in the initiation of the compensatory VOR that, in turn, produces an artificial and nonphysiologic VOR delay that was never intended. This often leads to aberrant results that fail to adequately reflect true physiology of the vestibular system. This concept will be revisited later when discussing the timing relationship of the VOR response (known as phase) in relation to certain rotational frequencies. High frequency rotations greater than 1 Hz are more often confined to research trials or within animal studies where unwanted dermal slippage can be negated through the use of bite blocks, molded face restraint devices, or surgically implanted head posts.

It is critical to keep in mind that the rotational stimuli applied during SHA testing are unique, insomuch that the acceleration of the rotating chair is always changing. That is, the rotation of the chair is under constant acceleration until the target velocity of rotation is achieved (most often 60° per second), at which time the rotation of the chair immediately begins decelerating until the chair returns to a velocity of 0° per second (i.e., no movement). At this *instantaneous* moment of zero movement velocity, the chair reverses rotational directions and once again is subject to constant acceleration until the target rotational velocity is reached, at which time the chair is once again decelerated back to 0° per second. This process of acceleration followed by deceleration repeats itself both in the rightward (or clockwise) and leftward (or counterclockwise) directions for a predetermined series of back and forth oscillations. Sinusoidal harmonic acceleration testing is always

---

Performing *Sustained* Rotations during Rotational Testing . . . A Peek into Chapter 7 Using Velocity Step Accelerations

In addition to SHA testing and its unique oscillatory stimulus, a VOR response can also be recorded following *sustained* rotations in both the CW and CCW directions. This form of vestibular stimulation is known as velocity step acceleration and is discussed in Chapter 7. Both the SHA and VST tests are critical to the RVT test battery and comprise the essential components of RVT testing. Fundamentally, it is the measurement and analysis of the VOR response during both SHA and step testing that is most relevant during a RVT assessment.

---

performed with the chair moving (or oscillating) back and forth in such a sinusoidal fashion.

The omnipresent acceleration and deceleration stimuli associated with SHA testing are absolutely critical for effective stimulation of the vestibular system. We are reminded of the principal mechanics of the vestibular system, more specifically the cupulae; that cupular *deflection* and subsequent saltation of an afferent neural response is entirely dependent on *acceleration*, not velocity. Simply put, the cupulae are accelerometers that detect changes in movement, not necessarily movement itself, and cupular deflection is completely reliant on such *changes* in motion.

So, it is the ubiquitous acceleration and deceleration of the rotational stimulus during SHA that creates the subsequent VOR due to ever-present cupular mechanics. It stands to reason then, that the stronger (or quicker) the acceleration, the greater the cupular deflection and stronger the subsequent VOR response. Simply put, the stronger the input, the more robust the output. That being said, it is then critical to remember that the opposite is true. Because the cupulae *are* accelerometers, the weaker the stimulus input, the less effective the vestibular system will be at generating an output response. If you recall from our discussions on the anatomy and physiology of

> ### Velocity Versus Acceleration: What Exactly Is the Difference?
>
> *Velocity vs. Acceleration.* To better understand the difference between velocity and acceleration, imagine yourself traveling in a car with your eyes closed. Your cupulae are designed exquisitely to detect accelerations and decelerations as you speed up or slow down. However, if it were possible that the car's motion was constant, say traveling at 60 mph with absolutely no change in acceleration or deceleration, your cupulae are not designed to detect the constant motion of the car traveling at 60 mph. Of course, other cues will tell your brain that you are moving, such as bumps in the road, and possibly wind noise or even road noise. However, if all other variables were removed, your vestibular system would be oblivious to the constant (non-changing) velocity of the car's movement—until it decelerated or accelerated. This is the difference between the cupulae being accelerometers and not velocitometers (if such a word exists!). This concept will again be revisited during our discussion on velocity step testing (Chapter 7) where cupular deflection actually dampens to their resting state despite ongoing constant-velocity chair rotation.

the vestibular system, this is indeed true as the efficiency of the vestibular system (acceleration detection) suffers dramatically below 0.1 Hz. We will see this reflected later when we review the differences in VOR output with respect to the various frequencies employed during SHA testing.

SHA STIMULUS PROPERTIES

The oscillation stimulus delivered during SHA testing can be characterized by a variety of parameters, most notably: frequency, cycle duration or period, angular acceleration, angular displacement, and number of oscillations (or rotations). Table 6–1 lists the relative rotational properties for each given frequency of rotation during SHA testing as well as some of the parameters for the caloric stimulus commonly employed during videonystagmography (VNG) testing.

Stimulus Frequency

As mentioned earlier, the *frequency* of chair rotation is defined as the number of oscillations (or cycles) competed per second. This is depicted by the equation:

$$Hz = \frac{\text{cycles of rotation}}{second}$$

That is:

1 hertz = 1 cycle of rotation completed
in 1 second of time

Frequency can, therefore, be simplified and expressed as the quotient between one (1) and the time (T) it takes to complete a single cycle of rotation, or:

$$\frac{1}{T} = \text{Frequency (Hz); or}$$

$$\frac{1}{100 \; secs} = 0.01 \text{ Hz; and}$$

$$\frac{1}{50 \; secs} = 0.02 \text{ Hz; etc.}$$

SHA testing is generally performed in octave frequencies between 0.01 and 0.64 Hz (and sometimes higher). The most common octave frequencies performed during SHA testing are provided in Table 6–1.

Table 6–1. Relative Rotational Properties by Frequency of Rotation

Stimulus (Hz)	Cycle Duration (s)	Velocity (ω)	Acceleration (α)	Angular Displacement (½ cycle)	Cycles of Oscillation (# of rotations)
0.004	250		~ 1.2°/sec²		
0.01	100	60	2.4°/sec²	1500°	4⅓
0.02	50	60	4.8°/sec²	750°	2⅙
0.04	25	60	9.6°/sec²	375°	1¹⁄₁₂
0.08	12.5	60	19.2°/sec²	187.5°	~ ½
0.16	6.25	60	38.4°/sec²	93.75°	~ ¼
0.32	3.125	60	76.8°/sec²	46.875°	~ ⅛
0.64	1.5625	60	153.6°/sec²	23.4375°	~ ¹⁄₁₆
1.28	0.78125	60	307.2°/sec²	11.71875°	~ ¹⁄₃₂
2.0	0.5	60	480°/sec²	7.5°	¹⁄₄₈

Stimulus Period

Although the term *"period"* is not frequently discussed in the clinical literature, it is significant in determining other parameters during the analysis of SHA data. The period of rotation is simply the time (T) it takes to complete one cycle of rotation. One complete *cycle* is defined as a single acceleration and deceleration of chair rotation to the right followed by acceleration and deceleration to the left. This is illustrated in Figure 6–3. However, because acceleration is frequency dependent (acceleration increases as frequency increases, see Table 6–1), the period of time (T) it takes to complete one cycle of rotation will vary depending on the rotational frequency being administered. For example, when conducting rotations at 0.01 Hz, the lowest common rotational frequency performed during SHA testing, the chair will complete one full cycle of rotation in 100 seconds (Figure 6–4). The period (T) of this cycle is simply the inverse of the frequency of chair rotation, and is expressed by the equation:

$$Hz = \frac{1}{T\ (sec)}$$

$$\text{Solving for T; } T = \frac{1}{Hz}$$

$$\text{Therefore, } T = \frac{1\ cycle}{0.01\ Hz}$$

$$T = 100 \text{ seconds}$$

In contrast, when conducting SHA testing using a higher rotational frequency of 0.32 Hz, the time needed for the chair to complete one full cycle of oscillation is only 3.125 seconds. This is depicted in Figure 6–5 and is determined by the equation:

$$T = \frac{1\ cycle}{0.32\ Hz}$$

$$T = 3.125 \text{ seconds}$$

The stimulus period for each of the frequencies performed during SHA testing is provided in Table 6–1.

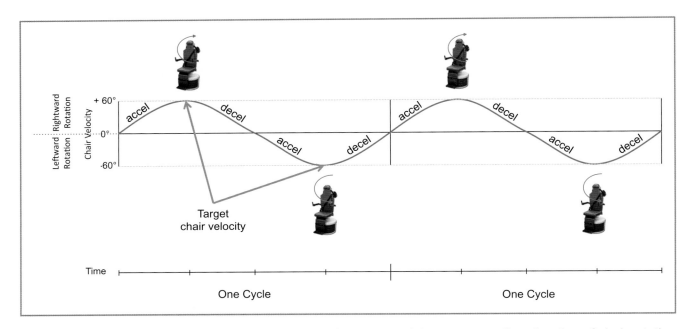

FIGURE 6–3. Rotational plot showing two cycles of rotation and the corresponding direction of chair rotation during each one-half cycle of rotation.

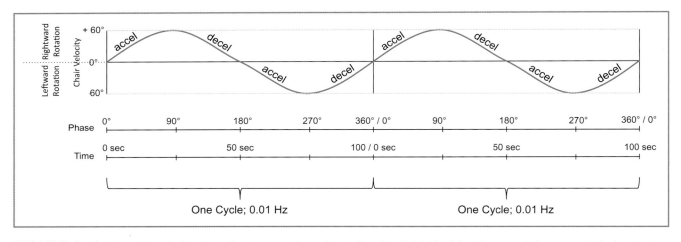

FIGURE 6–4. Rotational plot showing two cycles of rotation for 0.01 Hz. The time and degree of chair rotation are plotted for each cycle of rotation.

Angular Acceleration

As already mentioned, acceleration is frequency dependent and increases as frequency increases. When discussing acceleration is terms of a rotational stimulus, it is known as *angular acceleration* (α). Angular acceleration can be thought of as how many degrees the chair rotates in a certain period of time. Angular acceleration can be mathematically defined as the quotient of the change in angular velocity (ω) divided by the change in time (t), and is expressed by the equation:

$$\alpha = \frac{\Delta\omega}{\Delta t}$$

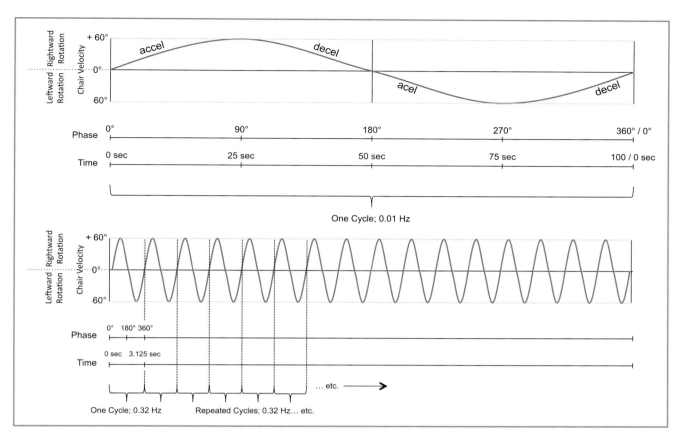

FIGURE 6–5. Comparison of rotational characteristics for 0.01 Hz and 0.32 Hz. *Note: The time scales between both examples are not relative to one another.*

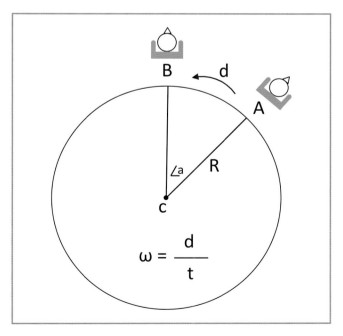

FIGURE 6–6. Angular velocity of chair rotation; (d) Equals distance in degrees traveled (A → B) in a known period of time (usually one second); ω = angular velocity; when R = 1; d = ∠a. *Note: cartoon of chair rotates at point "c". Chair is depicted off center of axis for illustrative purposes.*

In this equation, change in angular velocity is equal to the target velocity of chair rotation during SHA testing (a constant value either 50°/s or 60°/s), and change in time is equal to 1/4 duration of one full cycle of rotation, which is the time needed to accelerate to the stimulus target velocity before decelerating back to 0°/sec (see Figure 6–5). Using 0.01 Hz as an example, the angular acceleration of the chair is as follows;

$$\alpha = \frac{\Delta\omega}{\Delta t}$$

$$\alpha = \frac{60°/sec}{25\ sec}$$

$$\alpha = \frac{2.4°}{sec^2}$$

The angular acceleration for each of the stimulus frequencies performed during SHA testing is provided in Table 6–1.

Number of Required Cycles of Oscillation

One can quickly determine that the number of cycles conducted can have a significant impact on the overall time required to complete each rotational frequency, and ultimately impacting the total time required to conduct a complete range of frequencies during SHA testing. It stands to reason that a greater number of oscillations (or cycles) will invariably produce more compensatory VOR data during the test, which would undoubtedly result in greater reliability, validity, and repeatability of data. If one were to randomly assign a minimum number of ten cycles to be conducted for each rotational frequency, the total test time to complete 0.32 Hz would be 31.25 seconds (3.125 seconds times ten cycles). This is not unreasonable in a clinical setting. However, the time needed to complete ten cycles of 0.01 Hz would be 1,000 seconds, or 16 minutes and 40 seconds for a single frequency, which *is* clinically unreasonable. So how does one determine the best number of oscillations to administer?

To answer this question, we must first be cognizant that collection of a "bad cycle" of VOR response data has traditionally been highly prob-

lematic. This was due to the forced "deletion" of the *entire* cycle of data when "bad" data was collected, even if only a *portion* of a cycle was "bad." This was often secondary to the limitations of some analysis algorithms. This limitation has traditionally plagued rotational testing, as the deletion of an entire cycle of "bad" data, when only two cycles of data are collected, can be disastrous for data analysis and subsequent clinical interpretation, particularly if both cycles have periods of bad data and you are forced to delete both cycles or, worse, analyze "bad" data. Thankfully, this problem is becoming less of an issue as data analysis algorithms continue to improve in their ability to detect and remove discrete spurious data points/regions within distinct portions of any particular cycle. This eliminates the "forced deletion" of an *entire* cycle of data due to a small portion of the cycle containing "bad data."

Second, and perhaps the most important factor when determining the number of oscillations needed for reliable data, is that the test time must be long enough to allow for the characterization of the steady-state response of the vestibular system (Wall, 1990). For the lower frequencies of rotation (0.01 to 0.02 Hz), this will generally occur after 45 seconds of slow oscillatiory stimulation (Wall, 1990). In general, the *minimum* number of cycles for any frequency should be two full cycles for frequencies less than 0.04 Hz, with a higher number of cycles for frequencies above 0.02 Hz. For the lower two frequencies, this would equate to a testing time of 200 seconds for 0.01 Hz and 100 seconds for 0.02 Hz. If you are to add in the 45 seconds of test time needed prior to initiation of the steady-state response, this would calculate to 245 seconds for 0.01 Hz (or 4 minutes, 5 seconds) and 145 seconds for 0.02 H (or 2 minutes, 25 seconds). Although more data during these low frequencies of rotation is seldom discouraged, one must be cognizant of the added test time required and subsequent mental tasking demand placed on the patient, which could potentially lead to poorer data, secondary to reduced mental alertness. The tradeoff between a limited amount of robust clean data, and more data that are less robust, is undoubtedly important and can often be patient-dependent with respect to how adept they are performing mental tasking as well as each patient's relative fatigue. Most SHA rotational protocols typically present two to three cycles of rotation for 0.01 Hz and 0.02 Hz, and up to 10 cycles for the remaining frequencies between 0.04 and 0.64 Hz. To account for adaptation of the steady-state response, most current analysis paradigms delete a portion of, or the entire first and last half of, the beginning and ending cycle, respectively.

Chair Rotation Versus Chair Revolution

Finally, it is important to make a distinction between the rotational chair completing one full cycle of *rotation* versus making one full *revolution*. This distinction is relevant as one quickly realizes that the rotational chair no longer completes a full 360° revolution for stimulus frequencies above 0.04 Hz. This can clearly be seen when critically examining the video for each SHA frequency on the companion website. The reason for this lies in the test's terminal target velocity of 60° per second. Recall that as soon as the acceleration of the chair reaches the target velocity of 60° per second (which is achieved at 1/4 of one full cycle), the chair immediately begins to decelerate back to 0° per second (full stop at 1/2 cycle) before changing directions and completing the second half of the cycle (Figure 6–7). For SHA test frequencies greater than 0.04 Hz, the increased acceleration stimulus achieves this target velocity rather quickly and is able to both accelerate to the target velocity and decelerate back to full stop prior to completing a full 360° revolution. That is, the time needed to complete one-half a cycle of oscillation (acceleration and deceleration in the rightward or leftward direction) at a rotational frequency of 0.08 Hz is approximately 180° of rotational displacement, or just one-half a full revolution.

When considering the example using a rotational frequency of 0.01 Hz, where the rotational acceleration is slow (2.4°/sec²), the chair will take 25 seconds to accelerate to the target velocity of 60° per second (1/4 cycle) and another full 25 seconds to decelerate back to 0° per second (full stop at 1/2 cycle) before reversing direction of rotation. During these 50 seconds of rightward (or leftward) rotation, the chair will actually travel (or rotate) a full 1500°, or 4⅓ revolutions in 1/2 cycle before coming to a full stop and reversing directions. During the next 50 seconds of acceleration and deceleration in the leftward direction, the chair will once again make 4⅓ revolutions during this second, 1/2 cycle. However, during a rotational frequency of 0.16 Hz, because the rotational acceleration is much faster (38.4°/sec²), the chair will only take 3.125 seconds to accelerate to the target velocity of 60° per second and only another 3.125 seconds to decelerate back to 0° per second (full stop) before reversing direction of rotation. During these 6.25 seconds of rightward (or leftward) rotation, the chair will actually travel (or rotate) only 93.75°, or approximately ¼ of one revolution during this ½ cycle before coming to a full stop and reversing directions. The angular displacement and revolutions for each of the frequencies performed during SHA testing is provided in Table 6–1.

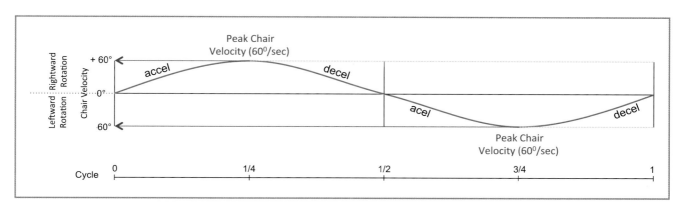

FIGURE 6–7. One cycle of rotation showing peak target chair velocity for both rightward and leftward rotations. Chair velocity always peaks at predetermined target velocity (60°/second in the example).

NORMAL PHYSIOLOGICAL RESPONSE DURING SHA TESTING

In response to chair rotations, specifically chair acceleration and deceleration, an intact vestibular system will generate a slow compensatory eye movement (i.e., the VOR) in the opposite direction to that of chair rotation. The constant-varying cupular deflection creates the excitatory and inhibitory peripheral afferent response that is integrated by the central vestibular nuclei, cerebellum, and various brainstem structures reviewed in earlier chapters. Central efferent signals are sent to the appropriate efferent ocular motor neurons resulting in the compensatory slow-phase vestibular nystagmus that is generated in the opposite direction of chair rotation (Figure 6–8).

The vestibular slow-phase occurs until the eye reaches an eccentric position within the orbit and is then followed by a fast resetting of the eyes back to the primary position (fast-phase), which is initiated by the brainstem. This pattern continues as long as the chair is accelerating or decelerating in a single direction. The resultant nystagmus (named for the fast-phase) is, therefore, always in the same direction of chair rotation: right-beating nystagmus with rightward rotation and left-beating nystagmus with leftward rotation. As the chair decelerates back to a velocity of 0° per second (full stop), the chair immediately reverses direction and begins accelerating and then decelerating in the opposite direction. The nystagmus switches directions in response to the change in the direction of chair rotation. This process is repeated until the predetermined number of oscillations has been

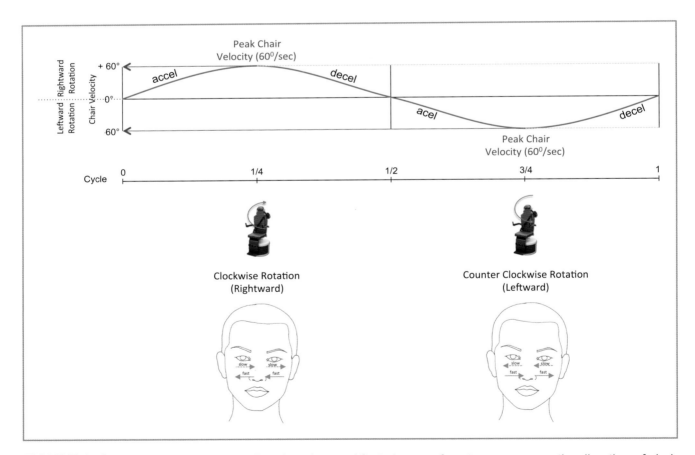

FIGURE 6–8. Relationship between direction slow and fast phases of nystagmus versus the direction of chair rotation. Direction of nystagmus fast phase is always in the direction of chair rotation. Vestibular slow phase is always in the opposite direction of chair rotation.

completed for each respective frequency. The observed nystagmus is captured and "traced," or "charted," in real time through a computer software program. A series of rightward and leftward chair oscillations and the respective right-beating and left-beating nystagmus can be seen in Figure 6–9. Notice how the nystagmus increases in its slope as the rotation of the chair increases to its peak target velocity, at which time the slope of the nystagmus begins to diminish as the chair decelerates back to a velocity of 0°/second.

From the resulting nystagmus, software programs delete the fast-phase components of the VOR response leaving only the slow-phase vestibular components remaining (Figures 6–10 and 6–11). The reason for this is simple but should, nevertheless, be stated. It is the vestibular response that is of interest during rotational testing and therefore only the slow phase that is of primary concern. After the slow-phases are parsed from the response, the degree of each slow-phase is measured and plotted in relation to chair oscillation. Because the plot of slow phase velocity of vestibular nystagmus is in the opposite direction to chair rotation and the

degree of nystagmus increases and decreases with the acceleration and deceleration of the chair rotation, the resultant nystagmus velocity and chair velocity data always appear as opposing (or mirror) sinusoids; that is, 180 degrees out of phase from one another (Figure 6–12). The peak velocity of the slow phase component of the vestibular nystagmus will generally increase and peak near the same time the chair reaches peak velocity prior to beginning deceleration (Figure 6–12). Once the degree of the slow-phase nystagmus has been plotted, various algorithms are applied to the data in order to characterize the vestibular response with respect to its response gain, phase, and symmetry.

SHA ANALYSIS PARAMETERS

Analysis of the VOR in response to sinusoidal chair rotations produces three principle measurement parameters: gain, phase, and symmetry (Brey et al. 2008a; Shepard, Goulson, & McPher-

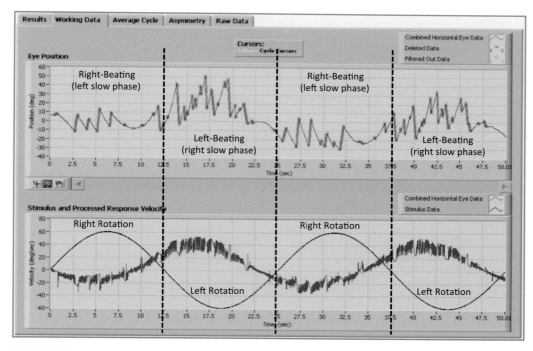

FIGURE 6–9. Relationship between direction of chair rotation versus slow and fast phase of nystagmus. Raw tracing of nystagmus (*top plot*) shows right-beating and left-beating nystagmus in relation to rightward and leftward chair rotation, respectively.

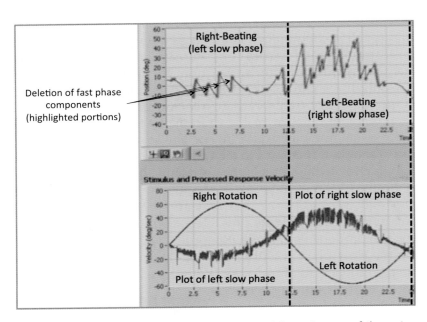

FIGURE 6–10. Close up view of slow and fast phases of the rotational nystagmus during one-cycle of rotation (*top graph*). Fast phases are deleted from the nystagmus (*orange*), leaving only the slow phase component of the nystagmus remaining for analysis.

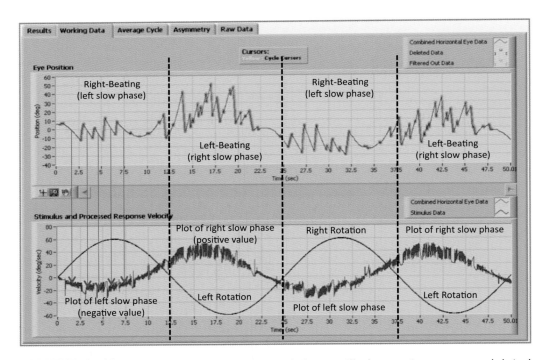

FIGURE 6–11. Fast phase components of the vestibular nystagmus are deleted (*orange*), and the degree for each slow phase component of the vestibular nystagmus is plotted below on the eye velocity plot (*green arrows to the lower graph*) for each one-half cycle of rotation.

son, 2016; Shepard & Telian, 1996). Comparison of the peak ocular response to that of peak chair rotational velocity can be easily determined (Figure 6–13). This ratio of peak eye velocity to peak chair velocity is known as the sensitivity (or gain) of the vestibular system and, through a series of rotations (accelerations and decelerations), the gain of the vestibular system can be effectively determined across a wide range of frequencies during SHA testing.

In addition, as the chair begins to accelerate in one direction and the eye begins to slowly deviate in the opposite direction due to the vestibular response, the timing relationship between the exact moment chair rotation begins and the exact moment the eyes begin to move in the opposite direction can also be determined. This timing relationship is known as the phase of the VOR response, and is simply the temporal (timing) relationship between the move-

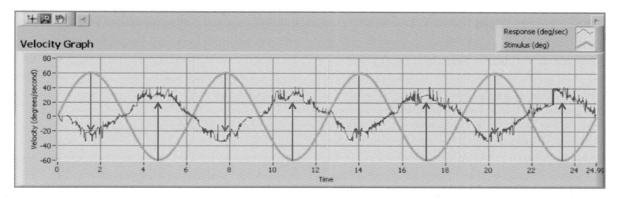

FIGURE 6–12. Plot of chair velocity and corresponding vestibular slow phase velocity data. Arrows identify the peak target velocity of the chair rotation in relationship to the peak vestibular slow phase component of the eye velocity data. Data show a strong temporal relationship between peak eye data and peak chair data. As dictated by the vestibular ocular reflex, the slow phase velocity data will always be in the opposing direction of chair rotation, thus forming a mirror eye velocity sinusoid in relation to the chair velocity.

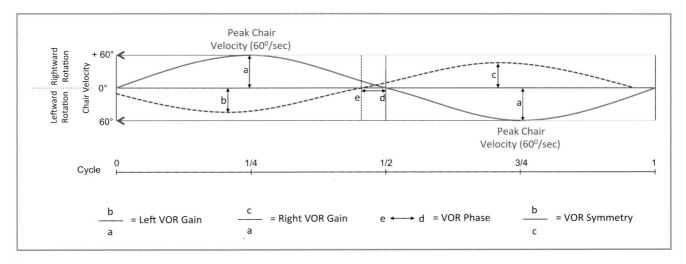

FIGURE 6–13. Single cycle of chair rotation, illustrating how the various analysis parameters of SHA testing (gain, phase, and symmetry) are determined.

ment of the eyes in relation to the movement of the head (chair).

Finally, the degree of peak eye response can be compared from rotations in the clockwise direction to those from the counter-clockwise direction. The ratio between these two peak responses is known as the symmetry of the VOR. Therefore, three primary measures are specifically analyzed during rotational testing; VOR gain, phase and symmetry (see Figure 6–13). Each parameter has unique characteristics, strengths, and limitations.

VOR Response Gain

Gain defines the relationship between peak eye velocity and peak chair velocity (Brey et al. 2008a; Shepard & Telian, 1996; Shepard et al., 2016). It is simply the sensitivity, or responsiveness, of the vestibular system to a particular stimulus (or rotational frequency). A *perfect* compensation of eye movement to that of chair rotation would produce a VOR response that was truly *equal* (and opposite) with respect to chair movement. That is, the relationship between peak eye and peak chair velocity would be exactly the same, which is expressed as the ratio 1:1, or simply a gain of 1.0. A perfect response is often referred to as *response unity*. VOR response gain is calculated for each stimulus rotational frequency performed during SHA testing.

Because the exact acceleration and velocity stimulus being delivered to the vestibular system is known, simple calculations of the slow-phase eye velocity in relation to chair velocity can be precisely determined. If the VOR were truly an equal and opposite response to head acceleration, then the degree of ocular reflex (slow-phase velocity slope calculation) would exhibit an equivalent increase or decrease in relation to an increase or decrease in chair rotational frequency. That is, as the frequency of chair rotation is increased, so too would the response velocity of the peak eye response. Although this is generally the case, we will discover that for the frequencies assessed during rotational testing (0.01 to 0.64 Hz) the response of the VOR is *always opposite* the direction of head (chair) rotation; however, it is seldom, if ever, truly *equal* to the intensity of the chair rotation. This concept is especially true for the slower rotational

frequencies below 0.08 Hz and, to a lesser extent, also true for the mid-to-high rotational frequencies above 0.04 Hz. This is not surprising as the frequency stimuli used during SHA testing remain below the vestibular system's optimum operating range of 1 to 5 Hz. Most physiological systems fail to exhibit sufficient responses for stimuli that do not adequately stimulate their ideal operating range, (visual acuity in darkness is one such example). However, if one could adequately and reliably assess the vestibular system using rotational stimuli between 1 to 5 Hz, the data would show that the degree of VOR response would not only continue to be opposite (this is always the case) but would also be truly equal (or nearly equal) to the degree of stimuli input. That is, response unity would be present within our functional operating range of 1 to 5 Hz.

Analyzing Raw VOR Gain Data

Figure 6–14 depicts the raw nystagmus response of the VOR during a rotational stimulus. The slow-phase responses are plotted against the rotational stimulus for 0.04 Hz. The figure depicts right-beating nystagmus in response to rightward rotation and left-beating nystagmus in response to leftward rotation. It can clearly be seen that the VOR nystagmus response (i.e., the slope of the nystagmus) crescendos and decrescendos in relation to chair acceleration and deceleration. A healthy VOR nystagmus response will, therefore, have a peak response that is often associated with, or occurs near, the peak response of chair rotation.

The gain of the VOR is determined by comparing the peak eye velocity response to peak chair velocity response. The peak velocity of chair rotation is always held constant, most often 50° or 60°/second, depending on the predetermined stimulus parameters of the rotational paradigm or chair protocol. The peak eye (VOR) response, however, will often vary with respect to the frequency of chair rotation and physiology of the vestibular system. For lower frequencies of rotation, like that in Figure 6–15, the peak VOR response crescendos to approximately 30°/second in response to a 0.02 Hz rotational stimulus, whereas the peak eye (VOR) response crescendos to a much more robust peak response at 35° to 38°/second in re-sponse to a 0.32 Hz rotational stimulus (Figure 6–16). Identify-

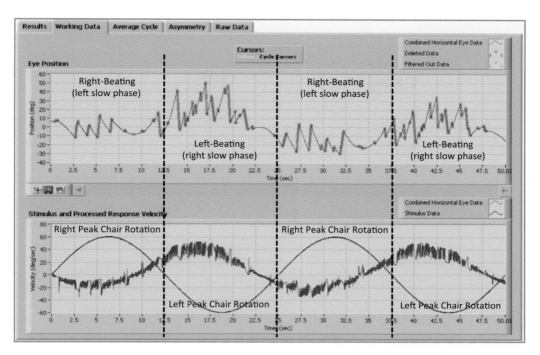

FIGURE 6–14. Data plot for two cycles of chair rotation and the corresponding slow and fast phases of the vestibular nystagmus.

FIGURE 6–15. Complete data for 0.02 Hz rotation. Top graph shows raw nystagmus tracing. Middle graph shows a plot of the slow phase component of the vestibular data in relation to chair velocity. Bottom graph shows averaged slow phase data in relation to chair velocity. Peak eye velocity data is determined and VOR gain for rightward and leftward rotation is calculated.

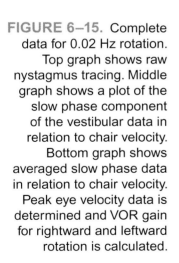

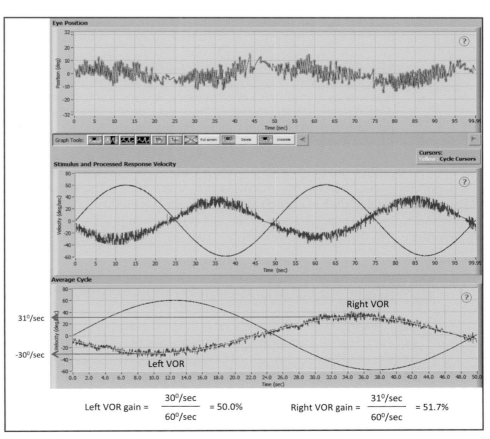

$$\text{Left VOR gain} = \frac{30^0/\text{sec}}{60^0/\text{sec}} = 50.0\% \qquad \text{Right VOR gain} = \frac{31^0/\text{sec}}{60^0/\text{sec}} = 51.7\%$$

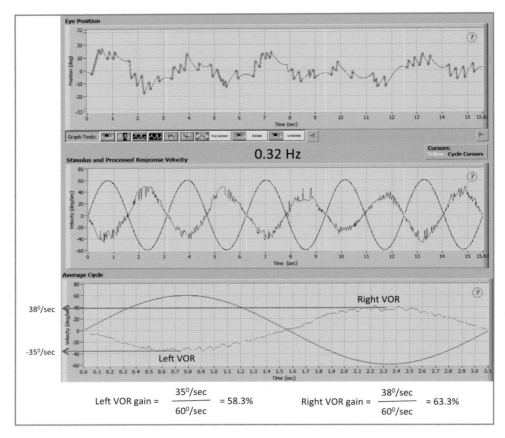

Left VOR gain = $\dfrac{35^0/\text{sec}}{60^0/\text{sec}}$ = 58.3%   Right VOR gain = $\dfrac{38^0/\text{sec}}{60^0/\text{sec}}$ = 63.3%

FIGURE 6–16. Complete data for 0.32 Hz rotation. Top graph shows raw nystagmus tracing. Middle graph shows a plot of the slow phase component of the vestibular data in relation to chair velocity. Bottom graph shows averaged slow phase data in relation to chair velocity. Peak eye velocity data is determined and VOR gain for rightward and leftward rotation is calculated.

ing the "peak" slow-phase velocity during rightward and leftward rotation is critical as it is this response parameter that is compared against the peak chair velocity response of 60°/second when determining the gain of the vestibular system.

Simply put, the VOR gain of the vestibular system is the ratio between the peak slow-phase eye velocity compared to (or divided by) the peak chair velocity (which is always 60°/second or 50°/second). The gain of the VOR is determined for

Calculating the VOR Response Gain from Sinusoidal Accelerations

Depending on the frequency or rotational being tested, the number of oscillations will vary. Recall that for higher frequencies of rotation, a total of 10 (or more) oscillations may be performed. However, for low rotational frequencies, a few as two oscillations may only be performed. However, whether it is two or 10 oscillations performed, the calculation of VOR gain is seldom made from a single cycle of rotation. Responses from each cycle are usually combined and averaged together to form a single "averaged" slow-phase VOR response plot. That is, all the right slow-phase responses obtained during each leftward rotation are averaged together, and all the left slow-phase responses obtained during each rightward rotation are averaged together. These averaged VOR slow-phase responses are then plotted against the averaged chair stimulus (which should be identical to a single period of chair rotation given the precise nature of the rotational stimulus—this is why the average chair stimulus continues to appear as a single data line). Figure 6–17 depicts data from the individual oscillations as well as after each cycle is combined to form an "average response plot." A best-fit line is then determined through the averaged slow-phase VOR data from which the averaged "peak" slow-phase velocity can be determined in response to both rightward and leftward rotations. Figure 6–17 illustrates such an example. The best-fit line identifies a peak slow-phase eye velocity (PSEV) response of 40°/second during rightward rotation and a peak slow-phase eye velocity response of 38°/second during leftward rotation. Each of these averaged PSEV responses is then divided by 60°/second (peak chair velocity is always the same independent of rotational frequency) and a VOR gain of 67% and 63% are determined for rightward and leftward rotation, respectively, for 0.16 Hz. Finally, averaging the two PSEV values and dividing by 60°/second generates a grand average VOR gain for this particular rotational frequency.

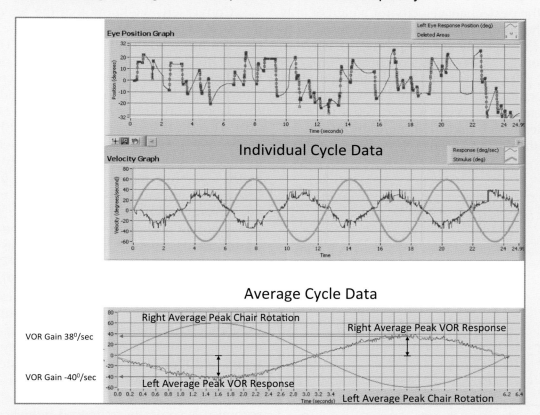

FIGURE 6–17. Complete data for 0.16 Hz rotation. Top graph shows raw nystagmus tracing. Middle graph shows a plot of the slow-phase component of the vestibular data (*blue sinusoid*) in relation to chair velocity (*green sinusoid*). Bottom graph shows averaged slow phase data in relation to chair velocity. Peak eye velocity data are determined and VOR gain for rightward and leftward rotation is calculated. A light-blue, best-fit line can be seen within the averaged VOR response data, from which the peak eye response is obtained for each rotational direction.

both rightward and leftward rotations, as well as combined for an averaged VOR response gain for each frequency of rotation.

Insight from VOR Gain With Respect to the Efficiency of the VOR

As previously mentioned, the sensitivity (or gain) of the vestibular system below 1 Hz is rarely *equal* to the stimulus velocity and is, in fact, often only one-half the gain (0.5 or 50%) of the actual chair velocity (Brey et al., 2008a; Shepard et al., 2016). Moreover, depending on the frequency of chair rotation, the sensitivity or gain of the vestibular system will vary. This can be fully appreciated when analyzing the normative reference ranges (Figure 6–18). As can be seen in Figure 6–18, the *mean* VOR peak eye velocity approximates only one-half the peak chair velocity for a gain of only 50% as the rotational frequency increases from 0.01 to 0.64 Hz. Only as we approach 1 Hz does the gain of the VOR begin to approach unity, or 1 (that is, peak eye velocity begins to equal peak chair velocity). This makes sense as we know that the efficiency of the VOR is best suited for those frequencies which occur during daily life activities; specifically 1 to 5 Hz. Only when consider-

ing the upper limits of two standard deviations for the frequencies testing during SHA does the VOR gain approach 1.0, and this is primarily confined to the mid-to-high frequencies. Although stated earlier, the reason for the gain of the VOR to, on average, only approach 50% stands repeating. Because the cupulae respond to acceleration, it is only from more robust accelerations experienced during faster frequency rotations that an adequate afferent neural response is able to produce a more robust VOR. One other factor for the lack of unity in the VOR response for frequencies administered during SHA testing is because the test is conducted in darkness. The VOR response is supplemented and often brought closer to unity by the visual system. This can be appreciated by the visual-vestibular interaction (VVI) test that is discussed in Chapter 8.

Conversely, we know that the sensitivity of the VOR is far less efficient for the low frequencies administered during SHA testing. This is primarily due to such impuissant stimuli producing insufficient cupular deflection, which creates too weak of an afferent neural response to adequately drive the compensatory VOR (Baloh & Honrubia, 2001; Hirsch, 1986; Leigh & Zee, 2006; Shepard & Telian, 1996). However, this low-frequency VOR inefficiency is acknowledged and easily detected by the CNS. Key central neurons are triggered by low threshold neural fibers, which in turn recruit key central mechanisms that activate a central network that augments the weak response. This central neural mechanism is known as velocity storage (Raphan, Matsuo, & Cohen, 1979; Robinson, 1976, Robinson, 1971) (Figure 6–19). Velocity storage plays a critical role in the processing and augmentation of the VOR response during low-frequency stimulation below 0.04 Hz. Through a network of commissural fibers and specialized type I and type II central neurons located within the vestibular nuclei (reviewed earlier in Chapter 3), the efficiency of the low-frequency VOR response is centrally enhanced, which produces an increased level of neural activity that is only now increased to a level sufficient to drive the VOR. Without velocity storage, the gain of the VOR for low frequencies would be significantly poorer (or even possibly non-existent), even with intact peripheral sensory end organs.

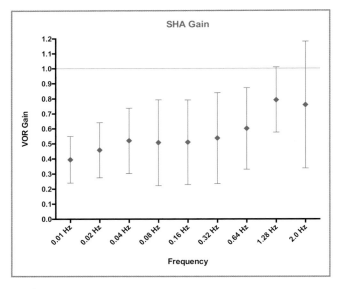

FIGURE 6–18. Normal reference range for VOR gain showing mean and two standard deviations for octave frequencies from 0.01 to 2.0 Hz.

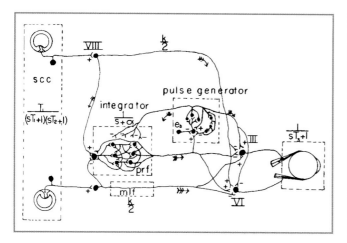

FIGURE 6–19. The central neural integrator converts semicircular canal afferent input to velocity position information to be used by the extraocular muscles. The concomitant pulse generator circuit is responsible for generating the fast-phase component of the vestibular nystagmus. From *Models of oculomotor neural organization* by D. A. Robinson, 1971. In P. Bach-y-Rita, C. C. Collins, and J. E. Hyde (Eds.) *Control of Eye Movements*, New York, NY: Academic Press. Reprinted with permission.

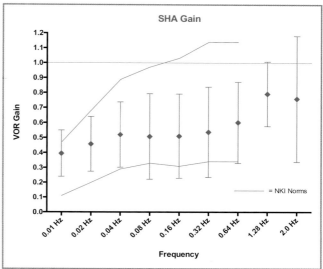

FIGURE 6–20. Comparison of normal reference range for VOR gain showing mean and two standard deviations for octave frequencies from 0.01 to 2.0 Hz. Mean and two standard deviations are compared from data collected at the National Institutes of Health against those from Neuro Kinetics, Inc. (*red lines*).

Interpreting VOR Gain

By examining and comparing the normative reference ranges across various sites, one can also acknowledge the high variability in the gain of the VOR (Figure 6–20). This high variability is best appreciated by acknowledging the large standard deviations contributing to a wide range of normal values, particularly when compared to the narrower normal reference ranges of VOR phase and symmetry. In fact, of the three parameters measured during SHA testing (gain, phase, and symmetry), VOR gain is easily the most variable (Cyr, 1991). This is secondary to a number of factors, which we will review later in the chapter when discussing factors that can impact your SHA results. Given the wide variability often observed with VOR gain, categorization of VOR gain is best assigned according to individual clinical site normative reference ranges. Site-specific norms will account for individual testing protocols (number of oscillations, head restraint device idiosyncrasies, individual site tasking paradigms, etc.).

Other than classifying patient VOR gain response as falling within normal limits, patient results are often categorized with respect to either abnormally high or low VOR gain. Abnormally low gain is certainly the more common of the clinical findings. When impacting all test frequencies, its interpretation is generally restricted to a bilateral reduction of vestibular reactivity. Although this is often associated with a bilateral *peripheral* pathology, a central pathology can also less frequently cause a bilateral reduction in VOR gain (Shepard & Telian, 1996; Wall, 1990). Therefore the site-of-lesion value for reduced rotational VOR gain is bilateral peripheral unless purely central indicators are suggested (Shepard & Telian, 1996). In addition, abnormally low VOR gain is often frequency dependent. Incomplete damage to the vestibular periphery causes reduced VOR gain that often occurs first in the low frequencies. This is juxtaposed to audiometric hearing loss, where loss often occurs first in the high frequencies. As vestibular pathology progresses, a loss of mid-to-high frequency vestibular reactivity ensues. This also helps to explain why caloric irrigations (comparable to a rotational frequency of 0.004 Hz) are so often reduced or absent with even slight peripheral vestibular damage. Moreover, this also sheds some light as to why rotational testing can be critical to the evaluation of a dizzy patient. Because VOR is frequency dependent, verifying intact, or even reduced but viable VOR gain for the higher frequencies is imperative when determining the potential for vestibular rehabilitation. This is similar to verifying usable hearing for the low to mid frequencies when determining the potential success for hearing aid outcomes.

Abnormally high VOR gain is a less seldom occurrence. The interpretation of this finding is similar to abnormally high caloric responses, and is usually associated with a central site of lesion that localizes to the cerebellum (Shepard & Telian, 1996). This finding is certainly uncommon, just as hypercaloric responses are uncommon. Less information is also known about hyperactive VOR gain during SHA testing. Hyperactive VOR gain has most often been reported in central pathologies, most often implicating the cerebellum (Baloh, Sills, & Honrubia, 1979; Hirsch, 1986; Shepard & Telian, 1996). Migraine and traumatic brain injury (TBI) have been implicated in producing high VOR gain results (Brey et al., 2008a, 2008b). Both of these pathologies have strongly implicated abnormal processes within the central nervous system.

Intra-Test Correlations

Jacobson, McCaslin, Grantham, and Shepard (2016) have reported a strong correlation between adjacent SHA frequencies, suggesting acute differences in VOR gain for neighboring frequencies are not common. In addition, Jacobson and colleagues (2016) further reported a significant correlation between reduced caloric response and reduced VOR gain at 0.01 and 0.02 Hz, as well as significant negative correlations between VOR phase lead for nearly all rotational frequencies through 0.16 Hz. Data from the normative reference range reported by this author corroborate this conclusion. A repeated ANOVA identified no significant differences in VOR gain between adjacent SHA frequencies. Such data are useful, insomuch that *patterns* in data interpretation often prove to be highly useful when analyzing within rotational test measures as well as across different vestibular test measures. One such example is that a normal caloric response is not likely going to occur in the presence of abnormal SHA data (gain and phase) keeping in mind that the caloric stimulus frequency of 0.004 Hz is roughly one octave, or one harmonic frequency, below 0.01 Hz.

A similar conclusion was corroborated by Kaplan and colleagues (2001) who reported that the probability of documenting abnormal rotational test results increased from only 0.8% in a group with normal caloric findings to 40% in a group with abnormal caloric findings. That is, if there exists an abnormal caloric response, the probability of having significantly reduced VOR gain is fifty times more likely than if the caloric response was normal. Although Kaplan and colleagues cited only a 6.7% occurrence rate of abnormal rotational VOR gain when a mild-to-severe unilateral caloric paresis was identified, they conceded that their analysis did not account for any abnormal phase or symmetry findings, which would have likely increased the probability for abnormal rotational results in the presence of unilateral caloric abnormalities. On the other hand, Kaplan and colleagues were able to effectively exclude the possibility of bilateral vestibular loss based solely on normal rotational chair VOR gain in 93% of their patients. These data would suggest that using rotational data to "screen" for bilateral vestibular loss might be more efficient and tolerable for patients than caloric testing.

Finally, the strong correlational data between adjacent SHA frequencies would also suggest that having a single SHA frequency exhibiting significantly lower (or higher) gain than the frequencies adjacent to the abnormal frequency is quite rare. For this reason, many clinicians refrain from classifying a response as abnormal unless a minimum of two adjacent frequencies (or multiple borderline abnormal frequencies) are abnormal. The exception to this is abnormally low VOR gain identified solely at 0.01 Hz, of which the clinical relevance could be significant in much the same way as a hearing loss confined to 8000 Hz is clinically relevant and not uncommon.

Relevance of VOR Gain to Phase and Symmetry

There is one more final comment to consider regarding VOR gain. Although not discussed yet, VOR phase and VOR symmetry are both calculated from VOR gain, and thus, when there is an absence of VOR response for either one or all SHA frequencies (i.e., zero gain), phase and symmetry values cannot be determined for any frequency where gain is absent. Figure 6–21 shows an example of a patient with a complete absence of VOR gain. Moreover, when there exists a situation where VOR gain is minimal, phase and symmetry should be interpreted with caution. Anytime VOR gain values are weak, there is a higher probability that physiological noise (e.g., blink artifact, ocular wandering, ocular vertical drift, etc.) has significantly reduced the validity of the weak VOR response. As such, VOR gain between 0.10 and 0.15 has been suggested as the lowest acceptable cutoff value when reliably calculating VOR phase and symmetry (Shepard & Telian, 1996). Therefore, when VOR gain values are near or below 0.15, it is highly recommended that the raw data be scrutinized to determine its signal-to-noise ratio in order to decide if the quality of the recording is "clean" enough to warrant calculation of phase and symmetry.

Although it is good practice to always review the raw nystagmus response, it is even more imperative when analyzing reduced signal-to-noise conditions that are common to low frequencies (given the inherent low gain naturally present at these frequencies) as well as during conditions of overall poor VOR gain where the response is minimal.

VOR Phase

In its simplest definition, phase refers to the timing relationship between head (chair) movement and eye movement (Shepard & Telian, 1996; Shepard et al., 2016). It can be thought of as the degree to which eye movement lags behind the applied stimulus, which is this case is head acceleration. By definition, the VOR dictates that an equal and opposite compensatory eye movement must occur in response to head movement. The exact time in which the eye begins to move in the opposite direction (in relation to head movement) is known as phase. Phase is the least intuitive of the three SHA mea-

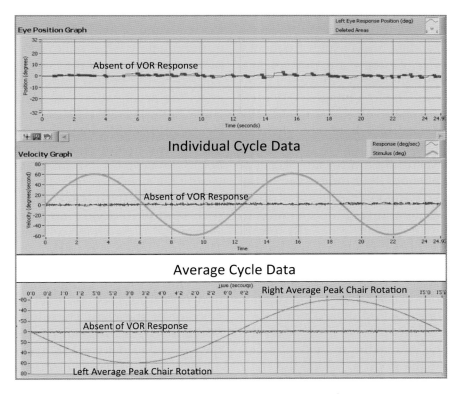

FIGURE 6–21. Example illustrating an absence of VOR response.

sures, but has the greatest clinical significance in its ability to document peripheral and/or central vestibular system dysfunction (Shepard & Telian, 1996). To put it bluntly, phase is something few clinicians like to discuss in terms of rotational testing, as its analysis is often thought of as very nonintuitive. However, the confusion surrounding an adequate understanding of VOR phase lies more in *how* the data are plotted and analyzed, rather than in *what* the phase data (erroneously) suggest—that the eyes actually *lead* chair movement.

Understanding Phase-Matching for Mid-To-High Frequency Stimuli

In order to gain a better understanding of VOR phase, it is first critical to understand the relationship between acceleration and velocity. To do this, let us first break down the basics of the chair SHA stimulus and VOR response. During this discussion, it is important to keep in mind that the VOR phase response is frequency dependent, with two basic response characteristics: one for low frequency stimuli (0.01 to 0.04 Hz) and one for mid-to-high frequency stimuli (>0.04 Hz). That being said, we will compare and contrast VOR phase as it relates to low versus mid-to-high frequency stimuli. Figures 6–22A–D depict the normal construct of a mid-to-high frequency sinusoidal stimulus (such as 0.16 Hz). The first image (A) depicts the classic stimulus of chair velocity as it normally occurs during SHA testing. Chair movement in the rightward direction is charted in the positive direction with increasing and decreasing acceleration to the target velocity. Chair movement in the leftward direction is charted in the negative direction with similar acceleration and deceleration to the target velocity. The second image (B) simply depicts the addition of the acceleration stimulus as it relates to the velocity stimulus. The point at which the chair is at 0° velocity marks the point when the chair begins accelerating to the right or is changing directions from rightward to leftward rotation. It is also at this precise time when the chair is experiencing its maximum peak of acceleration. Conversely, the point at which the chair has achieved its maximum velocity, the chair is at zero acceleration as it transitions from acceleration to deceleration. Thus one can see that the acceleration stimulus is 90° out of phase with the velocity stimulus.

At this point in time of our discussion, we are again reminded that the cupulae respond to *acceleration*, not velocity. However, the output of the ocular motor system is measured and plotted by the *velocity* of eye movement, not by the acceleration of the eye movement. Therefore, we must plot eye velocity as it relates to chair velocity. In a precise VOR response (those stimulus frequencies above 0.1 Hz), the vestibular slow-phase occurs nearly in perfect timing with head movement only in the opposite direction. Therefore, when plotting eye velocity, it is depicted as a mirror sinusoid with a near perfect temporal relationship to chair velocity (Figure 6–22C). Now, for simplicity of discussion and visual clarity, Figure 6–22D, has simply flipped the mirror eye velocity response 180° and is shown overlaying the chair velocity response. As illustrated, the now flipped and perfectly compensated 180° eye velocity response is clearly seen to lag the acceleration stimulus by 90° (exactly like chair velocity).

We now must account for this 90° phase shift (lag) between the detection of acceleration and the encoding of eye velocity. The observed lag of approximately 90° is believed to occur as a result of a series of second order vestibular interneurons known as the neural integrator, which assist in encoding acceleration into velocity (Baloh, Honrubia, & Kerber, 2011; Leigh & Zee, 2006). The efficiency of this 90° central processing time is only in response to stimulus frequencies greater than approximately 0.1 Hz (as discussed earlier, the vestibular system responds with much less efficiency for low frequency stimuli, and processes such stimuli in a very unique way through the assistance of the velocity storage mechanisms). Therefore, when accounting for the 90° lag time after the detection of the acceleration stimulus, the velocity output of the ocular motor system is now observed to be in direct alignment with the velocity of the chair stimulus. This is depicted in Figure 6–22D. In reality however, because the slow-phase velocity of the nystagmus response is opposite that of chair velocity, keep in mind that the actual eye velocity plot is a mirror image of chair velocity as we routinely see in our SHA data analysis (Figure 6–22C).

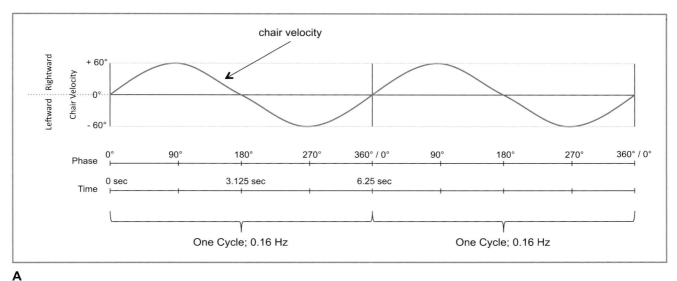

A

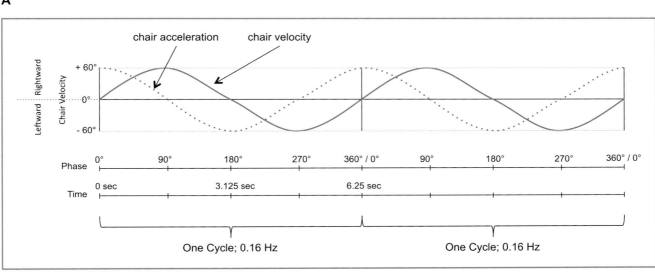

B

FIGURE 6–22. Individual graphs **A–I** illustrate the temporal (phase) relationship between chair acceleration and velocity to eye response velocity. **A.** Depicts the standard chair stimulus velocity for 0.16 Hz. **B.** Depicts the relationship between chair acceleration and chair velocity. Chair acceleration is greatest at the exact moment when chair is beginning to move in the opposite direction and least (zero) when chair velocity is at its peak velocity prior to slowing down. *continues*

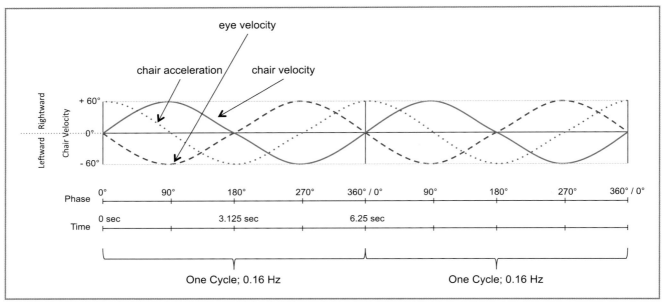

C

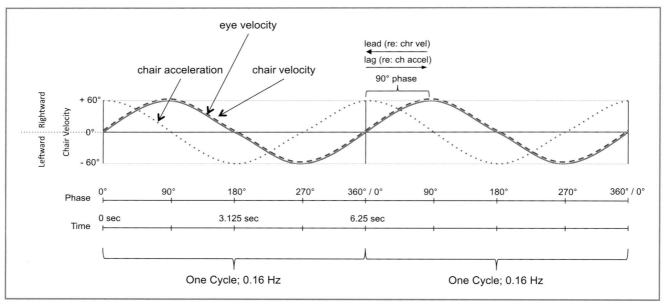

D

FIGURE 6–22. *continued* **C.** Depicts the relationship between eye velocity and chair velocity. When perfect, eye velocity is exactly opposite chair velocity (VOR is in the opposite direction to that of head or chair movement). **D.** Simply inverts the eye velocity response to more easily demonstrate its "temporal" relationship to chair velocity. In this view, eye velocity can be seen to lag chair acceleration by 90 degrees. *continues*

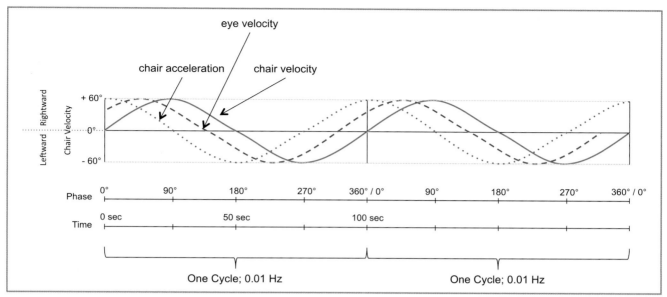

E

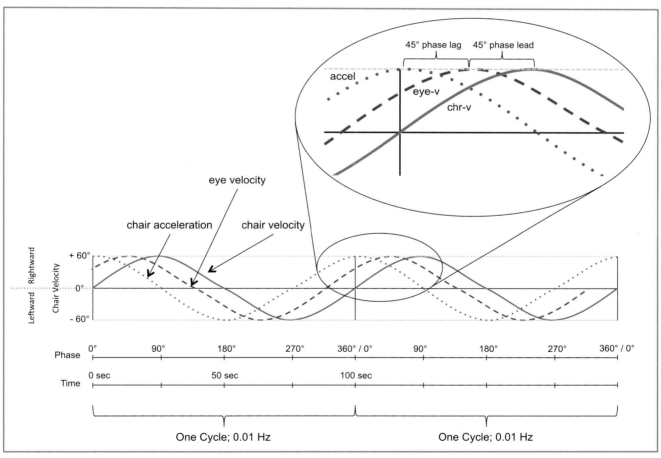

F

FIGURE 6–22. *continued* **E.** Depicts an earlier shift in the eye velocity plot. Depending on the reference point, the peak eye velocity can be seen to "lead" chair velocity or have a reduction in the lag time with respect to chair acceleration. **F.** Enhanced section showing a 45-degree phase lag (with respect to chair acceleration), or 45-degree lead (with respect to chair velocity). *continues*

177

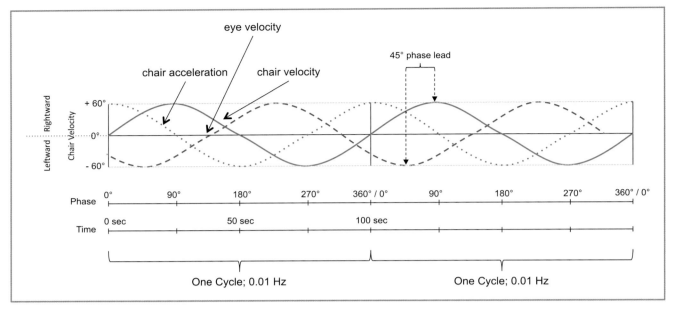

G

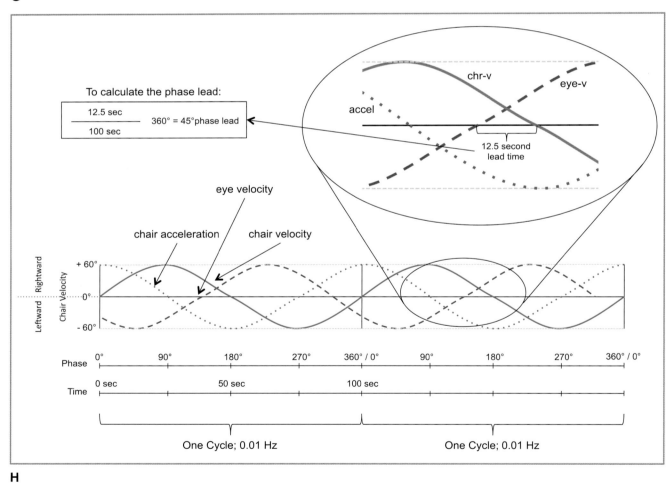

H

FIGURE 6–22. *continued* **G.** Image of plate "F" inverted to show actual plot of eye velocity data with respect to chair velocity depicting a 45-degree phase-lead (re: chair velocity). **H.** Enhanced section illustrating the 12.5-second eye-velocity lead time with respect to chair velocity and the conversion calculation to phase degrees. *continues*

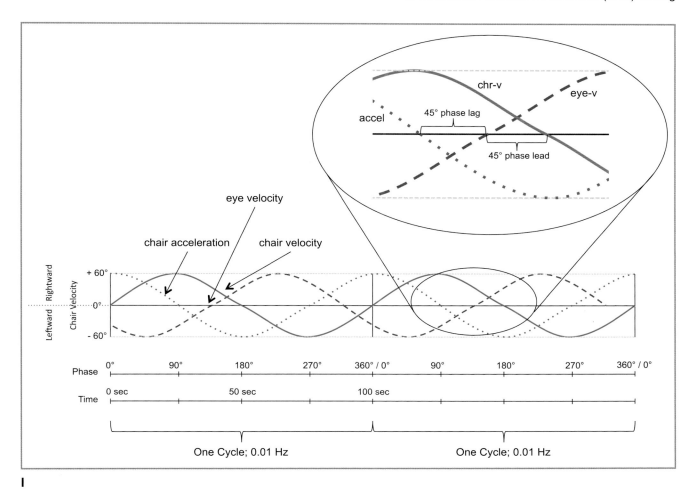

I

FIGURE 6–22. *continued* **I.** Final data plot of eye velocity data depicting a 45° VOR phase lead with respect to chair velocity data or a 45° VOR phase lag with respect to chair acceleration.

Understanding Phase-Matching for Low Frequency Stimuli

This exact phase velocity-matching of the VOR is essential, as it continuously strives to respond in a pure compensatory manner, always attempting to achieve response unity (gain of 1.0), as well as striving to produce a precisely timed response that is not only opposite to head movement, but occurs with little or no delay in relation to the velocity of head movement. So, given the inherent or "naturally" occurring 90° delay between acceleration and velocity, the vestibular system actually does an incredible job at "matching" eye velocity to head movement velocity, all because of this intrinsic 90° central processing time needed

between detection of acceleration and the production of the ocular motor [velocity] output. This is certainly true for frequencies that we experience in daily life (1 to 5 Hz), and is generally true for those SHA frequencies near or greater than 0.1 Hz (between 0.08 and 1.28 Hz). For these frequencies, the temporal relationship between the peak eye velocity response and the peak chair velocity stimulus does, in fact, approach unity, (although precisely 180° out of phase from one another as the slow-phase vestibular response is opposite in direction to that of chair [head] movement). This perfect temporal relationship of being precisely 180° out of phase is assigned a phase shift of "0°" for reasons related to how the phase shift is calculated. (See VOR phase calculation below.)

The idea of perfect "phase-matching," however, is frequency dependent. The exact phase "velocity-matching" is not the case for the lower frequencies applied during SHA testing (0.01, 0.02, and to a lesser extent 0.04 Hz). To understand this, we are back to recalling that: (1) the cupulae are accelerometers and the detection of low-frequency rotational stimuli is increasingly poorer below 0.1 Hz, and (2) the subsequent afferent neural response is therefore concomitantly weak. Because the afferent response is considerably weaker than that produced during higher frequency accelerations, there is concomitantly less neural information to be "managed" by the central processors. This central processing is composed of a sub-network of commissural fibers and cerebellar neurons that comprises a neural feedback loop that mediates and augments vestibular afferent input. We have discussed this "neural feedback loop" before as the neural integrator and subsequent velocity storage mechanism. The neural integrator and velocity storage mechanisms are critical and normal processes that provide much needed augmentation of the weak afferent input produced by low-frequency stimuli to sufficient levels, which is required to deliver an appropriate VOR output. Without such intervention, the low frequency stimulation (rotation in our case) is simply not sufficient enough to elicit an efficient ocular response and the typical VOR gain of the system for such low-frequency stimuli would likely be significantly weak, and, possibly even, unappreciable (Hirsch, 1986). Consequently, loss of the velocity storage mechanism due to peripheral or central pathology can lead to a significant reduction of VOR gain for low frequency stimuli (to be discussed later in this chapter).

So What Is Happening with "Phase-Matching" for Low Frequency Stimuli? Is It a Phase-Lag or a Phase Lead?

Actually it is both. It merely depends on whether you reference the recorded eye velocity response in relation to chair *acceleration* or chair *velocity*. With such impuissant stimuli delivered during low frequency SHA testing, the afferent neural drive from the periphery is (in the simplest of terms) insufficient to drive the secondary interneuron processing that occurs in response to higher frequency stimuli (Hirsch, 1986). As a result, the secondary interneuron 90° lag time between the detection of acceleration and the processing of the compensatory vestibular slow-phase eye *velocity* is *shortened*. This can graphically be depicted (see Figures 6–22E–I). Referring back to Figure 6–22D, the phase-matched eye velocity response is occurring with the inherent 90° phase lag from the detection of acceleration. However, by shortening the lag time due to the less robust low-frequency stimuli, the ocular response occurs with less than the standard 90° (velocity-matching) lag time. That is, peak eye velocity is occurring earlier than the peak chair velocity. This is illustrated in Figure 6–22E. This can easily be interpreted as a *phase-lead* in relation to chair velocity. This can be uncomfortable to think about, as it would seem that the eye "movement" is actually leading chair "movement." In reality, the eyes are not moving earlier than the chair, they are simply responding with less lag time in relation to a weaker acceleration stimulus. This is the fundamental confusion with understanding phase lead. We are not plotting eye displacement against chair displacement. We are plotting velocity against velocity—and velocity is very different from displacement (or movement). Since we plot eye velocity to chair velocity, it would "appear" that the eyes are, in fact, leading the chair. However, if we were to plot eye velocity to that of chair acceleration, we would see that the eye response is simply responding with less secondary interneuron processing lag time (i.e., not using the full 90 degrees of central processing time for perfect velocity-matching). When analyzing the normative data provided in Figure 6–23, one can see that the average phase lead for healthy (normal) vestibular systems is approximately 40 and 20 degrees for 0.01 and 0.02 Hz, respectively. In others words, in lieu of the 90-degree central processing time present at higher frequencies, there is a reduced but, *normal* phase lag of only 60 and 70 degrees postacceleration at 0.01 and 0.02 Hz, respectively. It is not until 0.08 Hz and above, that a "perfectly matched" phase lead of near zero degrees (90-degree lag time from acceleration) is achieved. In fact, phase lead sys-tematically increases with decreasing frequency below 0.08 Hz, reaching a 90° full phase lead around 0.005 Hz (i.e., near or at the caloric frequency) (Wall, 1990).

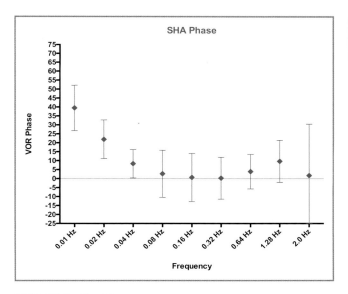

FIGURE 6–23. VOR Phase normative reference range in degrees for 0.01 to 2.0 Hz. Diamonds represent mean VOR phase for each frequency. Error bars denote ± standard deviations from the mean.

A Historical Point of View for Plotting VOR Phase

Interestingly, at one time, eye velocity data was actually plotted against chair acceleration data; however, it soon became conventional to plot chair velocity against eye velocity. This is primarily because it makes more sense to plot and compare similar measures (°/sec versus °/sec rather than °/sec versus °/sec^2).

It is true that a low-frequency phase-lead (or lag with respect to acceleration) is physiologically normal for acceleration stimuli less than 0.04 Hz. The reduction in the precision of phase matching can best be illustrated by comparing the VOR phase response against chair velocity across all the SHA frequencies (Figure 6–24). The progressively increasing VOR phase lead below 0.04 Hz

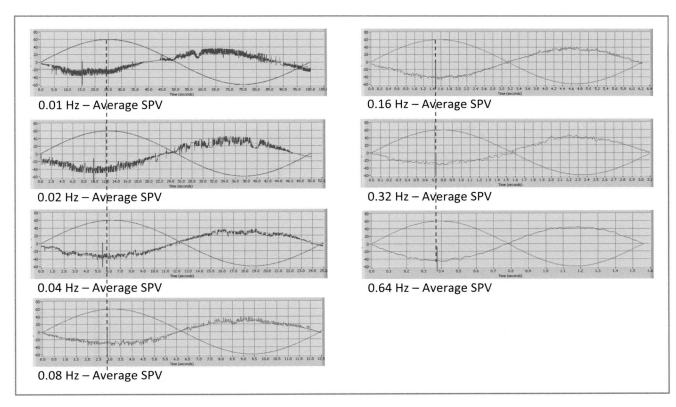

FIGURE 6–24. Average cycle slow-phase nystagmus plot data for all octave frequencies (0.01 to 0.64 Hz). Dashed line marks the approximate peak of the chair velocity data, whereas red solid line marks the approximate peak of the slow-phase nystagmus data. Note the advancing phase lead below 0.04 Hz.

can clearly be seen in this comparison of VOR responses by frequency. However, some have argued that there is seldom, if ever, a functional component that accompanies such a naturally occurring physiologic "deficiency," as our visual system is uniquely designed to compensate for this phase mismatch (Goldberg et al., 2012; Leigh & Zee, 2006). Honrubia, Jenkins, Baloh, Yee, and Lau (1984) also argued that velocity storage is likely inconsequential because visual input alone can provide eye stabilization at low frequencies of head motion. Conversely, others have argued of its functional importance. Jacobson, McCaslin, Patel, Barin, and Ramadan (2004) have argued that velocity storage and its role in augmenting the vestibular system's sensitivity to low frequency stimuli is intrinsically vital to an efficient vestibular response and its proper integration for subjective postural stability, particularly during low-frequency stance/postural sway (Jacobson et al., 2004). When a peripheral or central vestibular disorder disrupts velocity storage to where a significant-to-near theoretical maximum 90° VOR phase-lead occurs (i.e., zero phase-lag with respect to acceleration), the consequential phase mismatch becomes subtlety recognized by our central nervous system. When this happens, patients will often complain of poor postural stability, particularly at rest or when standing still, as these "postural resting movements" more closely match the low-frequency accelerations where such VOR phase abnormalities would predominate.

Calculating the VOR Response Phase from Sinusoidal Accelerations

Similar to calculating VOR gain, responses from each period are combined and averaged together to form a single "average" slow-phase VOR response plot. These averaged VOR slow-phase responses are then plotted against the averaged chair stimulus (single line as the chair stimulus should contain no noise to average out). Before we begin reviewing an example, it is a good to recall that because phase is calculated from gain, a thorough analysis of the signal to noise ratio (spectral purity) in the response must be considered whenever low gain (below 0.15) is present. Figure 6–25 depicts data from an "average response plot" showing averaged data in both the rightward and leftward rotations. A best-fit line is calculated through the averaged slow-phase VOR data. Although we talk about phase shift in terms of the temporal relationship between peak eye velocity data to peak chair velocity, the VOR phase is actually calculated from the difference between the point in time where the best-fit line and the chair velocity plot crosses 0° velocity. Since rotational cycles repeat themselves every 360 degrees, phase is, therefore,

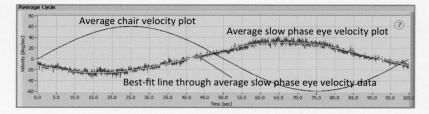

FIGURE 6–25. Average slow phase nystagmus data plotted against average chair velocity data, with a peak velocity at 60°/sec. Yellow best-fit line is plotted through the average of the slow phase eye velocity data.

expressed in terms of degrees. In Figure 6–26, the best-fit line identifies a peak slow-phase eye velocity response crossing 0° velocity at 40 seconds, whereas the chair velocity data crosses 0° velocity at 50 seconds. This difference in phase shift (time) is then divided by the time needed to complete one full cycle at the respective frequency. This difference is then multiplied by 360 degrees, which expresses the VOR phase shift in terms of degrees. That is, the VOR phase shift for this example would then be 10 seconds divided by 100 seconds (the time required to complete a full cycle at 0.01 Hz) multiplied by 360 degrees. This would yield a VOR phase lead of 36 degrees. A VOR phase lead of 36° means that only 54° of central processing occurred following detection of chair acceleration. So we can think of this as either a 36° VOR phase lead with respect to chair velocity or a 54° VOR phase lag with respect to chair acceleration. Again, a phase lead of 0° means that there was a full 90° of central processing that occurred following detection of acceleration.

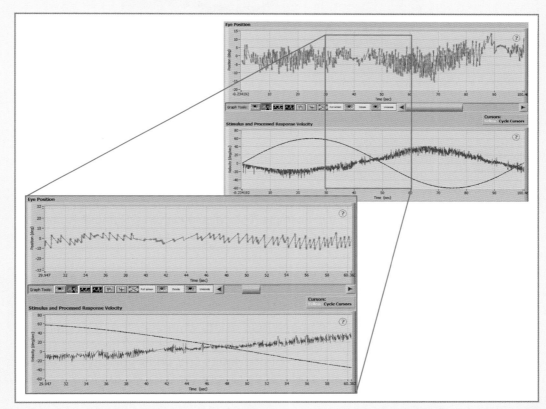

A

FIGURE 6–26. Individual graphs illustrate the phase lead calculation for a VOR response to a 0.01 Hz SHA stimulus. **A.** The top panel depicts the entirety of the 0.01 Hz raw averaged response showing both the nystagmus tracing and the plot of the slow phase eye velocity. The boxed insert and bottom panel depict a magnified look at the response between 30 to 60 seconds. The change over from right-beating to left-beating nystagmus can be more easily visualized in relation to the timing of the chair as it transitions from rightward to leftward rotation. *continues*

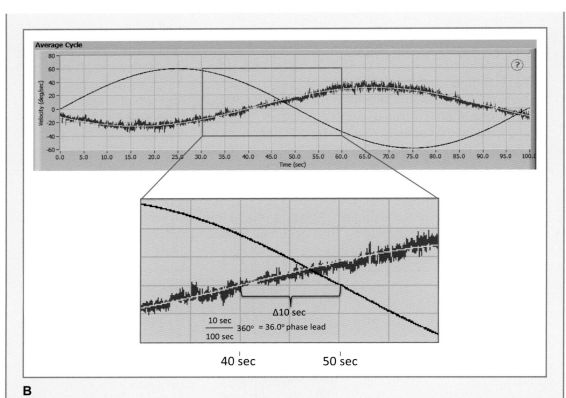

B

FIGURE 6–26. *continued* **B.** The inset box and bottom panel provide a magnified view of the transition point between rightward and leftward rotation, and the point in time where the best-fit line eye-velocity data crosses zero velocity (40 seconds) in relation to the point in time where the chair transitions from rightward to leftward rotation (50 seconds). The VOR phase lead can clearly be seen in this example. The calculation of VOR phase is shown.

A perfect compensatory response would then calculate as 0°, as a time difference of zero divided by the total cycle time multiplied by 360 would equal "0." Figure 6–27 shows the calculation of a 14.4° phase lead for a 0.02 Hz rotational stimulus.

As a point of nomenclature, a phase *lead* exists whenever the VOR gain best fit line crosses 0° velocity *before* the chair velocity crosses 0°. This could be 75° or 20°. Both examples are considered phase leads (re: chair velocity). However, when comparing against normative reference ranges for 0.01 Hz the former would be classified as a significantly *prolonged* phase lead, whereas the later would be considered a significantly *shortened* phase lead. It is not considered a phase *lag* until the VOR phase best-fit line crosses 0° velocity *after* the chair velocity crosses 0°. Figure 6–27 compares a prolonged VOR phase lead and a VOR phase lag. Figure 6–28 illustrates the graphical differences between a *prolonged* phase lead, a *shortened* phase lead and a phase *lag* with respect to normative data.

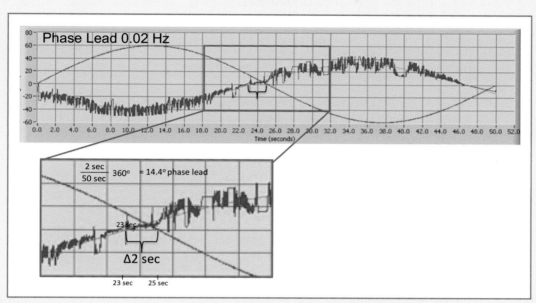

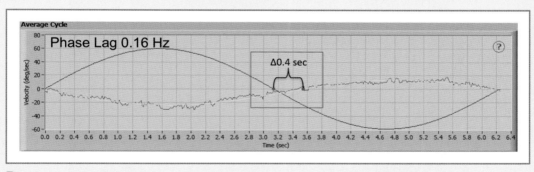

FIGURE 6–27. Magnified view of a close-up comparison of a VOR phase lead response (**A**) against a VOR phase lag response (**B**). Most VOR phase lag responses do not exhibit a lag of more than 1 to 2 seconds, which is often in stark comparison to some phase leads, which can extend well beyond a few seconds.

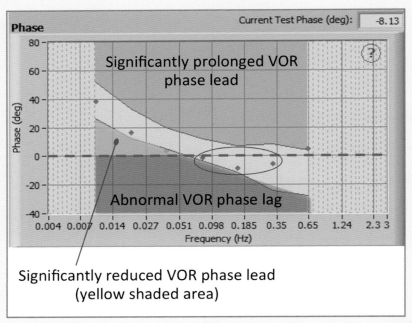

A

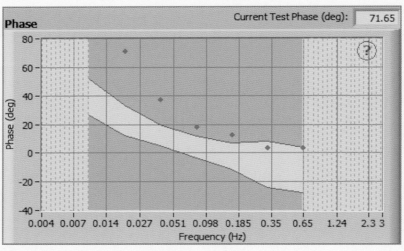

B

FIGURE 6–28. **A.** Differentiation between VOR phase leads and VOR phase lags. Green dashed line represents 0° VOR phase. Any data points *above* this line represent a phase lead. Any data points *below* this line represent a phase lag. Data points lying within the yellow shaded area are not a phase lag, they are a significantly reduced phase lead. Whereas the data points from 0.16 Hz to 0.32 Hz that are below 0° (*circled in blue*) represent a true phase lag (albeit within normal limits). **B.** Depicts significantly prolonged VOR phase leads for the low-to-mid frequencies. *continues*

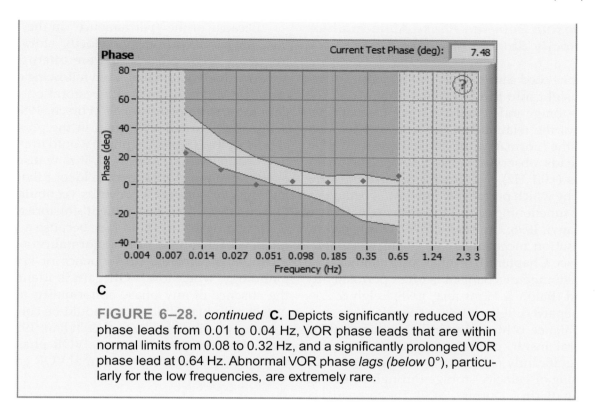

C

FIGURE 6–28. *continued* **C.** Depicts significantly reduced VOR phase leads from 0.01 to 0.04 Hz, VOR phase leads that are within normal limits from 0.08 to 0.32 Hz, and a significantly prolonged VOR phase lead at 0.64 Hz. Abnormal VOR phase *lags (below* 0°), particularly for the low frequencies, are extremely rare.

VOR Phase Interpretation

Now that we have a better understanding of how VOR phase is processed, let us consider how it is interpreted. Because VOR phase is a measure of the timing in the processing of the compensatory ocular response to vestibular stimulation, it is a measure of both the peripheral and central processing that occurs within the vestibular nerve and the central processors (i.e., the neural integrator and velocity storage mechanism). As such, a loss or reduction in afferent neural drive, or a loss in the efficiency of the velocity storage mechanism or the secondary interneuron commissural network, will cause abnormalities in VOR phase.

When a VOR phase abnormality is observed, it is nearly always a significant *prolongation* in the phase *lead* (when compared against chair velocity). This is most often due to a reduction of peripheral input secondary to peripheral pathology and subsequent loss of central processing that is normally present from the detection of acceleration to the output of ocular velocity (i.e., the 90° processing time needed for velocity-matching of the compensatory ocular response to head movement) (Hon-

rubia, Baloh, Yee, & Jenkins, 1980). A reduction in VOR gain due to a peripheral vestibulopathy (or, less frequently, a central pathology) will produce a shorter lag-time from the detection of acceleration, which is plotted as even a greater phase *lead* with respect to chair *velocity*. The primary loss of central processing time leading to longer phase leads is thought to be secondary to a reduction in the number of neural synapses leading to a decrease in neural processing within the neural integrator and velocity storage mechanism (Honrubia et al., 1980). Because of this, abnormalities in VOR phase most often occur in the low frequencies during SHA testing, where this central augmentation process is almost entirely dependent upon the velocity storage mechanism. In fact, a low-frequency VOR phase lead in the presence of normal (compensated) VOR gain is the most common SHA abnormality (Stockwell & Bojrab, 1997b). Conversely, given the greater velocity-matching efficiency of the VOR to acceleration stimuli >0.1 Hz, as well as the low demand placed on the velocity storage mechanism for higher frequencies, VOR phase abnormalities for the mid-to-high frequencies during SHA testing are far less common.

Relationship Between Phase Abnormalities and Velocity Storage Mechanisms

For reasons cited earlier, VOR low-frequency phase offers insight into the functional integrity of the velocity storage and neural integrator mechanisms. In light of the relationship between velocity storage and the (normal) predictable increase in VOR phase leads observed during lower frequency rotations (<0.1 Hz), it is possible to determine the capacity by which peripheral and central pathology alter the functioning of this mechanism (Curthoys & Halmagyi, 1996; Highstein, 1996). Due to central compensation mechanisms following peripheral insults (see Chapter 3), normal functioning of the velocity storage mechanism is often permanently modified (Baloh & Honrubia, 1998; Leigh & Zee, 2006; Shepard & Telian, 1996;). In order to restore and rebalance central vestibular gain following peripheral insult, central compensation mechanisms significantly reduce (or even negate) normal functioning of velocity storage through cerebellar clamping (Barin & Durrant, 2000). The consequence of altering the normal function of velocity storage, however, is the loss of central processing from the velocity storage mechanism, which we have already discussed. This leads to a significant-to-near complete loss of the secondary interneuron 90-degree phase lag that is normally present postdetection of acceleration, which is reported as a significant phase lead (re: chair (head) velocity). Therefore, the normal mechanisms underlying velocity storage are essentially "sacrificed" in order to restore and centrally rebalance vestibular gain. Because of this sacrifice, phase abnormalities for the low frequencies are often permanent. However, as mentioned earlier, the functional consequence of this is minimal and likely less damaging to one's balance phenotype than the alternative; a loss of low frequency vestibular gain. What if, however, the central compensation mechanisms were to correct for the abnormal phase lead by reinstituting normal operation of velocity storage mechanisms? The most probable answer is that the low frequency gain of the VOR would likely be sacrificed instead. This is the vestibular compensation "tradeoff"; the sacrifice of abnormal gain for normal phase, or the sacrifice of abnormal phase for normal gain. Thankfully, our central compensation mechanisms choose the latter, which is likely the more attractive of the two options.

Because of the "permanence" in the "clamping," or modification, of velocity storage, low frequency VOR phase leads are often the only abnormality that remains, even following effective central compensation and a restoration of VOR gain to within normal levels (Hirsch, 1986). That being said, normal VOR gain in the presence of abnormal low frequency phase would imply effective compensation. Moreover, it may also be the only "remaining" rotational evidence that would highlight or support a previous vestibular insult that could corroborate a patient's historical report of vertigo or dizziness. In fact, because a low frequency VOR phase lead abnormality is almost a certain predictable consequence of vestibular pathology, when low VOR gain is identified in the absence of any phase abnormality, technical or test administration error should be considered a strong possibility (Shepard & Telian, 1996). In a way, abnormal low frequency VOR phase leads validate the presence of abnormal VOR gain.

High Frequency Phase Abnormalities

For higher frequencies, the phase shift (or compensatory timing) of the VOR is nearly perfect (0°) as eye velocity is precisely in-sync with chair (head) velocity, only in the opposite direction (Curthoys & Halmagyi, 1996; Highstein, 1996). Secondary to the increased phase-efficiency of the VOR for the mid-to-high frequencies (greater than 0.1 Hz), the deleterious impact from acute peripheral vestibulopathologies impacting velocity storage is of less consequence for this frequency range (Leigh & Zee, 2006). As a result, phase abnormalities for the mid-to-high frequencies are seldom observed from peripheral lesions. However, phase abnormalities are not devoid in this frequency range and, when present (particularly in isolation), are often associated with central lesions (Shepard & Telian, 1996). Figure 6–29 depicts two examples illustrating significant prolongations in VOR phase leads for the mid-to-high frequency range.

Abnormally Reduced Phase Leads and Phase Lags

Abnormally reduced (or significantly shortened) VOR phase leads are certainly uncommon with respect to phase abnormalities. Moreover, abnor-

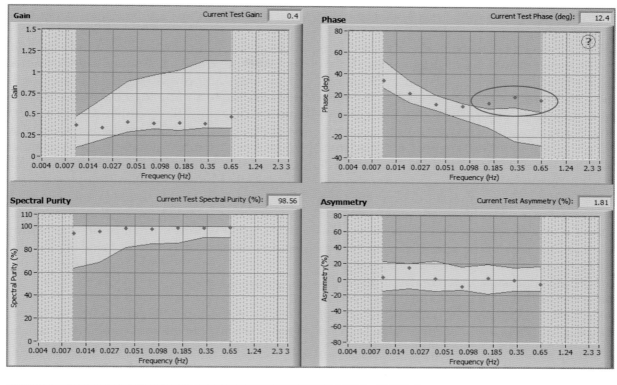

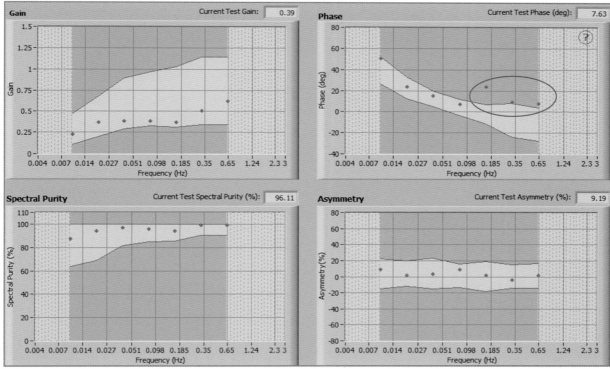

FIGURE 6–29. Two examples illustrating VOR phase leads isolated to the mid-to-high frequency range (*green ovals*). **A.** Patient with a Chiari malformation Type I. **B.** Patient with Lyme disease. Both patients exhibit VOR gain values that are within the normal range. The increased VOR phase leads extending to the mid-to-high frequencies, particularly in the presence of normal VOR gain, is suggestive a central component to the abnormal VOR findings (as well as their chronic uncompensated dizziness). Both patients had concomitant findings of abnormal saccadic smooth pursuit (results not shown here).

mal VOR phase *lags* are extremely rare (see Figure 6–28). By extension of our previous discussion regarding *prolonged* phase leads, an understanding of a shortened VOR phase lead or a phase lag would suggest an *increase* in the normal processing time following the detection of acceleration. This process would suggest an abnormal propagation or continuance of central processing of the secondary interneuron commissural network beyond the normal 90-degree lag-time (from detection of acceleration), and could be consistent with a lesion associated with the velocity storage mechanism, or possibly even higher up in the neural process. Although less is known about the mechanisms that create abnormally *shortened* phase leads or phase lags (Shepard & Telian, 1996), lesions in the nodulus region of the cerebellum have been shown to be critical

in the processing of the velocity storage integrator (Waespe, Cohen & Raphan, 1985). Shortened phase leads and phase lags have been associated with migraine, a pathology having central implications that may have down-regulating effects on the velocity storage mechanism from higher brainstem structures, namely, the amygdala or the locus ceruleus (Johnson, 1998). Figure 6–30 shows an example from a patient exhibiting significantly shortened VOR phase leads, while Figure 6–31 illustrates an example of a phase lag (albeit the phase lag is within normal limits - an abnormal example is extremely rare to come by).

Stability of Phase

Finally, of the three SHA parameters, phase has been shown to be the most stable and repeatable

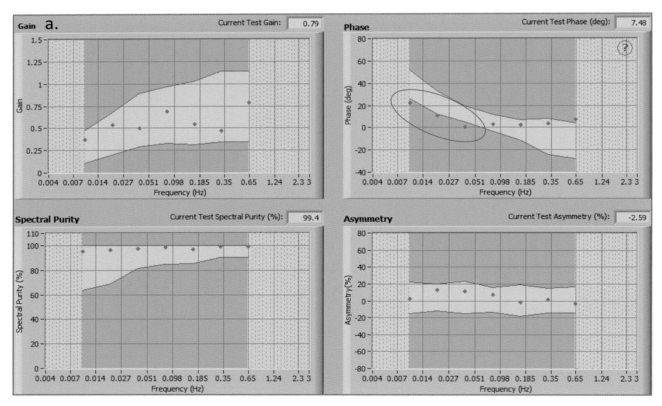

FIGURE 6–30. Significantly reduced low frequency VOR phase leads. (a) Presented data are from a patient with a cerebellar tumor. Note the VOR gain values that are within the normal range. The occurrence of significantly decreased low frequency VOR phase leads, particularly in the presence of normal VOR gain, suggests a central site-of-lesion; particularly those structures that comprise the neural integrator and play a key role in velocity storage. These data may further help to explain the patient's reports of chronic uncompensated dizziness. This patient also had concomitant findings of abnormal saccadic smooth pursuit and prolonged time constants (Chapter 7) (results not shown here).

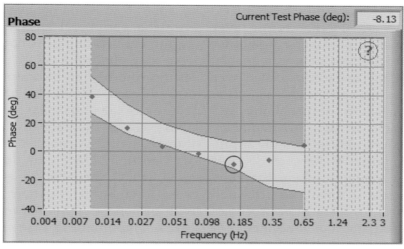

A

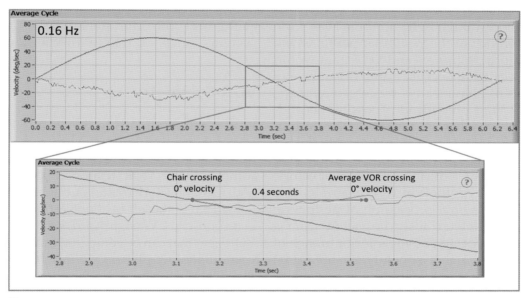

B

FIGURE 6–31. A. VOR phase response from a patient with Chiari malformation. Although the VOR phase lag from 0.08 to 0.32 Hz is within normal limits, this example illustrates the timing relationship between the VOR response to that of the chair (head) response. **B.** Using 0.16 Hz as an example, the ocular response is "lagging" the head response by approximately 0.4 seconds, which contributes to a −8.3° VOR phase lag. Although reduced VOR phase leads are possible, abnormal VOR phase *lags* are extremely rare.

measure during rotational assessment (Shepard & Telian, 1996; Shepard et al., 2016). VOR phase is an extremely repeatable and reliable measure with significantly less variance when compared against the other SHA parameters (Hirsch, 1986). This can be best appreciated when analyzing the normative reference range depicted in Figure 6–23. The two standard deviations that define the normal range of VOR phase are considerably narrower than those associated with VOR gain. The exception to this is during high frequency rotations (2 Hz), as the degree of dermal slip becomes a significant impediment to capturing precise time-locked head movement in relation to chair movement. Given its repeatability, VOR phase is an excellent parameter to monitoring over time. Progression of slow peripheral vestibular disease causing a progression of low-frequency VOR phase prolongation can be appreciated over time, despite the slow mechanistic compensation that keeps VOR gain within normal limits and largely stable over time. In fact, low-frequency VOR phase prolongations may be the only appreciable progressive abnormality for such diseases like vestibular schwannomas where the slow decrement of VOR gain is "matched" through highly efficient central compensation processes over time. This clinical pattern of abnormal VOR phase in the presence of normal VOR gain suggests subtle pathology that would otherwise go undetected. This is particularly true even if the origin of the vestibular schwannoma was from the inferior branch of the vestibular nerve, where effects on caloric responses and SHA gain would be spared. Recall that because approximately one-half of the VOR phase lead is processed *centrally*, an abnormal VOR phase lead is possible secondary to lesions anywhere in the vestibular periphery (even if the pathology does not directly impact the peripheral structures or neural pathway being assessed, e.g., h-SCCs during rotational or caloric testing). In this hypothetical case example, it is possible that the *central* processing of peripheral input could be deleteriously impacted from a peripheral lesion located on the inferior branch of the vestibular nerve. Subsequently, the abnormal VOR phase lead in this example could be a manifestation of a *central* processing error caused by an abnormal *peripheral* input that, interestingly,

is caused by a lesion not even directly associated with the peripheral structures being assessed during SHA testing. It is not impossible to suggest that abnormal VOR phase during SHA testing could be an indicator of *indirect* peripheral disease. Moreover, this could also be true of isolated macular disease, where VOR phase could theoretically be impacted even though neither maculae is assessed during SHA testing. This is an interesting phenomenon, which, theoretically, could also cause the most common SHA pattern; normal VOR gain with prolonged abnormal low frequency phase leads. Hypothetical case examples illustrate the complexity of the vestibular system as well as the challenges that accompany its assessment, particularly if the clinical assessment evaluates both the peripheral *AND* central systems, such as that with rotational testing.

VOR Symmetry

VOR symmetry refers to the equality of the VOR gain when stimulated during rightward (CW) rotations versus leftward (CCW) rotations. The compensatory VOR response occurs following both CW and CCW rotations, but in opposite directions. That is, the left-beating vestibular slow-phase in response to CW (rightward) rotations produces a VOR gain that can be compared to the right-beating vestibular slow-phase gain from CCW rotations. The relationship between the generated VOR gain from CW and CCW rotations represents the symmetry of the vestibular system.

Calculating the VOR Response Symmetry from Sinusoidal Accelerations

Similar to VOR gain and phase, responses from each period are combined and averaged together to form a single "average" slow-phase VOR response plot. These averaged VOR slow-phase responses are then plotted against the averaged chair stimulus. Similar to the calculation of phase, it is a good to recall once again that, because symmetry is also calculated from gain, a thorough analysis of the signal to noise ratio (spectral purity) in the response must be considered whenever VOR gain is below 0.15. Figure 6–32 depicts the best-fit line through the averaged slow-phase VOR data from which the averaged "peak" slow-phase velocity (VOR gain) can be determined in response to both rightward and leftward rotations. The best-fit line identifies a peak slow-phase eye velocity (PSEV) response of −40°/second during rightward rotation and a peak slow-phase eye velocity response of 38°/second during leftward rotation. VOR symmetry is determined by calculating the ratio between the two PSEV values for each particular rotational frequency. VOR symmetry is the quotient between the difference from the absolute peak nystagmus values divided by the sum of the absolute peak nystagmus values multiplied by 100 (see Figure 6–32). A positive asymmetry will reflect a stronger right compensatory slow-phase in response to leftward rotation (i.e., left-beating nystagmus), whereas a negative asymmetry will reflect a stronger left compensatory slow-phase in response to rightward rotation (i.e., right-beating nystagmus).

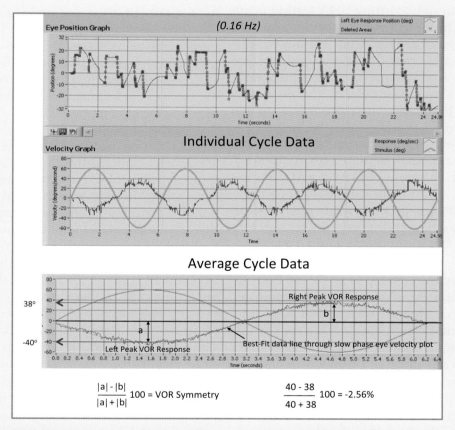

FIGURE 6–32. VOR response to a 0.16 Hz SHA stimulus. Top panel shows the individual cycle data depicting the raw nystagmus tracing (*top*) and slow phase eye velocity plot (*middle graph*). Bottom panel shows the averaged cycle data depicting the chair rotation and the averaged slow phase eye velocity data. A faint (*light blue*) best-fit line traces through the averaged slow phase eye velocity data. VOR gain for rightward and leftward stimulation is shown and the symmetry calculation is provided.

VOR Symmetry Interpretation

Because both labyrinths are actively providing an excitatory and inhibitory response during head rotations, laterality should not always be inferred from the symmetry measure. VOR asymmetry, therefore, does not directly reflect a state of weakened laterality in the peripheral system. Rather, it reflects a physiologic *preponderance* within the vestibular system (Shepard & Telian, 1996). A vestibular preponderance merely indicates that the system has a preferential bias toward a particular direction of rotation (movement) or, more precisely, a preference toward the production of a particular slow-phase VOR response. The measure of VOR symmetry during SHA testing is, in fact, analogous to directional preponderance calculated during caloric irrigations. However, it is important to realize that directional preponderance calculated from caloric irrigations is determined from the slow-phase velocity component of the nystagmus, but named in accordance with the fast phase (i.e., right-beating or left-beating directional preponderance). Rotational asymmetries, on the other hand, are calculated *and* named in accordance with the slow-phase velocity component. Therefore, a *right* caloric directional preponderance (i.e., left slow-phase velocity component) is analogous to a *left* rotational asymmetry (i.e., left slow-phase velocity component) and vice versa.

VOR Asymmetry Secondary to an Acute Peripheral Vestibulopathy. Rotational asymmetries most often occur in the presence of an acute peripheral vestibular lesion that has yet to be *fully* compensated, that is, both statically and *dynamically*. As a result, the postacute unilateral peripheral lesion continues to produce a *dynamic* asymmetry during rotations secondary to incomplete (dynamic) compensation from the central nervous system. In fact, the simplest explanation for most rotational asymmetries is due to an acute (or postacute) unilateral peripheral vestibular lesion. During an acute unilateral lesion, a rotational asymmetry occurs secondary to the presence of a spontaneous nystagmus as well as a rotational dynamic labyrinthine bias. Under the acute (and semi-postacute) lesioned status, the intact labyrinth will contribute a stronger slow-phase velocity component under dynamic rota-

tional conditions that is contrasted against the weaker slow-phase component produced from the lesioned labyrinth. Moreover, the spontaneous nystagmus will add to a particular direction of rotation and produce an even greater asymmetry, courtesy of the intact ear. For example, a patient with an acute unilateral left ear peripheral lesion will generate a greater left slow-phase velocity component than a right slow-phase velocity component. This is due to the intact right labyrinth's ability to produce a greater left slow phase velocity component while rotating toward the right. In addition, the underlying acute right-beating spontaneous nystagmus (if present) will also contribute to a larger left-slow-phase velocity component, thus augmenting an even greater left rotational asymmetry (recall that unilateral peripheral weaknesses produce an acute spontaneous nystagmus that beats toward the intact ear). The opposite is, of course, true when rotating toward the lesioned left ear (lower right slow-phase velocity component).

In the acute lesioned status, the presence of a spontaneous nystagmus will generally force an asymmetry until central compensation occurs and tonic neural symmetry is once again restored. In time, central compensation effectively resolves both the static (spontaneous nystagmus) as well as the dynamic (rotational) asymmetry. It is important to note, however, that such conditional asymmetry will only exist during a unilateral peripheral *weakness*. Everything discussed at this point regarding asymmetry and the direction of the slow-phase velocity component will be reversed in the presence of an *irritative* lesion, such as Ménière's disease. Thus, a rotational asymmetry can be secondary to *either* peripheral system and care should be given to ensure the underlying etiology and laterality of the vestibulopathy. In light of this, a comprehensive vestibular assessment is essential to elucidate a more complete peripheral vestibular phenotype for such patients. In addition, corroborating evidence suggesting incomplete compensated VOR gain, low frequency VOR phase leads and even a caloric asymmetry should also be apparent during this acute (and semi-postacute) stage.

VOR Asymmetry Secondary to a Central Pathology. The presence of a significant VOR asymmetry can also occur from a lack of effective central compensation long after the onset of an acute peripheral lesion. Less common is an asymmetry that occurs in the *absence* of any unilateral peripheral weakness or irritative lesion. These conditions are far less common than the transient lack of dynamic compensation for an acute peripheral lesion and, as such, these rotational asymmetries can be quite perplexing. Such chronic or "idiopathic" VOR biases have been reported from lesions affecting both the peripheral and/or central vestibular system (Brey et al., 2008b; Shepard & Telian, 1996; Shepard, et al., 2016). For this reason, such VOR asymmetries should be interpreted with caution. However, in the presence of normal VOR rotational gain, as well as the absence of any unidirectional spectral impurity (noise) and spontaneous nystagmus, such VOR asymmetries often suggest the presence of a chronically uncompensated vestibular asymmetry secondary to an isolated, or diffuse central nervous system pathology (Shepard & Telian, 1996). Similar to asymmetries attributed to peripheral lesions, corroborating evidence for central pathology should be evident in such cases, as central pathologies rarely produced isolated findings.

Figure 6–33 illustrates a case involving a persistent uncompensated unilateral peripheral pathology due to a progressive central nervous system degenerative disease. These data depict a stronger rightward (positive) vestibular slow-phase VOR asymmetry that occurs in response to leftward rotation for essentially the entire rotational frequency range. In this example, VOR gain is observed to be within normal limits, spectral purity was excellent, (discussed in the next section) and no spontaneous nystagmus was present at the time of evaluation, despite a known right labyrinthine weakness previously identified using caloric irrigations (data not shown). For such cases involving chronic unilateral peripheral weaknesses, the observed rotational asymmetry should not be merely interpreted as reflecting *only* a right labyrinthine weakness. Rather, these data indicate that a CNS bias likely contributes to the production of a vestibular slow-phase nystagmus that is considerably more robust following leftward rotation. This interpretation is suggested particularly given the presence of normal rotational VOR gain and the absence of any spontaneous nystagmus. Moreover, other rotational data including signifi-

cantly prolonged VOR phase lead involving the mid-to-high frequencies, failure of VOR fixation suppression (discussed in Chapter 8; data not shown) and concomitant abnormal ocular motor findings provide additional data that are consistent with this patient's degenerative CNS disease. All things considered, these data collectively suggest a *chronic* uncompensated right vestibular asymmetry, secondary to this patient's degenerative CNS pathology, that is likely restricting full compensation of a previous right peripheral vestibulopathy. Moreover, these data also support this patient's complaint of unremitting vertigo and dizziness.

VOR Symmetry Reference Ranges. Finally with respect to VOR symmetry, Figure 6–34 depicts normal reference ranges (means and two standard deviations) for symmetry using a 60° peak velocity stimulus (note the exceptionally large variance for 2.0 Hz consistent with the larger variance inherent to this frequency).

Spectral Purity

Signal to noise ratios are important in nearly every behavioral and physiological measure. Unfortunately, biological systems are inherently noisy (Wall, 1990). VOR gain is no exception to this and, because both VOR phase and symmetry measures are dependent upon VOR gain, all three parameters of SHA are highly dependent on a good signal to noise ratio. The signal to noise ratio for SHA testing is known as spectral purity.

Spectral Purity Calculation

The determination of spectral purity is usually expressed as a percentage of noise with reference to the signal. In short, it is simply the signal-to-noise ratio between the ocular response and the rotational stimulus. It is not calculated form the averaged VOR tracings as is VOR gain, phase, and symmetry. Rather, spectral purity is calculated as the ratio between the fundamental power of the ocular response against the total power of the frequency stimulus. To illustrate this, consider two extremes. On one hand, during poor VOR responses, where there is minimal to no VOR gain,

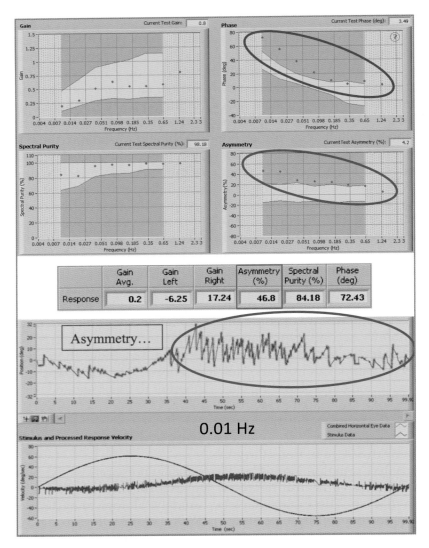

FIGURE 6–33. Case example showing a significant VOR asymmetry with a more robust right slow phase vestibular response to leftward rotation for the entire frequency range, (*highlighted by the green ovals*). The significant asymmetry for 0.01 Hz is calculated to be +46.8%, suggesting the rightward slow phase component is 46.8% stronger than the left slow phase component, (*bottom graph* and *red square*). The percent asymmetry varies depending on the rotational frequency tested, (*green oval in the top graph*). Normal VOR gain, excellent spectral purity, and a low-to-high frequency VOR phase lead (*blue oval*) are concomitantly identified (*top graph*). Collectively, these data are most likely consistent with a persistent, uncompensated right vestibular lesion, (previously identified). Lack of complete compensation is most likely secondary to this patient's underlying progressive CNS degenerative disease. The CNS pathology is further supported by significantly prolonged VOR phase leads involving the mid-to-high frequencies, (*blue oval, top chart*), failure of rotational VOR fixation suppression, (data not shown), and abnormal ocular motor findings (data not shown).

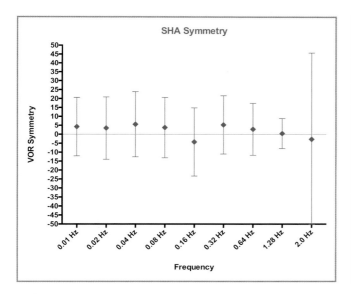

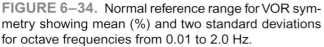

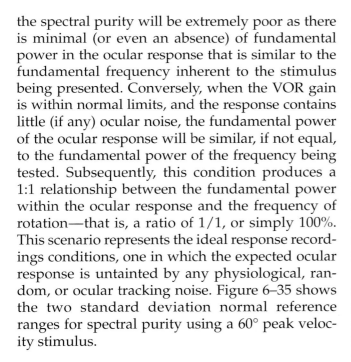

FIGURE 6–34. Normal reference range for VOR symmetry showing mean (%) and two standard deviations for octave frequencies from 0.01 to 2.0 Hz.

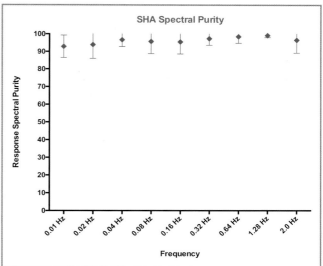

FIGURE 6–35. Normal reference range for SHA spectral purity showing mean (%) and two standard deviations for octave frequencies from 0.01 to 2.0 Hz. Upper limits for standard deviations are limited to 100% where upper limit error bars are not shown.

the spectral purity will be extremely poor as there is minimal (or even an absence) of fundamental power in the ocular response that is similar to the fundamental frequency inherent to the stimulus being presented. Conversely, when the VOR gain is within normal limits, and the response contains little (if any) ocular noise, the fundamental power of the ocular response will be similar, if not equal, to the fundamental power of the frequency being tested. Subsequently, this condition produces a 1:1 relationship between the fundamental power within the ocular response and the frequency of rotation—that is, a ratio of 1/1, or simply 100%. This scenario represents the ideal response recordings conditions, one in which the expected ocular response is untainted by any physiological, random, or ocular tracking noise. Figure 6–35 shows the two standard deviation normal reference ranges for spectral purity using a 60° peak velocity stimulus.

Spectral Purity Interpretation

In general, the greater degree of noise relative to the signal, the larger the error of estimate for the true response. There are many factors that can deleteriously impact the spectral purity of a nystagmus recording. The number one factor is usually excessive eye movements, primarily because they introduce energy outside the fundamental energy of the rotation frequency being tested (Cyr, 1991). This factor becomes even more amplified when the underlying VOR gain response is low, either due to reduced physiology from pathology or is fundamentally inherent to a lower frequency being tested. Because low frequencies have an inherent reduction in physiologic gain, spectral impurity becomes a greater concern at these frequencies, particularly if the mental tasking is too inappropriate or ineffective.

Specifically, poor spectral purity (below 75%) may negatively introduce artifact in the phase and symmetry "best-fit" data calculations even if VOR gain is normal (Cyr, Moore, & Möller, 1989). Other minor factors that introduce excessive noise during SHA testing are arbitrary ocular muscle activity, noise that is inherent to electrode recordings (if EOG is being used to measure the corneal retinal potential), fluctuations in synaptic activity, and simple variability in ocular muscle performance, such as ocular position (Wall, 1990). Ocular and head deviation have also been shown to dramatically reduce VOR gain (Fetter, Hain, & Zee, 1986). Specifically, vertical ocular deviation (similar to Bell's phenomenon) is well known to substantially decrease VOR gain.

Factors Impacting Spectral Purity

Excellent spectral purity should always be the goal of any rotational assessment. In Chapter 5, we discussed many factors that can negatively impact response data. When a good signal-to-noise ratio is in doubt, one should consider repeating each rotation in question and every attempt should be made to improve the quality of the recording. I am reminded of the old saying "garbage in, garbage out." The number one priority when collecting data is always to achieve the cleanest ocular response possible, otherwise the interpretation will be subject to an analysis based on spurious data. Whether this is improving patient factors (boredom, eye closure, fatigue, stress, deviation of eyes upward), or recording parameters (eye tracking threshold), clean data are always critical for a more valid analysis and interpretation.

To Repeat or Not to Repeat: A Case Example

Mental tasking is critically important during SHA testing, just as it is during caloric testing. Inappropriate tasking techniques can either reduce the spectral purity of the response due to the introduction of physiological artifact into the signal, or it can reduce the VOR gain response due to increased VOR suppression. Recall our discussion involving the importance of mental tasking on the VOR in Chapter 5. Figure 6–36 shows results from a patient who received SHA testing twice. In Figure 6–36A, the patient was tested using infrequent and simple tasking procedures. Secondary to a suspicion of inappropriately low VOR gain, the patient was re-examined later in the day using a higher level of tasking procedures in order to better challenge the patient to decrease the level of suspected suppression of VOR gain. As can be clearly seen, the gain obtained during repeat testing is significantly higher (Figure 6–36B) when compared to the VOR gain initially documented earlier in the day (Figure 6–36A).

The determination of whether or not to retest a patient is seldom straightforward. In the absence of any corroborative clinical evidence suggesting the reduced VOR gain response is reliable, such data should always be questioned and possibly reacquired. In this case example, serial testing had previously identified a healthy VOR response during SHA testing, and the absence of any clinical abnormalities or historical evidence of vestibular symptoms, suggested such a decrease in VOR reactivity was unlikely. As a result, it was decided that the patient should be re-examined later in the day. In addition, the patient's educational background was highly technical, and the type of mental tasking (simple naming task) may have been insufficient. Follow-up testing clearly reveals a significant increase in VOR gain (Figure 6–36B). VOR levels on reexamination were more in line with historical VOR gain responses. This case example clearly illustrates the importance of appropriate tasking and the deleterious impact that can sometimes result from insufficient or inappropriate tasking methods. It also clearly illustrates how fickle VOR gain can be, and provides a good case to characterize the high variance that can be inherent to VOR gain during any vestibular measure.

Finally, this example can be used to demonstrate how the clinical interpretation of patient data should always be made with some caution. If this patient had not previously received serial testing, and the results obtained in Figure 6–36A were not questioned because of a historical incongruence, these results could just as easily been accepted as valid. This certainly would have provided evidence to support this patient's history of nonspecific dizziness. However, we as clinicians must always keep in mind that a reported history of dizziness does not always guarantee or predict abnormal results. Finally, there is one additional piece of key evidence to suggest low gain was questionable in this case. Even if historical results were unavailable, these data neglected to reveal any associated low-frequency VOR phase abnormalities (<0.04 Hz). As mentioned earlier, low-frequency VOR phase abnormalities are almost invariably associated with a loss of VOR gain. In the absence of any concomitant phase abnormalities in the presence of low VOR gain, the validity of SHA results should always be questioned.

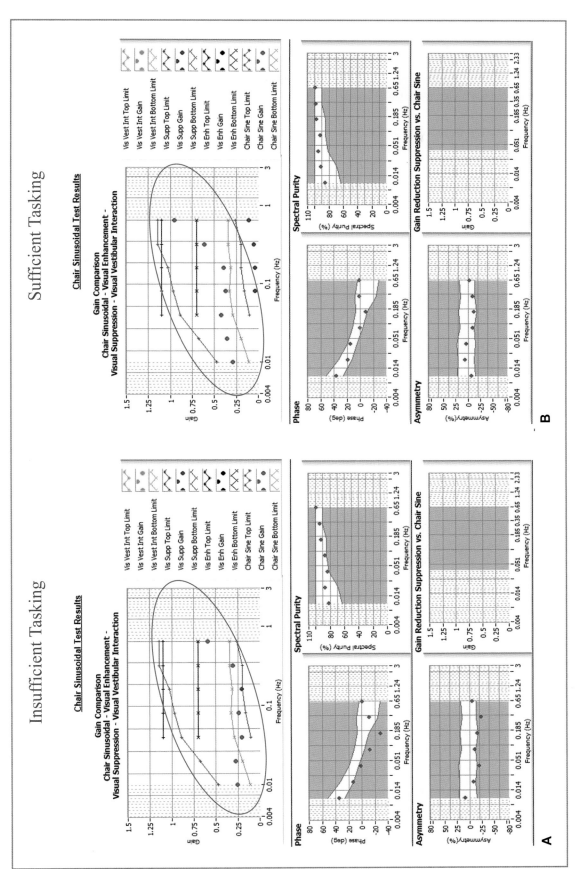

FIGURE 6–36. Example illustrating the effects of mental suppression on the VOR for the same patient tested approximately three hours apart. Top chart for both graphs displays VOR gain for the octave frequencies (0.01 to 0.64 Hz) (*green ovals*). Red lines depict normative reference ranges for this manufacturer at the time. Note how the VOR gain increased from below normal limits to within normal limits for the mid-frequency range on follow-up testing with sufficient tasking. VOR phase and symmetry measures also improved on follow-up testing with a concomitant improvement in the spectral purity (*lower graphs for both charts*).

THE CLINICAL APPLICATION OF SHA TESTING

The clinical use of SHA testing is a fundamental component to rotational testing. Identification of certain SHA "patterns" can help facilitate a vestibular diagnosis, as well as provide valuable insight into the peripheral and central physiology of the vestibular response. Patterns in VOR phase (particularly low frequency phase leads) can be very powerful in the interpretation of vestibular function and, more importantly, vestibular compensation. Patterns in VOR phase can provide insight into the integrity of velocity storage as well as provide subtle clues as to any historical vestibular pathology. As mentioned earlier, isolated low frequency VOR phase leads are, in fact, the most common SHA abnormality. When present in association with normal VOR gain and symmetry, abnormal prolongation of low frequency VOR phase leads are almost always consistent with a previous unilateral peripheral vestibulopathy that has been effectively compensated. Although a bilateral vestibulopathy will also produce a low frequency VOR phase lead, the bilateral nature of the peripheral disease will also cause a concomitant low frequency reduction in VOR gain that may extend into the mid-to-high frequencies. This is often one of the first differentiating signs of bilateral versus unilateral disease. Although the laterality of the unilateral disease cannot directly be inferred from the SHA results, other clinical indicators can provide that knowledge. Ultimately, SHA testing will help to determine the extent or severity of the vestibular pathology. Although categorical labels are not traditionally assigned to vestibular disease (i.e., mild, moderate, severe, profound), the extent of disease with respect to the affected frequency range is important to differentiate, as residual vestibular response in the high frequencies can offer significant potential for the possibility of vestibular rehabilitation.

Effect of Unilateral Peripheral Vestibulopathies

Unilateral peripheral vestibular disease can produce SHA results that place the VOR gain near the lower range of normal, but rarely does even a complete unilateral labyrinthectomy cause a severe reduction in VOR gain below normal limits. As expected, unilateral peripheral lesions have their greatest impact on VOR phase (Honrubia, Baloh, Yee, & Jenkins, 1980). Figure 6–37 is an example of SHA results from a long-standing left ear vestibular nerve resection. Since SHA rotations stimulate both labyrinths simultaneously, the gain of the entire system can effectively be compensated over time. Think of ocular output in terms of the response from the entire vestibular system rather than individual labyrinths. Given the fact that the central system can undergo effective compensation and modify how the central vestibular nuclei process the asymmetric peripheral input, the inhibition and excitation from a single healthy reflexive labyrinth can be sufficient, given enough time, to produce an ocular output, which not only falls within the normal range of vestibular reactivity, but is also symmetrical. Also note that in this example the VOR phase is significantly prolonged for the low frequencies (see Figure 6–37). This is precisely the expected pattern as we have previously discussed. VOR phase returns to within (or near) normal limits as the demand placed on velocity storage becomes less significant near and above 0.08 Hz. Again, this is often the most common VOR phase pattern seen from SHA testing and also provides evidence to suggest a compensated unilateral vestibular lesion.

When assessing *acute* peripheral vestibulopathies, the VOR can show a dramatic decrease in VOR gain; however, the most striking abnormality will usually be a significant asymmetry that is biased in the direction of the spontaneous nystagmus. A concomitant low frequency VOR phase lead will likely also be present. Over time, the gain responses will gradually improve to within normal limits as will the asymmetry slowly adjust to within normal limits. However, the abnormally prolonged VOR low frequency phase leads will remain.

Effect of Bilateral Peripheral Vestibulopathies

Conversely, a bilateral vestibular lesion will have a significantly more deleterious impact on the output of the system, as some peripheral input (even if it is only one-half that of normal, as with a

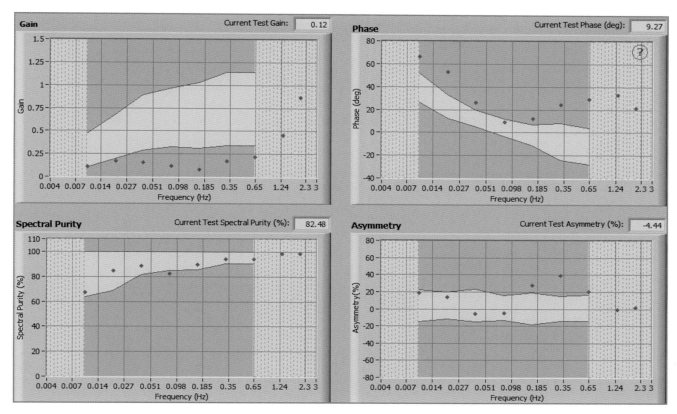

FIGURE 6–37. Chronic loss of VOR gain following a patient with a unilateral VIII Nerve resection due to a sporadic acoustic neuroma.

unilateral peripheral lesion) is requisite to be processed by the central system to drive the ocular output. Figure 6–38 is an example of a bilateral vestibular lesion. Note the complete absence of VOR gain. Here, the determination of phase and symmetry would not be considered valid, and any results that the analysis algorithm calculates should be ignored. This is an example of a complete loss of vestibular reactivity. Figure 6–39 is another example of a bilateral vestibular lesion. Note the near to complete loss of low frequency VOR gain that improves to within normal limits for the mid and high frequencies. This is also a common pattern of SHA testing. This pattern suggests an incomplete or partial loss of bilateral vestibular function. Similar to the auditory system having frequency dependent loss of sensitivity, the vestibular system can experience a similar frequency dependent loss, only in the opposite manner. Depending on a sufficient amount of low frequency gain from which to analyze phase and symmetry, the phase will likely be significantly

prolonged, and the degree of reduction in peak eye response will likely be symmetrical, with the exception of an asymmetric acute lesion.

Effect of Central Pathologies

Figure 6–40 is an example of a *shortened* VOR phase lead. In these cases, VOR gain can be normal, reduced, or even high. Many times, the VOR gain will be on the higher end of normal limits if not above the upper limit of the normal range as in Figure 6–40. As we discussed earlier, a shortened phase lead (or abnormal phase lag) may suggest an abnormal perpetuation of central processing, which could suggest an abnormality in how the central control of the VOR response is mediated. As we previously discussed, this facilitated control is often performed though the central processors and, most notably, the cerebellum. In the absence of any regulation by the cerebellum, VOR phase and gain is believed to exhibit an

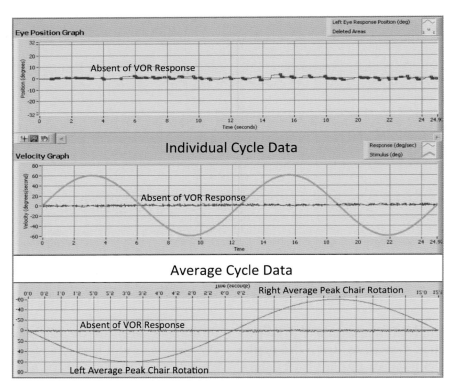

FIGURE 6–38. Example illustrating the absence of a VOR response to sinusoidal stimulation. There is the presence of a slight left-beating spontaneous nystagmus present in the raw top tracing. The absence of any VOR response (slow-phase eye velocity plot) is depicted by a straight line in both the individual cycle data (*middle graph*) and the average cycle data (*bottom plot*).

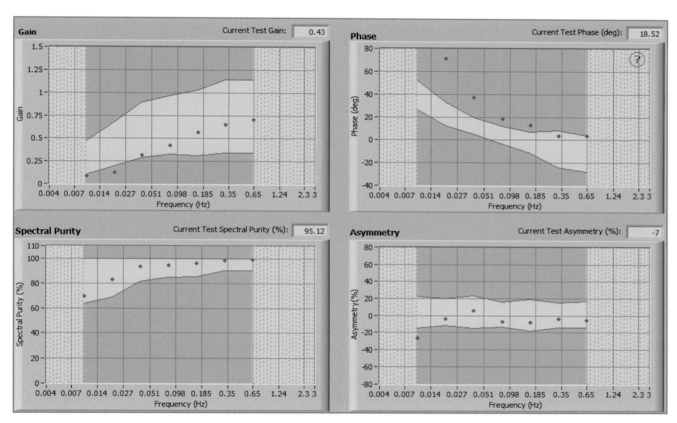

FIGURE 6–39. Partial bilateral vestibular loss with near complete loss of VOR gain from 0.01 to 0.02 Hz, and VOR gain that recovers to within normal limits for 0.04 to 0.64 Hz. These data are from a patient with neurofibromatosis II with concomitant loss of bilateral caloric response.

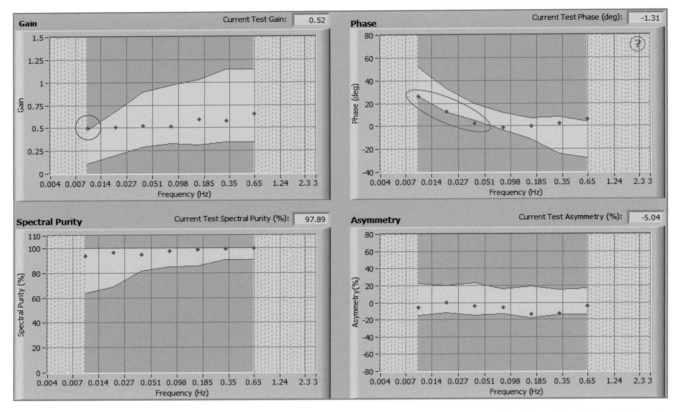

FIGURE 6–40. Summary data for a patient with a progressive cerebellar atrophy. Note the high VOR gain isolated to 0.01 Hz (*blue circle*) with a concomitant abnormal *reduction* in VOR phase lead (*green oval*). Both of these findings are commensurate with this patient's central pathology.

unregulated increase in gain, similar to hyperactive caloric responses. Although certain irregularities in secondary interneuron processes likely contribute to this process, namely, dysfunction of the neural integrator, this process has been localized to the nodulus of the cerebellum (Waespe et al., 1985). Another possible central finding may be an increase in VOR phase leads that are isolated to the mid-to-high frequencies (or may include the entire frequency range). An abnormal increase in VOR phase for the mid-to-high frequencies would suggest an inappropriate engagement of central processing neurons associated with the velocity storage mechanism. Recall that velocity storage is needed to extend the efficiency of the VOR for *low* frequencies. Central pathologies may inappropriately mediate such mechanisms and create a central processing environment that improperly extends VOR phase for the mid-to-high frequency range with respect to head velocity, (or inappro-

priately shortens the VOR phase lag with respect to acceleration), within a frequency range where the peripheral system is adequately designed to function *without* the need for central augmentation of the VOR response. Figure 6–41 depicts two examples showing VOR phase lead prolongations involving the entire frequency range, one in a patient with Chiari malformation and the other with Lyme disease.

Summary of Clinical Findings

Unilateral and bilateral peripheral vestibular lesions often produce generalized patterns that become evident from a comprehensive evaluation. With respect to SHA gain, bilateral lesions can most often be clearly distinguished from unilateral lesions. Moreover, unilateral lesions can often be differentiated from both normal and bilateral

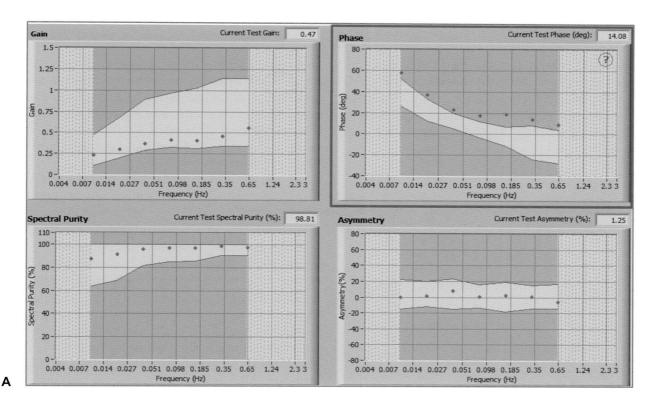

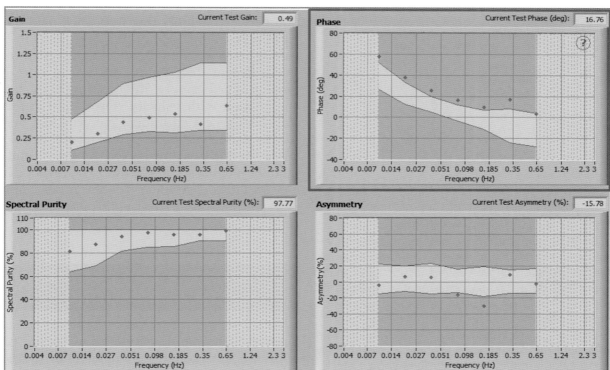

FIGURE 6–41. Two examples illustrating VOR phase leads involving the entire frequency range. **A.** Patient with a Chiari malformation Type I. **B.** Patient with Lyme disease. Note that both patients exhibit VOR gain values that are within the normal range. The increased VOR phase leads (*green rectangles*) extending to the mid-to-high frequencies, particularly in the presence of normal VOR gain, is suggestive of a central component to the abnormal VOR findings as well as their chronic uncompensated dizziness.

lesions, particularly for low frequency gain and phase parameters. A comparison of mean SHA gain and phase data between a group of normal, unilateral, and bilateral vestibular lesion patients has been previously reported by Baloh and

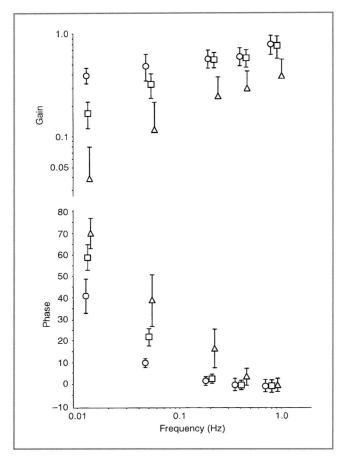

FIGURE 6–42. Rotational mean and ±1 standard deviation VOR gain and phase data comparing unilateral vestibular dysfunction versus bilateral vestibular dysfunction versus normal vestibular function. Circles (O) represent data for 10 normal subjects; Squares (□) represent data for 20 patients with compensated unilateral vestibular lesions (absent unilateral caloric); and Triangles (△) represent data for 22 patients with bilateral peripheral vestibular lesions (symmetrically decrease caloric responses). Velocities shown are for 0.0125 Hz at 100°/sec; 0.05 and 0.2 Hz at 60°/sec; 0.4 and 0.8 Hz at 30°/sec target velocity. From *Baloh and Honrubia's Clinical Neurophysiology of the Vestibular System* (4th ed.) by R. W. Baloh, V. Honrubia, and K. A. Kerber, 2011, New York, NY: Oxford University Press. Reprinted with permission.

Honrubia (2001). These data are shown in Figure 6–42. These data present the relative means and standard deviations for each response parameter within each group, and successfully illustrate the generalized difference a clinician can expect given the presence of a unilateral or bilateral vestibular lesion.

Overall, it is important to interpret SHA test results in conjunction with other assessment data when available. Although SHA testing, by itself, may offer the most comprehensive evaluation of the vestibular system, a complete vestibular assessment that involves videonystagmography testing, ocular motor assessment, vestibular evoked myogenic potential testing, video head impulse testing, and/or dynamic posturography is best, as no single vestibular test evaluates the entire system. Finally, similar to the overall "pattern" interpretation of findings across vestibular tests, it is also important to look for and interpret patterns within rotational testing. Recall our discussion involving a strong relationship or correlation between neighboring frequency data points. Although a single abnormal data point in SHA testing may not definitively identify pathology, two adjacent data points are much more convincing. Furthermore, interpreting SHA data in conjunction with velocity step data (Chapter 7) can often reveal additional patterns that help to further define vestibular pathology. Table 6–2 provides a summary of expected abnormal findings that are often associated with SHA testing. Table 6–3 provides a summary of the more common SHA findings associated with peripheral versus central lesions.

STRENGTHS AND LIMITATIONS OF SHA TESTING

Sinusoidal harmonic acceleration testing could easily be considered the backbone to rotational assessment, but it is important to keep in mind its strengths and limitations. No other vestibular assessment tool is uniquely designed to evaluate vestibular physiology with such precision. It can often provide a wealth of information regarding peripheral and central vestibular function, and,

Table 6–2. Sinusoidal Harmonic Acceleration (SHA) Test Abnormalities

Parameter	Abnormal Result	Possible Interpretation	Rule Out
GAIN	Low VOR gain for low Hz's (<0.04–0.08 Hz)	1. With concomitant abnormal phase lead at low Hzs & asymmetry—uncompensated UVL on side of asymmetry 2. With no phase abnormalities but abnormal symmetry, possible irritative or stable lesion (side uncertain) 3. No other abnormalities & normal spectral purity, compensated UVL is likely	Insufficient alerting
	Low VOR gain for all Hz's	1. BVL given eyes open during test (symmetry and phase cannot be interpreted) 2. Vestibulotoxic medication, aging (usually >65–70 years), rare degenerative disorders of the brainstem and/or cerebellum (especially if caloric data are normal)	Insufficient altering, restricted EOM, fixation
	High VOR gain for all or most Hz's	1. Cerebellar lesion (associated ocular motor abnormalities) 2. Has been observed in migraine and hydrops	Medications; stimulants
PHASE	↑ Low Hz Phase lead	1. Peripheral vestibular end-organ lesion/ vestibular nuclei lesion 2. With concomitant asymmetry, uncompensated UVL (on side of asymmetry) 3. Acute vestibular end organ lesion; vestibular hydrops	Compare with Step Tests & calorics
	↑ High Hz Phase lead	1. CNS lesion; (look for associated ocular motor abnormalities)	Lateral medullary syndrome
	↓ Low/High Hz Phase lead/lag	2. CNS lesion; (associated ocular motor abnormalities); consider lesions involving brainstem or posterior cerebellum; cerebellar nodulus	
SYMMETRY	Asymmetric SPV	1. Two or more consecutive abnormal Hzs; similar to DP on caloric testing (non-localizing with respect to site-of-lesion unless secondary to spontaneous nystagmus) 2. With low Hz phase lead, uncompensated peripheral lesion on side of asymmetry	Unstable lesion with normal phase findings

when used in conjunction within a comprehensive vestibular test battery, can be an indispensable test when identifying vestibular disease. Some of its key strengths include its precision and rigidity of stimulus delivery for effective monitoring, its ability to identify and monitor successful

Table 6–3. SHA Abnormalities Associated with Site-of-Lesion

Site-of-Lesion	Possible Response	Rule Out
PERIPHERAL — UNILATERAL	1. Initial loss of VOR gain can involve low, mid, and high frequencies with a greater impact toward the lower frequencies. 2. VOR gain can return to normal, and often does for the higher frequencies over days or months. 3. Increased low frequency phase leads almost always remain even following compensation (secondary to a permanent change in central integrator processing). 4. Asymmetrical "bias" often is present due to afferent asymmetry. At first, fast-phase components of the vestibular nystagmus are ipsilesional, but may change over time and are, therefore, a poor indicator of laterality of lesion. 5. The severity of the abnormal response will often co-vary with the severity of the peripheral lesion. 6. SHA gain and symmetry may be entirely within normal limits with an isolated low-frequency VOR phase lead suggesting a compensated unilateral pathology.	Decreased spectral purity is often associated with the onset of a unilateral lesion, which may contribute to the initial decrease in overall gain; Rule out antidizziness medication effects if patient's remain on pharmacology treatment.
PERIPHERAL — BILATERAL	1. Low, mid, and high frequency gain is reduced below normal limits. 2. When gain is within normal limits, it almost is always confined to the higher frequencies suggesting an incomplete bilateral vestibular loss. 3. Phase leads are often randomly distributed, particularly at low frequencies. 4. Phase and symmetry data should be interpreted with caution when gain falls below 0.15 (15%). 5. Spectral purity is often poor, particularly for frequencies where gain is poor.	Insufficient altering, restricted EOM, fixation; Differentiate peripheral and central with concomitant results (ocular motor, etc.).
CENTRAL	1. Hyperactive gain may involve any frequency, but often occurs in the low frequencies where central control (velocity storage) is in higher demand (i.e., cerebellar site-of-lesion). 2. Hypoactive gain with no concomitant peripheral indicators (rare). 3. Isolated mid-to-low frequency phase leads, (or sometimes involving the entire frequency range), suggesting an inappropriate processing of central velocity storage mechanisms for frequencies where the neural integrator is not required. 4. Bias (asymmetry) may or may not be present.	Compare with step test and caloric data; Central pathologies rarely cause abnormalities isolated to a single test—identify concomitant abnormalities across tests (ocular motor, etc.).

Source: Adapted from Wall, 1990.

compensation, its ability to identify residual [high] frequency vestibular function when identifying the potential for vestibular rehabilitation, and its application to pediatric populations as previously discussed in Chapter 5. Despite these advantages, SHA testing does present with some frank limitations. Most importantly, since SHA testing stimulates both vestibular labyrinths simultaneously (providing both an excitation and inhibition response), its sensitivity for identifying and lateralizing unilateral vestibular disease is poor. This is truer for chronic unilateral disease than it is for unilateral acute disease, as acute disease will often produce a VOR asymmetry that will generally be congruent with the patient's spontanous nystagmus. Moreover, the localizing value of SHA testing for detecting the specific site-of-lesion can be poor, although one could argue that there are few, if any, vestibular tests that offer excellent site-of-lesion detection. This is often because both peripheral and central disorders can contribute to reduced VOR gain as well as provide abnormalities in phase and symmetry. The interpretation of peripheral versus central disease is generally performed with some caution, although certain patterns of SHA results can provide stronger insight for one or the other, as eluded to earlier. Site-of-lesion detection can also certainly be strengthened with a comprehensive vestibular assessment.

CHAPTER SUMMARY

All three parameters of VOR gain, phase, and symmetry are relevant to rotational assessment, and should be interpreted collectively. The means and standard deviations for VOR gain, phase, symmetry, and spectral purity are provided from 0.01 through 2.0 Hz in Appendix A. Identification of patterns in SHA analysis can often facilitate a better interpretation of rotational data. Understanding how results "work" together can often broaden the analysis and interpretation of SHA data. This is even truer when additional tests are performed, such as velocity step testing, VOR fixation suppression testing, and even visual-vestibular enhancement testing (Chapter 8).

We are reminded that phase and symmetry of the VOR are derived from gain and should be interpreted with caution when VOR gain is between 0.10 and 0.15 (10–15%), and considered noninterpretable when VOR gain is absent or below 0.10 (Shepard & Telian, 1996). We are also reminded that because VOR gain is calculated from the slow-phase vestibular nystagmus, it is vital to record the best physiologic response, and one that is void of any stimulus or patient artifact. If care is given to control spectral purity, excellent reproducibility of the three rotational analysis parameters has been previously illustrated (Maes et al., 2008). The advantage of excellent reproducibility makes rotational assessment an exceptional measure to monitor vestibular function over time. Brey and colleagues (2008b), emphasized this point stating that harmonic acceleration is the best test for monitoring the vestibular system over time because the stimulus is delivered in a consistent manner. More importantly, it is critical to highlight the use of rotational paradigms that not only monitor vestibular function when tracking loss of vestibular physiological response, but also monitor recovery of vestibular function, due to central compensation.

Examining the responsiveness of the vestibular system across a broad frequency range provides a more comprehensive evaluation of vestibular function, particularly in the presence of bilateral caloric areflexia, where preservation of high frequency vestibular function is not uncommon. Similar to an audiometric assessment, which identifies normal to near normal low frequency hearing with a concomitant profound high frequency hearing loss, the vestibular system is also subject to such frequency dependent damage. Assuming an absence of vestibular response based on an absence of caloric response would be similar to concluding anacusis based on an absence of hearing at 8000 Hz. This would, indeed, be a remarkably poor assumption.

Overall, SHA testing offers tremendous advantages in the clinical assessment of vestibular pathology. As more sensitive eye-tracking goggles and detection programs are developed and more sensitive analysis algorithms continue to emerge, the use of SHA assessment will undoubtedly offer even stronger and more precise methods by which vestibular pathology will be identified.

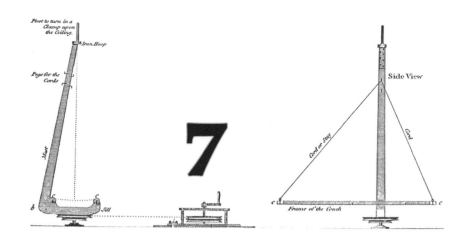

7

Velocity Step Testing

INTRODUCTION

As we discovered in Chapter 1, velocity step testing was the first clinical rotational paradigm used to assess vestibular function by Róbert Bárány beginning in 1907. Despite several attempts to modify and improve Róbert Bárány's rotational impulse paradigm, the basic principle of velocity step testing was used for decades. Velocity step testing of the modern era continues to remain an integral part of a comprehensive rotational vestibular assessment. Its ability to expand the knowledge of the vestibular system can be critical to the understanding of vestibular pathology. When used in conjunction with SHA testing, velocity step testing offers much added insight into the peripheral and central functioning of the vestibular system. The horizontal VOR and the velocity storage mechanisms can effectively be evaluated during velocity step testing. Velocity step testing can often confirm velocity storage and neural integrator deficits, identify peripheral asymmetries, as well as monitor or confirm vestibular central compensation. The test is generally well accepted by patients but has its limits for tolerance that is generally commensurate with stimulus (intensity)

velocity. Step velocities above 300°/sec are often encumbered with technical administration difficulties and are generally less tolerable, particularly for sick patients.

VELOCITY STEP STIMULI

During velocity step testing, abrupt computer-controlled accelerations of 120 to 200° per second squared are precisely delivered to an upright-seated patient in the yaw (horizontal) plane until a predetermined constant velocity is achieved and can be subsequently maintained for a given period of time. At this time, the reader is encouraged to review the videos on the companion website depicting two common velocity step rotations, one at a relatively low angular velocity and the other at a relatively high angular velocity. Sustained step target velocities usually fall into one of two categories: low velocity target step stimuli and high velocity target step stimuli. Low velocity step stimuli are usually performed at 60° per second, whereas high velocity step stimuli are performed at 240 to 300° per second (Brey, McPherson, & Lynch, 2008a, 2008b). The test begins with the rotational chair performing a very abrupt acceleration period to the target rotational velocity. Once achieved, the specific target rotational velocity is precisely maintained for sixty seconds before a rapid deceleration ($200°/sec^2$) back to a velocity of $0°/sec$ is applied. The acceleration and velocity stimuli are graphically illustrated in Figure 7–1.

Rapid accelerations and deceleration to and from a specific sustained target velocity are performed in both the CW and CCW directions. A period of sixty seconds is commonly applied to each constant velocity stimulus period of the VST, such that the test is composed of four distinct sections:

1. Abrupt acceleration to the right (clockwise), followed by 60 seconds of constant unchanging velocity rotation at a predetermined target velocity.

2. Abrupt deceleration from the target constant rightward velocity back to $0°/sec$, which is maintained for another 60 seconds.

3. Abrupt acceleration to the left (counterclockwise), followed by 60 seconds of constant unchanging velocity rotation at a predetermined target velocity.

4. Abrupt deceleration from the target constant leftward velocity back to $0°/sec$, which is maintained for another 60 seconds.

An example of the stimulus paradigm in its entirety is graphically illustrated in Figure 7–2. When an intact vestibular system is subjected to such rotational stimuli, a per- and post-rotary VOR nystagmus ensues following both acceleration and deceleration in each direction of rotation, respectively. The specifics of this physi-

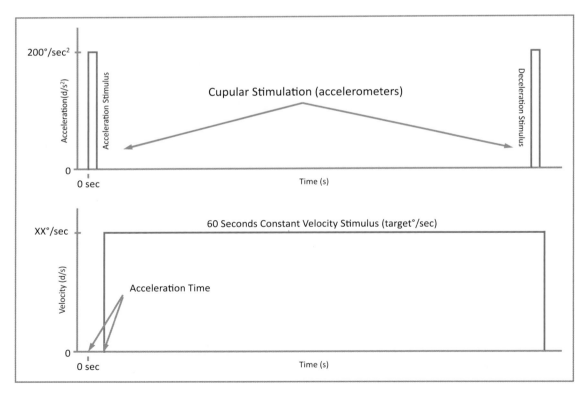

FIGURE 7–1. Stimulus characteristics for velocity step testing. Top graph illustrates the abrupt stimulus onset (acceleration) and offset (deceleration) to and from constant angular velocity. Duration of this stimulus is dependent on the target angular velocity. Bottom graph illustrates the ongoing, constant (unchanging) angular velocity stimulus that occurs immediately following the acceleration stimulus. The acceleration time and target velocity is arbitrarily depicted and is dependent on the selected test paradigm.

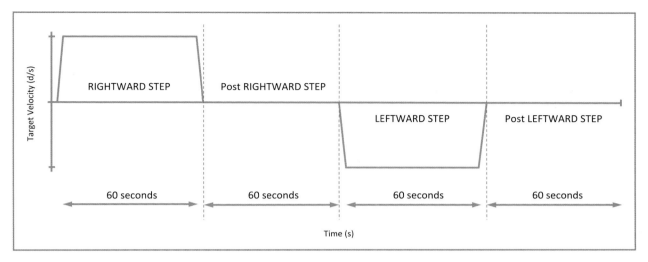

FIGURE 7–2. Step velocity paradigm showing each 60-second per and post, rightward and leftward step stimuli (*separated by vertical dotted lines*).

ologic response will be discussed later. First, let us review two of the step test's critical elements, the acceleration (and deceleration) stimulus as well as the velocity stimulus.

The Step Acceleration (and Deceleration) Stimulus

It is important to keep in mind that the fundamental principle of velocity step testing lies in the properties of the stimulus. First, it is critical to understand that the abrupt *acceleration* (or *deceleration*) is the critical component to the step stimulus. Recall our earlier automobile analogy presented in Chapter 6 explaining the distinction between acceleration and velocity. Acceleration is how fast the car gets from "0 mph" to some specified target speed (say 60 mph), whereas velocity is the target speed of the car (i.e., 60 mph). If the rate of acceleration is always constant, but the target speed of the car is increased to 100 mph, the car must spend more time accelerating to get to 100 mph. This is the basic principle of the velocity step stimulus. The rate of acceleration is always the same. What changes, is how much time the rotational chair spends *within* the acceleration phase. For lower target angular velocities, say 60°/sec, the chair only needs 0.3 seconds of time in the

acceleration phase to achieve the target velocity (provided the acceleration of the chair is held constant at 200°/sec²). However, for a higher target angular velocity, say 240°/sec, the chair requires 1.2 seconds of time in the acceleration phase to reach the higher target velocity (using the same constant acceleration of 200°/sec²). Because a target velocity of 240°/sec is 180°/sec faster than 60°/sec, the rotational chair must spend an additional 0.9 seconds of time accelerating to the faster target "speed" of 240°/sec; and for the cupulae under the load of such an acceleration force, the additional 0.9 seconds of time spent under the influence of this acceleration force is an eternity.

The acceleration period is, therefore, the critical component to velocity step testing. The following equation is used to determine how much time is spent during acceleration versus any target velocity:

$$t = \frac{Vf - Vi}{acceleration}$$

Where: Vf = final velocity (target velocity)
Vi = initial velocity (0°/sec)
$acceleration$ = 200°/sec²
t = time

Figure 7–3 shows the relationship between target velocity and time spent during angular

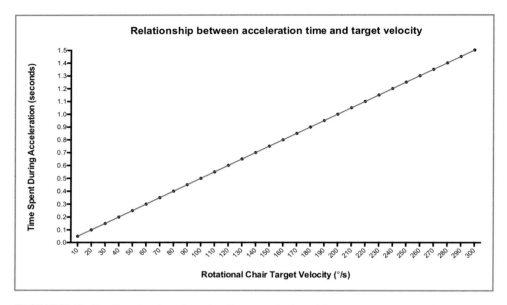

FIGURE 7–3. Graph showing the linear relationship between time of acceleration and chair target velocity. Rate of acceleration is held constant at 200°/second². Angular rotational velocity is expressed in degrees/second. Relationship is linear with an increase in velocity of 10°/sec every 0.5 seconds.

acceleration given a common acceleration stimulus of 200°/sec². It can be clearly seen that the relationship is linear. Once this relationship between acceleration and velocity is understood, the concept of velocity step testing is easy to understand. One simply needs to determine how a longer duration of acceleration stimulus affects the viscoelastic properties of the cupulae and how this impacts the overall output, that is, the VOR nystagmus.

The Velocity Step Stimulus

The second critical point to understand when considering the velocity step stimulus is that it is a *sustained* target velocity stimulus. This is primarily different from the stimulus employed during SHA testing, as well at that in everyday life. During SHA and daily life activities, our vestibular system is almost always confronted with brief head turns and, therefore, brief and ever-changing accelerations. Our vestibular system is rarely, if ever, confronted with sustained, unchanging angu-

lar velocity stimuli (head rotations) during daily life activities, with the exception of amusement park rides, playground rides, and the occasional spinning of ourselves while holding our children, or playing dizzy bats. Sustained rotations are a relatively uncommon and unnatural stimulus for our vestibular system to encounter, but the use of such stimuli can be quite clinically relevant. The primary advantage is that sustained rotational stimuli allow for investigation of central velocity storage mechanisms. This becomes particularly relevant during lower target velocity step stimuli, which is discussed a little later in this chapter.

VELOCITY STEP PHYSIOLOGIC RESPONSE

Cupular Response

As noted earlier, cupular mechanics describe the deflection of the cupula in response to a *change* in acceleration; that is, either an acceleration or deceleration force. This is the same principle we learned in Chapter 6 regarding SHA testing. Specifically, cupulae are accelerometers not "velocilometers"; they respond solely to changes in acceleration, not velocity. As long as the velocity is unchanging and constant, and there is also no change in acceleration, the cupulae will naturally return to their resting position despite an ongoing, constant velocity rotation post acceleration (no matter how strong the velocity). Recall our earlier analogy of the moving car. As long as a car is moving at a constant speed and continues to move without altering its speed (accelerating or decelerating), your vestibular system will have a difficult time detecting any "movement" of the car; that is, until the car accelerates or decelerates due to increased gas or a change in the inclination of the road impacting the speed (velocity) of the car. This concept is, in fact, the fundamental principle underlying VST; an abrupt acceleration in one direction, followed by constant (unchanging) velocity, followed by an abrupt deceleration back to no rotation (0° velocity). This is then followed by a similar acceleration and deceleration in the opposite direction (see Figure 7–2).

In the case of low velocity step testing, the target velocity to which the chair quickly accelerates to and decelerates from is often 60° per second. As far as angular velocity stimuli go, this is a relatively weak stimulus. As mentioned above, the cupulae experience this angular acceleration force for only 0.3 seconds. Despite the robust acceleration stimulus, it is important to keep in mind that this is not a very long time for the cupulae to be undergoing an angular force and subsequently, there is only a modest degree of cupular deflection. Now compare this to a high velocity step target stimulus such as 240°/sec. With an acceleration stimulus period of 1.2 seconds, this represents a 300% longer period of time the cupulae must endure the acceleration stimulus, which (according to the pendulum model of cupular dynamics) subsequently produces a significantly greater degree of cupulae deflection (see Baloh & Honrubia 1990 and 2011 for a detailed explanation of the pendulum model). As already mentioned, this is the critical concept to keep in mind during velocity step testing, but we will discuss the implications of the longer versus shorter duration acceleration stimuli as we move through this chapter.

Afferent Response

A rightward step stimulus generates leftward deflection of the cupulae, which produces a leftward vestibular VOR slow phase with a quick resetting fast-phase component to the right. This nystagmus response is exactly like that discussed earlier during SHA testing; that is, the resulting nystagmus will beat in the direction of the rotational stimulus, (right-beating nystagmus in response to a rightward stimulus and left-beating nystagmus in response to a leftward stimulus). However, recall that because we are interested in the vestibular component of the nystagmus, it is the leftward *slow phase* in response to rightward step stimuli and the rightward *slow phase* in response to leftward step stimuli that we are interested in. The resulting nystagmus to both rightward and leftward acceleration stimuli is graphically illustrated in Figure 7–4. This nystagmus response is relatively straightforward to conceptualize and is no different than that used during the SHA stimulus discussed in Chapter 6. However, it is important to realize that everything is reversed when the rotational chair experiences abrupt *deceleration*. As Newton's first law states, an object will continue to move at a constant velocity, unless acted upon by an opposing force. In this frame of reference, when the cupulae are under constant velocity and the rotation of the chair suddenly stops, the cupulae are thrust in the direction of the previously ongoing angular velocity. That is, if the chair were under constant rightward velocity, the cupulae would be thrust in the rightward direction immediately following abrupt deceleration and produce a left-beating nystagmus. This cupular deflection is essentially equivalent to leftward acceleration. Under these circumstances, the underlying physiologic response is the same as an abrupt acceleration to the left and does, in fact, cause a brisk vertiginous subjective response despite the chair velocity being 0°/sec.

Therefore, there are two opposing *slow-phase* responses obtained in response to a single step

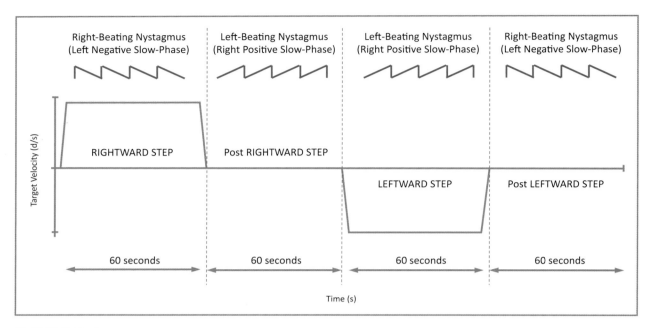

FIGURE 7–4. Step velocity paradigm showing each 60-second per and post, rightward and leftward step stimuli (separated by vertical dotted lines). For each per and post rotational step stimulus, the respective right- and left-beating nystagmus responses are shown.

stimulus in both the rightward or leftward directions, one following acceleration and another following deceleration. By extension then, a total of four *slow-phase* responses are obtained during a complete velocity step test (see Figure 7–4). They are as follows:

1. Left vestibular slow-phase (right-beating nystagmus) following rightward acceleration
2. Right vestibular slow-phase (left-beating nystagmus) following rightward deceleration
3. Right vestibular slow-phase (left-beating nystagmus) following leftward acceleration
4. Left vestibular slow-phase (right-beating nystagmus) following leftward deceleration

The appropriate nystagmus response for each of the two accelerations and decelerations can be seen in Figure 7–4. Always remember, however, that it is the *slow-phase* vestibular component of the nystagmus that is of interest during rotational testing. Subsequently, it is the slow phase component of each nystagmus beat that is plotted below each step response during the analysis of the data. This is precisely the same process by which the slow phase component is plotted during SHA testing.

Physiological VOR Response

Because of normal cupular deflection in response to the applied acceleration (or deceleration), the displaced stereocilia bundles polarize (or depolarize) the underlying hair cell, and, subsequently, produce an afferent neural response (Schwarz & Tomlinson, 2005). The subsequent opposing neural change from each periphery causes an imbalance in central vestibular neural symmetry, which produces an enduring nystagmus. The cupula(e) experience some degree of deflection for as long as an acceleration (or deceleration) stimulus is present. According to the pendulum model of cupular dynamics, the degree of cupular deflection is in direct relationship to the degree of acceleration stimulus (Baloh & Honrubia, 1990). During such time of extended acceleration step stimuli, afferent neural asymmetry, (and subsequent VOR), can be expected for as long as the horizontal cupulae remain deflected. In summary, the longer the cupulae remain under the influence of an acceleration or deceleration force, the greater the deflection of the cupulae and the stronger the afferent drive. Conversely, the less (or weaker) the deflection of the cupulae, the less the afferent drive. The resulting nystagmus is commensurate with the degree of cupulae deflection and neural asymmetry, such that higher degrees of slow phase eye velocities will result from higher velocity step stimuli, (due to a longer period of time under acceleration). In addition, the peak of the slow phase eye velocity response will likely occur immediately post acceleration, which is also the precise moment the cupulae achieve maximum deflection. Figure 7–5 illustrates an example of peak slow phase nystagmus response immediately post-rightward acceleration.

In the absence of any acceleration (or deceleration) force, the cupula(e) will slowly return to their natural position. During velocity step testing, this return to neutral position will occur immediately after the acceleration stimulus achieves the target velocity, even despite the presence of an on-going constant velocity stimulus. According to the pendulum model, in the absence of any acceleration, the viscoelastic forces of the cupula will return the

gelatinous mass to its resting position in 4 to 7 seconds in humans (Baloh & Honrubia, 2001, Baloh, Honrubia, & Kerber, 2011; Brey, McPherson, & Lynch, 2008b; Leigh & Zee, 2006). Given this, one could assume that the resultant nystagmus would quickly deteriorate (decay) in association with the viscoelastic return of the cupula back to its resting position (Baloh & Honrubia, 1998; Baloh, Honrubia, & Kerber, 2011). That is, as the cupulae return to their resting upright position, the resulting nystagmus gets progressively weaker as the deflection of the underlying stereocilia diminishes and the afferent drive gets progressively less. Theoretically, the nystagmus response should, therefore, completely dissipate when the afferent drive returns to baseline (its spontaneous neural firing rate). One could then possibly assume that if the viscoelastic restoring force of the cupulae is approximately 4 to 7 seconds, the complete dissipation of the nystagmus response would concomitantly occur at this time. However, the nystagmus response is clearly observed and recorded well

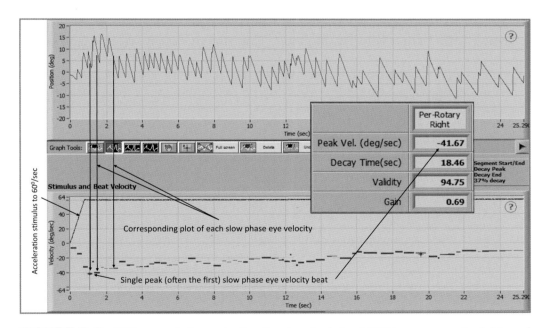

FIGURE 7–5. 60°/second step velocity stimulus depicting VOR in response to rightward acceleration and constant velocity rotation. Top chart depicts decay of raw nystagmus. Bottom graph depicts a temporally locked plot of the decaying slow-phase eye velocity response in relation to the decaying raw data tracing of right-beating nystagmus shown in the top chart. Solid black line represents chair velocity. Each plot below corresponds to an individual slow phase nystagmus beat above (downward facing arrows). Inset chart shows peak eye velocity response and decay time constant for this step response.

beyond the cupular return rate of 4 to 7 seconds (Stockwell & Bojrab, 1997a). This can be seen in Figure 7–6 where the right-beating nystagmus in response to a rightward step stimuli is clearly identifiable to 50 seconds. In reality, a healthy vestibular system will produce an enduring nystagmus that continues well beyond cessation of afferent signaling from the h-SCC peripheral end organ. What is the reason for this perpetuation of the VOR beyond that of cupular dynamics alone? As cited earlier, the persistence of the VOR response beyond afferent input is largely due to velocity storage mechanisms and the neural integrator (Curthoys & Halmagyi, 1996; Highstein, 1996). The persistence and slow decay of the VOR response beyond cupular mechanics is of significant clinical interest and has been termed the VOR time decay constant, often abbreviated as TC (Raphan, Matsuo, & Cohen, 1979). We discuss the properties of the VOR time decay constant later during our discussion of the low velocity step test.

Low Versus High Velocity Step Stimuli

The primary difference between low and high velocity step testing is the target velocity. In gen-

eral, velocity step testing is performed twice, using both a low and high target velocity. This would suggest there exists a clinically significant difference in the outcome measure between the two target velocities, and this would be correct. The fundamental difference lies in the degree of cupular deflection, which is fundamentally determined by the target velocity. As mentioned earlier, it is the target velocity that determines how long the acceleration period persists; the longer the period of acceleration, the greater the degree of cupular deflection. As previously stated, with a greater degree of cupular deflection comes a greater the degree of afferent drive. Subsequently, this creates a greater degree of labyrinthine asymmetry between the depolarized labyrinth (excited or leading ear) and polarized labyrinth (inhibited or trailing ear). For the lower target velocity step testing, the degree of cupular deflection causes a concomitantly lower excitatory and inhibitory response as both cupulae are only modestly deflected. However, during high velocity step testing, the period of acceleration is significantly longer allowing for a near-to-complete deflection of the cupulae to their maximally displaced position. This effectively causes a near-to-complete satura-

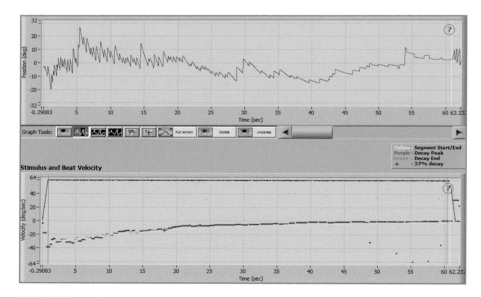

FIGURE 7–6. 60°/second step velocity stimulus depicting VOR in response to rightward acceleration and constant velocity rotation. Top chart depicts decay of raw nystagmus. Bottom graph depicts a temporally locked plot of the decaying (leftward) slow-phase eye velocity response in relation to the decaying raw right-beating nystagmus shown in the top chart. Solid black line represents chair velocity.

tion of the inhibitory afferent response from the trailing ear allowing for the resulting nystagmus response to more solely represent the prevailing excitatory response from the leading ear. In doing so, the excitatory response from each step stimulus (ear) can be compared to determine a gross measure of labyrinthine symmetry, or, conversely, asymmetry.

Due to the significant differences in the outcome measures between each test (low versus high velocity), each measure will now be discussed separately.

LOW VELOCITY STEP TESTING

Nystagmus Response

The primary purpose of a low velocity step test is to measure the rate of nystagmus decay in response to an abrupt angular acceleration (and deceleration) to the right (clockwise) and left (counterclockwise) (Brey et al., 2008b). Target step velocities of 60° per second are often considered standard for low velocity step testing, largely because normative reference data for nystagmus decay have been determined for this velocity. Figure 7–7 depicts a 60° per second rotational test paradigm. A step velocity to the right is followed by a step velocity to the left. Each period of per-

rotation and post rotation contains a 60 second interval during which the nystagmus response is recorded. Figure 7–8 depicts a normal nystagmus response to each step velocity. Figure 7–9 shows an enhancement of the nystagmus response in response to both rightward and leftward acceleration to the target velocity of 60°/sec (an enhancement of the deceleration response periods are shown later in Figure 7–10). A right-beating nystagmus can clearly be seen in response to *rightward* acceleration. Using rightward acceleration (top panel A) for this discussion, the left slow-phase component of each nystagmus beat is measured and plotted directly below the raw nystagmus tracing. Note how the strongest slow-phase component occurs almost immediately after or even during the final moments of the acceleration stimulus. In this example focusing on rightward step stimuli, (Figure 7–9) the strongest slow-phase component occurs at approximately one second and is measured at −41.67° per second. This is a vital data point to the velocity step analysis, and is known as the *peak* slow phase eye velocity. Following this data point, each subsequent slow-phase velocity component is plotted for the reaming nystagmus beats within the 60-second constant-velocity rightward interval. Note how the slow-phase components of the VOR response slowly decrease in intensity and are commensurate with the decline in the intensity of the raw nystagmus tracing. In this example, the nystagmus and corresponding vestibular slow-phases

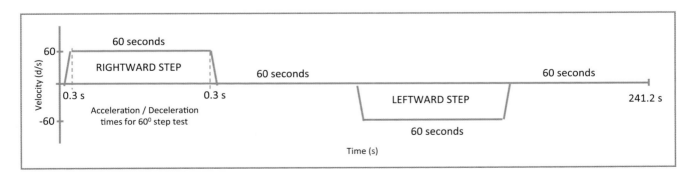

FIGURE 7–7. 60°/second step velocity paradigm showing each 60-second per and post, rightward and leftward step stimuli. Time (in seconds) is plotted on the x-axis and velocity (in degrees/second) is on the y-axis. Acceleration and deceleration stimuli are held constant at 200°/second², which produce an acceleration and deceleration period equal to 0.3 seconds. Total test time including the acceleration, deceleration, and constant velocity stimuli periods of 60 seconds each, equals 241.2 seconds.

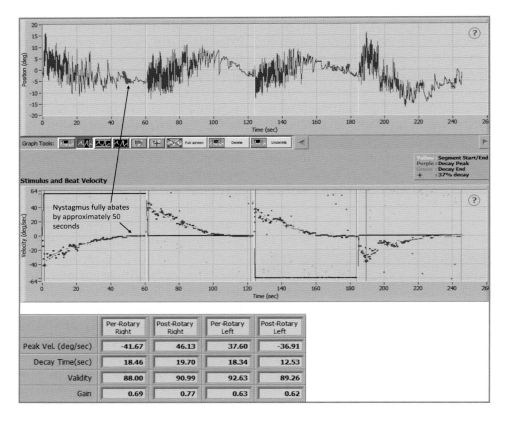

FIGURE 7–8. Normal 60°/second velocity step test (after correcting/deleting for noise). Bottom chart shows relative response parameters (e.g., peak slow phase eye velocity) for each stimulus condition. Solid black line represents chair velocity.

have essentially fully abated by approximately 50 seconds (see Figure 7–8), despite the ongoing constant rotational velocity. This nystagmus decay is the second vital data points to the velocity step analysis and has been termed the nystagmus time decay. A similar response is observed in response to leftward step acceleration, although the VOR response is now appropriately reversed.

Figure 7–10 now shows an enhancement of the nystagmus response following rightward and leftward deceleration back to 0°/sec. A left-beating response can clearly be seen following deceleration from rightward rotation. Plotting of the vestibular slow-phase components is performed in the same manner as post acceleration. Note a similar decaying of the nystagmus raw tracings and the corresponding plot of each slow-phase

vestibular component. The same is true for the right-beating response following deceleration from leftward rotation.

Low Velocity Step Response Parameters

Following an abrupt acceleration (usually 120° to 200° per second squared) to a low velocity target of 60°/second, a burst of peak nystagmus is generated and noted to slowly deteriorate in its slow-phase velocity over time. During a low velocity step test, the primary response parameter is the timed decay of the nystagmus response from the peak slow-phase component post acceleration/deceleration. We will explore this parameter shortly.

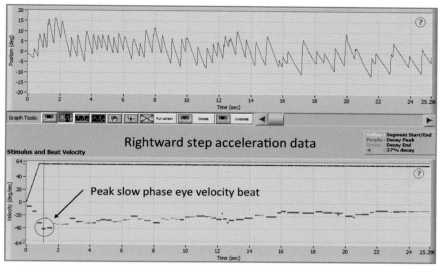

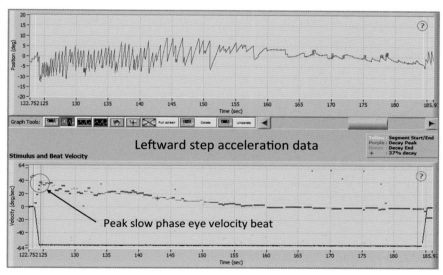

FIGURE 7–9. Right (**A**) and left (**B**) step acceleration stimuli and nystagmus responses. There is a right-beating nystagmus in response to a rightward step stimulus and a left-beating nystagmus in response to a leftward step stimulus. The respective slow-phase component for each nystagmus beat is plotted below each raw tracing of nystagmus. A leftward (negative) slow phase component decay is plotted in **A**, whereas a rightward (positive) slow phase component decay is plotted in **B**. The peak (maximum) slow-phase nystagmus component is identified by the pink vertical line immediately post acceleration. A best-fit (yellow) line is plotted through the decaying slow-phase component plots for each step stimuli.

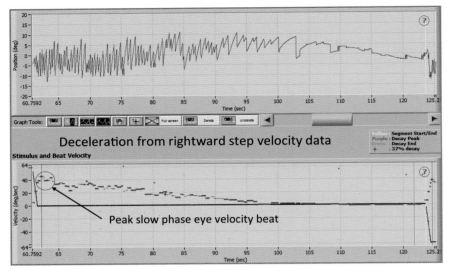

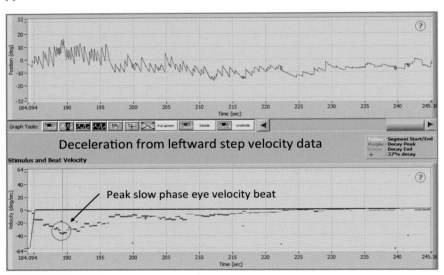

FIGURE 7–10. Right (**A**) and left (**B**) step deceleration stimuli and nystagmus responses. There is a left-beating nystagmus in response to deceleration from a rightward step stimulus and a right-beating nystagmus in response to deceleration from a leftward step stimulus. The respective slow-phase component for each nystagmus beat is plotted below each raw tracing of nystagmus. A rightward (positive) slow phase component decay is plotted in **A**, whereas a leftward (negative) slow phase component decay is plotted in **B**. The peak (maximum) slow-phase nystagmus component is identified by the pink vertical line immediately post acceleration. A best-fit yellow line is plotted through the decaying slow-phase component plots for each step stimuli.

In addition to the slow-phase nystagmus time decay, the peak gain of the VOR response can be calculated, but less emphasis is given to this parameter. The peak VOR response gain is determined in the same manner as gain is calculated during SHA testing. The peak slow-phase eye velocity response is divided by the target chair velocity (in this case, 60°/sec). For example, if the peak slow-phase component was 40°/sec, the response gain would be $\frac{40°/sec}{60°/sec}$ = (0.67), or 67%. Similar to the response gain during SHA testing, determination of VOR response gain during VST is important to determine if the response was sufficiently robust to validate calculation of the time of the decaying nystagmus response. As with SHA testing, if there is insufficient VOR gain per or post acceleration, calculation of a VOR time decay constant may be invalid or unreliable. This is largely due to the fact that the insufficient presence of nystagmus is likely inadequate to identify and calculate an appropriate decay of the response.

Similar to SHA testing, peak VOR gain values near or below 15% should be performed with caution only after reviewing the response spectral purity. There exist no clear agreed upon normative reference ranges for what constitutes normal low velocity step gain, and, as a consequence, little attention is given to this parameter. Some facilities have used low velocity step gain in conjunction with high velocity step gain to judge compensation status in unilateral peripheral vestibulopathies, but more will be discussed regarding this interpretation after we discuss high velocity step testing. Finally, like any near absence of VOR response, when significantly reduced VOR gain is identified following one or both acceleration step stimuli, and is free of any noise or artifact, any analysis of the response parameters (time decay constant) should be done with extreme care and precision - although the time decay response would also likely be abnormal in the presence of such low VOR gain.

VOR Time Constant

The low-velocity step test is primarily concerned with the rate of nystagmus decay; specifically the time, in seconds, for the nystagmus response to deteriorate by 63% from the peak slow phase eye velocity, or alternatively said; the time, in seconds, for the response to decline to 37% of its peak value (Stockwell & Bojrab, 1997a). Time decay constants are usually discussed in terms of a decline to 37% of the peak value—but the two interpretations are equivalent.

What Is the Significance of 37% When Discussing VOR Time Decay Constants?

Many students will often ask where the number 37% comes from when describing time decay constants. The reason for this is fairly straightforward. Time decay constants are used to define the deterioration of energy (or sometimes gain) of a logarithmic function such as those often encountered in physics, pharmaceutical, meteorological, neurophysiologic, and even electrical science. *Linear* decay is easy to define and even visualize. It is simply the rise over the run, which we know as the slope of the function (Figure 7–11). However, the decay of a natural logarithmic function (Figure 7–12) is more difficult to visualize and must be defined differently. As can be clearly seen in Figure 7–8, the decay of the nystagmus response is non-linear (curved). The decline (or "slope") of such non-linear functions is termed the time decay constant and is defined by the inverse of the base of the natural logarithmic function. Recall that the base of a natural log function is "*e*" or Euler's number ($\log X$ is actually written $\log_e X$, where the subscript "*e*" if often implied and often excluded

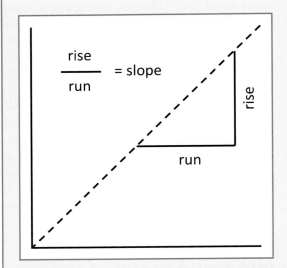

FIGURE 7–11. Calculation of the slope of a linear equation.

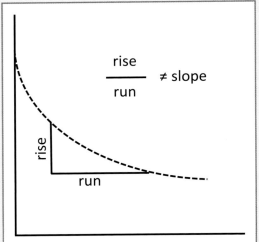

FIGURE 7–12. Calculation of the slope of a *non-linear* equation does not follow the same rules when determining the slope of a *linear* function.

when writing natural log equations). So the time decay of a natural logarithmic system (our nystagmus decline) is best defined by the period of time that a non-linear system declines (or decays) to the inverse of the base of the log, or simply:

$$\frac{1}{e}$$

Where *e* (Euler's number) = 2.718; therefore:

$$\frac{1}{2.718} = 0.37, \text{ or } 37\%$$

Natural log decay functions are commonly used to define such non-linear functions and are, in principle, very similar to the slope of a linear function (*rise/run*). One example of a non-linear time decay response that you may be familiar with is the half-life of a drug, which describes the non-linear decay constant of a drug's concentration levels in the body. Although the two decay processes are similar, in reality, one time decay constant is slightly longer than a pharmaceutical half-life decay constant. All things considered, one time decay constant does not describe the *complete* loss of energy within a nonlinear system, only a portion of it (specifically 63% of it). Most physiological systems natural time decay from the peak of the response to a near complete depletion of the response takes approximately three time decay constants (Leigh & Zee, 2006). However, most reports of time decay often imply "one" time decay constant and use of the word "one" when discussing any time decay constant is usually omitted, unless more than one time decay constant is being discussed.

Calculating the Time Decay Constant

Most computer software algorithms will calculate the VOR time constant automatically. However, prior to this, it is absolutely critical that the data be analyzed for its signal to noise ratio and any spurious data deleted.

To begin the analysis process, most software algorithms are designed to identify appropriate beating nystagmus by "looking" for the expected slope of the vestibular slow-phase, whether it is negative (in the case of right-beating nystagmus) or positive (in the case of left-beating nystagmus) (Figure 7–13). For example, when a step acceleration is performed to the right (clockwise), the software "expects" to analyze right-beating nystagmus (i.e., leftward moving slow phases) and subsequently filters out any and all portions of the raw nystagmus response that exhibits a positive slope, including all the fast-phases of the nystagmus response (as the fast-phase will invariably have an extreme positive slope as well). In turn, the software identifies and calculates the remain-ing portion of the raw nystagmus tracing that exhibits a negative slope. Although most software "filters" are quite refined at identifying and measuring the negative slow-phase of a right-beating nystagmus, at times, the software will mistake "noise" that contains a negative slope and interpret it as a potential slow-phase of a right-beat nystagmus. Figure 7–14 is an example of such an analysis. This can wreak havoc on your analyses as it significantly weakens the signal-to-noise ratio of your response, (not to mention such "analyzed noise" usually have relatively higher or lower degree values then the actual degree of the surrounding true nystagmus beats). Any spurious or extraneous noise that is being erroneously analyzed and subsequently included in the overall (decay) response should be modified or deleted.

The same rules and principles apply to a step acceleration to the left (counterclockwise), although the software "expects" to analyze *left-beating* nystagmus (i.e., rightward slow phases). During this analysis, the software filters out any and all portions of the raw nystagmus response that exhibits a negative slope including all the fast-phases of the nystagmus response (as, again, the fast-phase will invariably have an extreme negative slope as well). In turn, the software identifies and calculates the remaining portion of the raw nystagmus tracing that exhibits a positive slope.

Prior to interpreting the velocity step data, there is one additional key data analysis point that needs to be investigated, or, more precisely, needs to be *confirmed*. Because the time decay constant is calculated from the peak slow phase-eye velocity response, it is critical to determine that the correct peak eye velocity response is properly identified and selected. The peak VOR response usually occurs immediately after the acceleration (or deceleration) stimulus is finished. In the case of a 60° step acceleration, this would likely be near 0.2 to 0.5 seconds after the onset of acceleration (or deceleration). It is vital that the response during this time period have as high (good) a signal-to-noise ratio as possible. Peak nystagmus can often be obscured during this time period by spurious data caused by blink artifact, eye closure, or ocular noise. Identification of the correct and true slow-phase eye velocity peak response should be

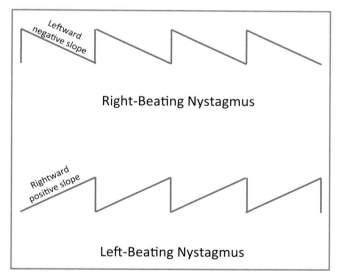

FIGURE 7–13. Simple cartoon of nystagmus illustrating the direction of slow-phase eye velocity component in relation to the nomenclature for which right-beating and left-beating nystagmus is identified. The slow phase component of nystagmus is always the portion of nystagmus that is analyzed during (vestibular) rotational testing.

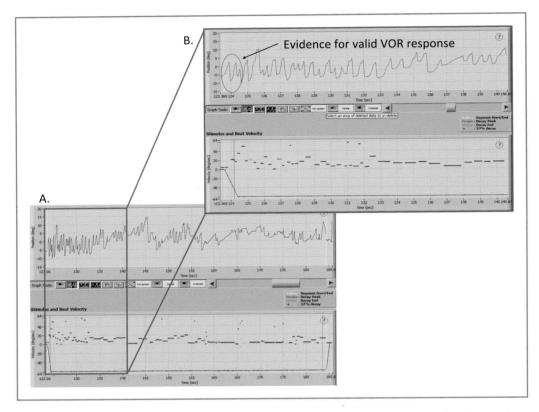

FIGURE 7–14. Example illustrating the deleterious effects of noise on the determination and calculation of the slow phase eye velocity response. **A.** Depicts the entire VOR response to leftward step acceleration. **B.** A magnified view from 123 to 140 seconds of the response. The circled portion of the response in **B** provides evidence to suggest that a VOR response is valid; however, the inclusion of the erratic noise (saccadic intrusions and ocular jitter) throughout severely limits the algorithms ability to determine what constitutes actual slow phase components versus positive sloping noise.

scrutinized closely and any cleaning or correction of the data should be performed at this point prior to further data analysis. We review some examples of noisy step responses in the next section. Recall our discussion in Chapter 5 regarding clinician intervention into data analysis as being a vital and critical factor to the correct interpretation of rotational data. This is never truer then when analyzing step data. Some critical errors during step analysis are discussed in the following section.

Once the VOR peak response has been confirmed, the time decay constant can be calculated (Figure 7–15). Simply subtract 63% from the peak response. As an example, let us say that the peak VOR nystagmus response immediately following rightward acceleration is 40°/second (for a VST

gain to rightward acceleration of 0.66$\overline{6}$ or 67%). Subtracting 63% from 40°/sec equals 14.8°/sec. Therefore, the time lapse at which the nystagmus response decays from the peak response (40°/sec) to 14.8°/sec equals one time decay constant. Using the example presented in Figure 7–15, this time would equate to 18.47 seconds. This process is then repeated for the three remaining step stimuli; rightward deceleration, leftward acceleration, and leftward deceleration.

To help identify or indicate the time decay through the declining nystagmus, most software algorithms plot a best-fit line from the point of peak slow-phase eye velocity through the remaining slow-phase velocity plots of the decaying nystagmus (this is shown in Figure 7–15 as the yellow

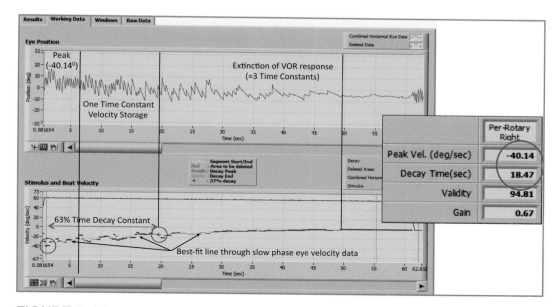

FIGURE 7–15. 60°/second step velocity stimulus depicting VOR in response to rightward acceleration and constant velocity rotation. Top chart depicts decay of raw nystagmus. Bottom graph depicts plotting of slow-phase eye velocity response. Inset chart shows peak eye velocity response and decay time constant for this step response. Response is parsed and identified by: the peak response, one VOR time-decay constant, and the extinction of the nystagmus response (which usually occurs after three time constants).

line). From this best fit line, the time between the peak response and 37% of the peak response is automatically determined and the time decay constant is reported. Figure 7–15 illustrates how the best-fit line approximates the decaying slow phase eye velocity data points.

Critical Errors in Calculating Time Decay Constants

There are a few critical errors that can occur when determining time decay constants. The first two have already been alluded to. First, extraneous noise in the slow-phase velocity plot can lead to a best-fit line that either underestimates or overestimates the proper decay. Figure 7–16 is an example of extraneous undeleted data points that aberrantly "elevates" the best-fit line above the primary slow phase eye velocity data points, which erroneously extends the decay. This can be problematic, particularly if the "uncleaned" response initially identifies the response as "normal" when, in fact, the "cleaned" response would otherwise calculate as abnormal. Although we have yet to discuss

what exactly constitutes an "abnormal" 60° step test, Figure 7–16 is such an example. Figures 7–17 and 7–18 are two more examples illustrating how deleting any extraneous noise and "cleaning" the overall data response can change the decay time constant. Moreover, Figure 7–18 is yet another example where the "cleaning" of the data changes a "normal" to an "abnormal" 60° step response.

A second error in the calculation of the VOR time constant is an inaccuracy in identifying the absolute peak of slow-phase eye velocity response, which can often significantly shorten (or lengthen) the time decay constant. One example of this can occur when the peak response is incorrectly identified later in the time domain rather than at the appropriate, "earlier," time just postcompletion of the acceleration or deceleration stimulus. In this case, the time decay constant would likely be incorrect (often shortened), as the logarithmic decay tends to calculate as a much steeper decline from the aberrant peak response and result in a much shorter time decay constant. Figure 7–19 illustrates this point. The opposite can also occur when the VOR step gain is significantly low.

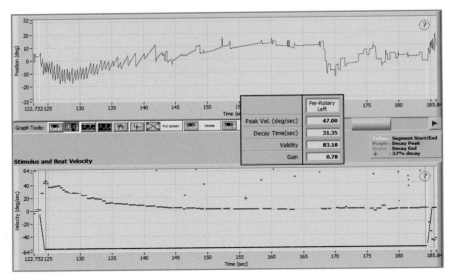

A

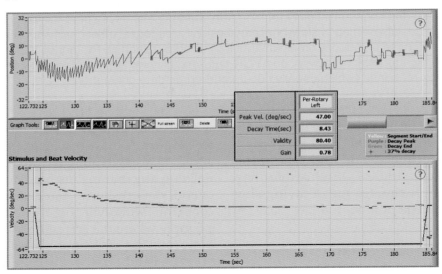

B

FIGURE 7–16. Example illustrating the effect of noise on the calculation of the time decay slow phase eye velocity plot. **A.** Shows a significant elevation in the slow phase velocity best-fit line secondary to the extraneous noise occurring in the mid-to-late portion of the step interval. This causes a consequential prolongation of the time decay constant, which is calculated at 31.35 seconds. **B.** Shows the corrected data with the extraneous noise deleted from the analysis. The slow phase velocity best-fit line now nicely approximates the data with a corrected time decay of 8.43 seconds. As a result of "cleaning" the data, the time decay constant now falls within the abnormal range. (In this example, the peak slow phase velocity did not have to be adjusted.)

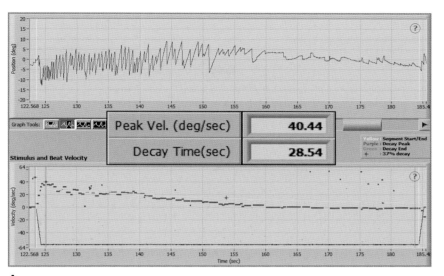

A

FIGURE 7–17. **A.** Uncorrected 60°/sec step response to leftward acceleration. **B.** Slow phase eye velocity data cleaned (noise deleted) during primary nystagmus portion from 122 through 160 seconds. Peak slow phase eye velocity adjusted from 40.44°/sec to 37.60°/sec. Extraneous occurring noise is elevating the best-fit line above the actual slow phase data plots. **C.** Corrected slow phase eye velocity data (cleaned for the remaining step portion), bringing the best-fit line into better match to the slow phase velocity plots, thus reducing the decay time constant from 28.70 seconds to 18.34 seconds.

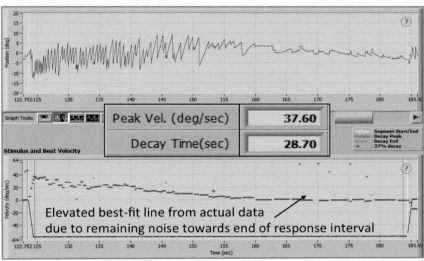

B

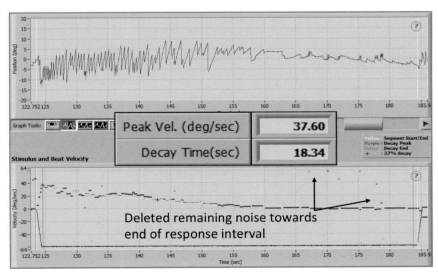

C

229

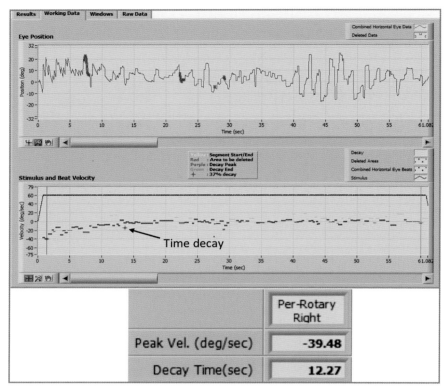

A

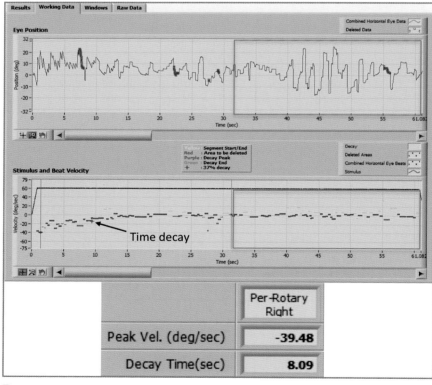

B

FIGURE 7–18. Identical response data from a rightward (clockwise) 60°/second step acceleration. **A.** Illustrates the best-fit line and resultant time decay constant when the response considers the entire portion of the 60-second constant velocity interval (less a few slow phase data; points that were determined to be noise and have been deleted). **B.** Illustrates the same data, however, only the data from the first 30 seconds are included in the analysis as the data from 30 to 60 seconds is judged to be noise. This effectively reduces the analysis period to 30 seconds and brings the best-fit line closer to the actual slow phase data plot within this time frame. Consequently, the time decay constant is reduced from 12.27 seconds (normal) to 8.09 seconds (abnormal), which is in agreement with concomitant vestibular data identifying a peripheral vestibulopathy. This example illustrates the importance of confining data analysis *only* to data that is relevant, and how *noise* (highlighted boxed areas) can inappropriately be accepted as actual response data, which can contribute to an incorrect interpretation.

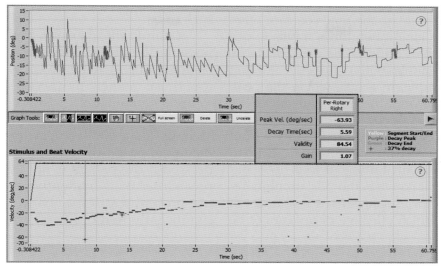

A

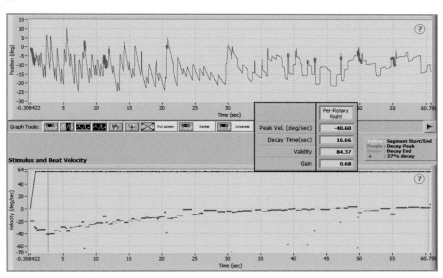

B

FIGURE 7–19. Example illustrating an inappropriate data analysis for a 60°/second step test where the peak slow phase eye velocity data point is inaccurately identified (**A**)—the algorithm will generally "look" for the strongest measured velocity during or post acceleration and assign it as the peak response. Consequently, the time decay is deleteriously impacted (shortened to 5.59 seconds). Correction of this error is thankfully quite straightforward as deleting the extraneous data point(s) will cause the analysis algorithm to identify the correct peak response (or the correct data point can manually be selected) and the time decay constant will recalculate accordingly. Following the correct identification of the peak slow phase velocity response (as shown in **B**), the time decay constant increased from 5.59 seconds (abnormal) to 16.66 seconds (normal).

Because the peak nystagmus on a low-gain response is inherently small, the time constant often appears incredibly long (often times it fails to calculate a time constant (infinity) as the 63% decay point cannot be identified within the 60 second step interval). For example, in a case where the peak nystagmus is 4°/second, the time constant of the response would not occur until nearly 1.48°/second, which may be difficult to identify within the 60-second poststimulus interval (due to background noise contributing to to a poor signal to noise ratio). Likewise, the poststimulus response may have produced only a few beats of nystagmus from which effective decay cannot be measured. Figure 7–20 illustrates two examples of such cases.

A third critical error not yet discussed is the possible "blunting" of the peak eye velocity step response due to inattentiveness or suppression at the critical moment the peak response is expected to occur immediately post acceleration. Because the period of acceleration stimulus is so brief (0.3 seconds for a 60°/sec velocity target stimulus), the initial peak response could be missed or suppressed if the patient is not attentive to the test procedures or is inattentive to the mental tasking procedures, respectively. The "blunted" or significantly reduced peak eye response would,

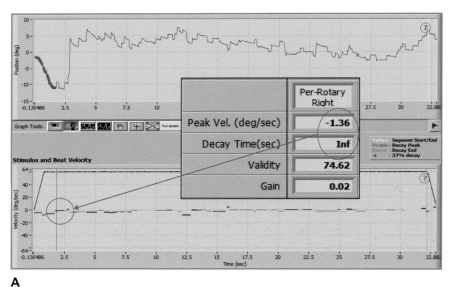

A

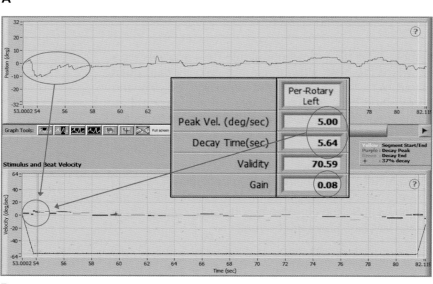

B

FIGURE 7–20. Two frequent 60°step results that often occur as a result of an absence or near-absence of VOR. **A.** 60° step response to rightward acceleration. A near absence of a peak slow-phase velocity response, or in this case, a slight underlying spontaneous is identified. This often creates a scenario which produces a best fit analysis of the slow-phase data that fails to reach the criteria for a 63% time decay, thus producing an infinite time decay response. In such a case, the time decay response should be disregarded as the response to the step stimuli is essentially absent. **B.** 60° step response to leftward acceleration showing a near absence of a peak slow-phase velocity response that produces only a few beats of nystagmus post acceleration. In such a scenario, a meaningful time decay cannot be determined. In such cases, identifying a precise time decay value is deferred in favor of reporting an absence, to near-absence of VOR response (note the gain of 8%).

therefore, underestimate the accurate peak slow phase velocity response and would subsequently produce an inaccurate time decay constant. An example of this is illustrated in Figure 7–21. This type of error may be difficult to detect or realize as the clinician may have no way of knowing if the true response could have been stronger. This is most often problematic when the tasking procedures are inappropriate or insufficient. It is clear that the best way to avert such error is often to task throughout the *entire* four-plus minutes of the test, with a task that is both appropriate as well as sufficiently difficult.

Finally, because the peak response is fundamentally the strongest part of the nystagmus response, it may be subverted by blinks and spurious data points that obscure and often inflates the correct identification of the "true" peak VOR response. Every effort should be made by the clinician to obtain as clean data as possible throughout the entire test.

Certainly, analyzing step results take great care and scrutiny. The response analysis algo-rithms are only as good as the program (or analysis filters) permit them to be. Each response must carefully be examined and the programming filters adjusted accordingly to ensure accurate and reliable results. Each rotational device and associated software will have its unique aspects of analysis that will often require a keen eye and experienced clinical judgment to determine the validity of the results. Take for example Figure 7–22. This example illustrates an extreme case of intrusive noise within the response recording. Upon careful examination (panel C) it is evident that a slow-phase eye velocity response exists and, moreover, there appears to have a vague collection of slow-phase velocity data points that seem to approximate a decaying nystagmus (panel A). The clinical challenge, however, is determining how to validate these data to ensure a reliable result and interpretation. Retesting this was likely not an option, as this origin of this noise was secondary to poor eye tracking due to significant blink artifact and mascara (although EOG recordings could be performed). Figure 7–23 depicts a more

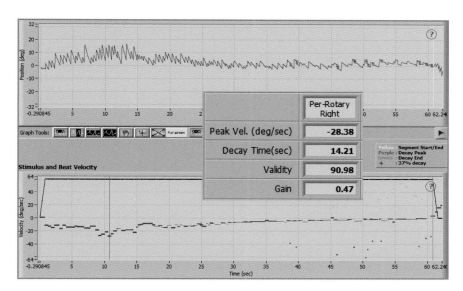

FIGURE 7–21. Example of a "blunted" VOR peak response during a 60° rightward acceleration step stimulus, due to either inappropriate tasking or inadequate tasking. The VOR slow phase eye velocity peak response should occur during or immediately post completion of the acceleration (or deceleration) stimulus. In this example, the peak response occurs at approximately 11 seconds, which is approximately 10 seconds post completion of the rightward acceleration stimulus. It is likely the peak response may have exceeded the −28.38°/sec if the appropriate tasking was conducted. As a result, these data should be interpreted with significant caution.

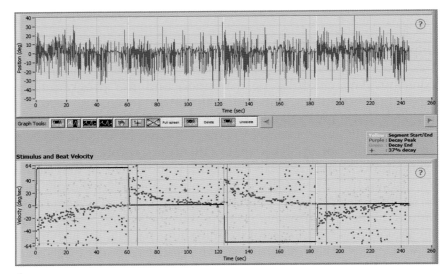

A

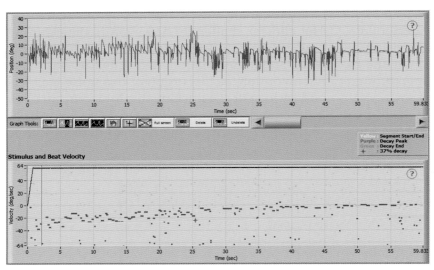

B

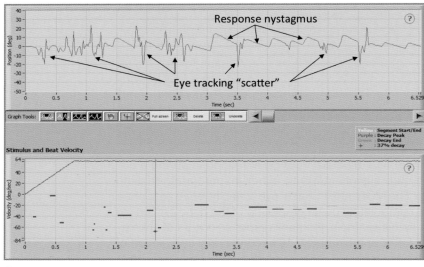

C

FIGURE 7–22. Example illustrating a 60° step test marked by an extreme degree of ocular noise. **A.** Represents the entire step response for all four-response intervals. **B.** Represents a magnified view of only the right step acceleration interval. **C.** Represents only the initial 6.5 seconds of the rightward acceleration interval. A gross decay of the response can be "visualized" for each interval (**A**), however, the extraneous noise must be isolated if the slow phase velocity best-fit line is to be determined. This noise was due to eye tracking "scatter" related to mascara as well as significant blink artifact. Response nystagmus can clearly be seen within the noise (**C**).

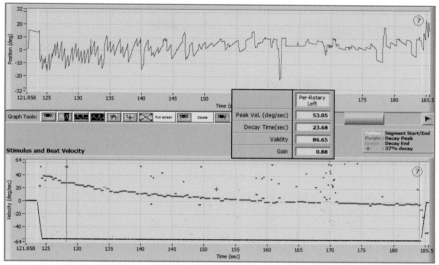

A

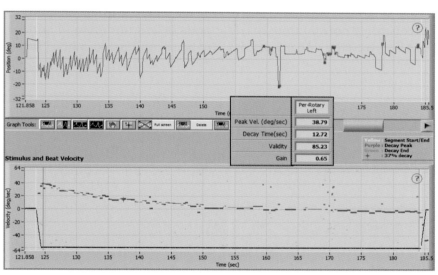

B

FIGURE 7–23. Example illustrating the effect of noise on the determination of the peak slow-phase eye velocity and the calculation of the time decay slow phase eye velocity plot in response to a leftward acceleration during a 60°-step test. **A.** Shows an incorrect peak slow phase velocity of 53.05°/sec and an erroneous prolongation of the time decay constant to 23.68 seconds. **B.** Shows the correct peak slow phase eye velocity immediately post leftward acceleration of 38.79°/sec and the correct time decay constant of 12.72 seconds after the raw data have been cleaned and all appropriate noise has been deleted.

common example of noise impacting a 60° step response. This example of leftward acceleration depicts an uncorrected 60° step velocity response versus the same data that have been "cleaned."

The peak slow phase eye velocity point has been correctly identified and the extraneous noise has been appropriately deleted from the analysis. In the corrected response panel (B), the slow phase eye velocity best-fit line intersects nicely with the slow phase eye velocity data. Finally, the corresponding time constants are shown for each step.

What Is a Normal Time Decay Constant?

We have already discussed that the persistence of the VOR response beyond that of cupular mechanics has been attributed to the velocity storage mechanism (Curthoys & Halmagyi, 1996; Highstein, 1996). The fundamental question, however, is how much longer is the velocity storage mechanism expected to propagate the response beyond the 4 to 7 seconds provided by the viscoelastic properties of the cupulae? The velocity storage mechanism extends the peripheral cupular time decay response to an average of 14 to 16 seconds (Goulson, McPherson, & Shepard, 2016). However, the consensus for a normal time decay reference range (±2SD from the mean) across

studies is between 10 to 30 seconds (Baloh & Honrubia, 2001; Brey et al., 2008b; Shepard et al., 2016). Therefore, time decay constants that are below 10 seconds are usually considered abnormal. Figure 7–24 depicts an abnormal 60° step velocity response. This example illustrates the sharp decline of the nystagmus response down to 5 to 7 seconds, which is no more than the time decay provided by simple cupular mechanics alone. That being said, the answer to the question of how much longer is the velocity storage mechanism expected to propagate the response beyond the 4 to 7 seconds provided by the viscoelastic properties of the cupulae, is approximately 3 seconds. Both peripheral and central pathologies can negate this 3-second propagation and shorten the time constant below 10 seconds. Conversely, the *prolongation* of time constants greater than 30 seconds is less understood and largely agreed upon to be secondary to central pathologies.

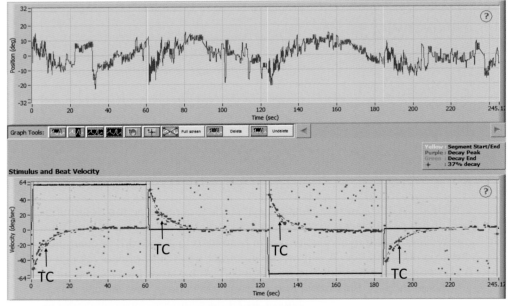

	Per-Rotary Right	Post-Rotary Right	Per-Rotary Left	Post-Rotary Left
Peak Vel. (deg/sec)	-51.96	53.27	45.65	43.13
Decay Time(sec)	6.49	6.04	5.69	6.72
Validity	71.31	68.53	82.36	72.67
Gain	0.87	0.89	0.76	0.72

Asymmetry	-1.97 %

FIGURE 7–24. Abnormal (corrected) 60°/sec velocity step test results. Abnormally shortened decay time constants are identified for each stimulus interval. Notice the sharp decline of each decaying nystagmus in the slow phase eye velocity plots. TC = One Time Constant.

Relationship Between Velocity Storage and the Time Decay Constant

We have discussed how the propagation of the VOR response beyond the 4 to 7 seconds provided by the viscoelastic properties of the cupulae is secondary to an intact velocity storage mechanism. We also know that one of the primary disadvantages of the vestibular system is its ability to integrate sustained rotational accelerations. Cupular mechanics, as well as the sharp onset and offset of the vestibular afferents, are ideally situated to detect transitory accelerations such as brief head turns encountered during daily life activities. The sustained afferent drive that accompanies sustained accelerations, causes a temporary "unrelenting" influx of afferent input to the central vestibular nuclei that far exceeds the required amount needed to drive the VOR. As a result, the solution is to simply "store" the afferent vestibular drive centrally and dispense it over time, hence the propagation and prolongation of the VOR response beyond cupular mechanics and the afferent drive.

The "storing" of this "unrelenting" afferent input is mediated by the velocity storage mechanism and the neural integrator. This process actually helps to explain the reason for the significant reduction in the time decay constant below 10 seconds following either a peripheral or central vestibular lesion. A reduction in the peripheral detection or conduction efficiency of the afferent response secondary to a peripheral vestibulopathy (e.g., vestibular schwannoma) would certainly reduce the amount of afferent input and subsequent recruitment of velocity storage. Similarly, a central pathology could affect the velocity storage mechanism's ability to effectively store the "unrelenting" afferent input and inappropriately "release" the stored neural response as quickly as it is received. This would also serve to reduce the decay time constant to that of cupular mechanics alone (<10 seconds). Therefore, both a peripheral and central pathology has the potential to reduce the time decay constant below the lower 10-second limit.

Conversely, a central pathology could also cause a significant *prolongation* of the decay time constant. In such cases, a central pathology can inadvertently cause the velocity storage mechanism to get "hung up" on itself and create a pro-

longation in the neural integrator's "feedback loop." As a result, the "release" of neural response is appreciably extended, and perpetuation of the VOR is significantly longer than the upper limits of the normal velocity storage propagated response (>30 seconds). Although this is uncommon, such prolongations in the VOR decay time constant have been suggested to be secondary to central pathology (Brey et al., 2008b).

These concepts are further illustrated in Figure 7–25. Let us first consider how a normal velocity storage mechanism manages step stimuli. By conceptualizing the afferent neural input as "incoming water" into a central neural "storage bucket," the bucket quickly fills up in response to the "unrelenting" step stimuli, as the outflow needed to drive the VOR is significantly less than the high neural input being supplied by the prolonged acceleration step stimuli. This is not the case with SHA testing, as the degree of acceleration is either constantly changing, is significantly less than 200°/sec², and/or the stimuli are too brief—which is also the reason that brief head movements during daily life activities do not follow this model. During a peripheral lesion, the afferent neural drive (incoming water) to the central storage neural integrator ("bucket") is significantly reduced and more closely matches the outflow required to move the ocular motor system, hence no central storage is needed, and a significant reduction in time decay constant is documented to be no longer than cupular mechanics alone (Figure 7–25B). Finally, during a central lesion, either the outflow of incoming neural activity is not "maintained" and the increased afferent drive during a step stimuli is released as quickly as it comes in (which can often produce a subsequent high, "uncontrolled" VOR gain), or the neural outflow is released too slowly and the VOR is subsequently extended beyond the normal storage time (i.e., time constants greater than 30 seconds) (Figure 7–25C).

Relationship Between VOR Phase and the Time Decay Constant

If you recall our discussion regarding VOR phase during SHA testing, the fundamental component that is responsible for the observed low frequency

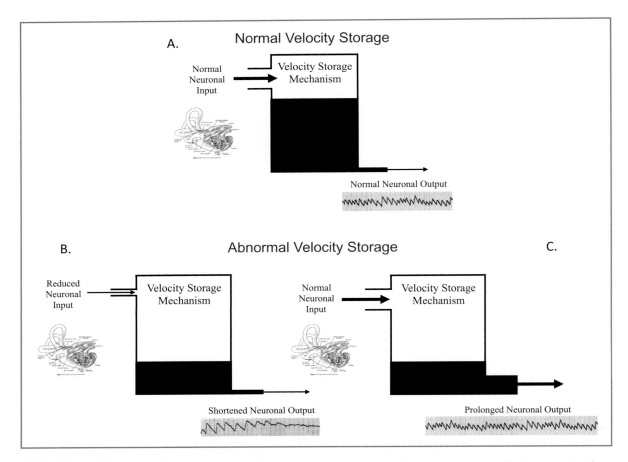

FIGURE 7–25. Illustrated depiction of the velocity storage mechanism during velocity step testing. The persistent afferent neural input during the step stimuli exceeds the limit needed to drive the output (VOR). Therefore in the normal system (A), the neural input is centrally "stored" and is slowly dissipated over time. In the abnormal system, the neural input fails to be "stored" either due to significantly decreased input (secondary to peripheral vestibular pathology). (B), or due to an uncontrolled, prolonged output (secondary to a central pathology). (C). *Source*: Adapted from Barin and Durrant, 2000.

phase lead is velocity storage. Therefore, if both the time-decay constant and low frequency phase leads are mediated by the velocity storage mechanism, then it would stand to reason that VOR phase and the time decay constant are related. This is, in fact, true. The VOR decay time constant is inversely related with the phase of the VOR response for low-frequency harmonic acceleration (SHA) between 0.01 and 0.04 Hz (Baloh & Honrubia, 1990; Brey et al., 2008; Shepard & Telian, 1996). This relationship is, in fact, *entirely* due to the fact that both phase and the VOR TC are mediated by the velocity storage mechanism (Raphan et al., 1979; Shepard & Telian, 1996). Mathematically, the relationship between VOR TC and phase can be expressed by the following equation (Baloh, Honrubia, Yee, & Hess, 1984):

$$TC = \frac{1}{\omega tan\Theta}$$

Where: $\omega = 2\pi f$
TC = time constant,
ω = angular frequency of rotation,
$\pi = 3.1416$,
f = frequency of rotation, and
Θ = phase angle in degrees

Figure 7–26 illustrates the inverse relationship between VOR phase lead and time decay constant.

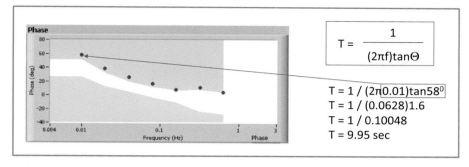

FIGURE 7–26. Example of determination of the theoretical nystagmus time decay constant of a patient with a VOR phase lead of 58° in response to a 0.01 Hz sinusoidal stimulus. The VOR phase and time decay constants have an inverse relationship by which an increase in VOR phase lead will cause a decrease in the VOR time decay constant.

This example depicts an abnormal VOR phase lead at 0.01 Hz of 58°. Results for rightward acceleration for a 60° step test for the same patient are presented in Figure 7–27. As can clearly be seen, the time decay constant in response to rightward acceleration is 9.965 seconds (Figure 7–27). The relationship between low-frequency VOR phase and time decay constant is clearly seen when the phase of 58° is applied to the inverse time constant equation:

$$TC = \frac{1}{2\pi f\, tan\Theta}$$

$$TC = \frac{1}{2(3.1416)(0.01)tan58°}$$

$$TC = \frac{1}{0.0628(1.6)}$$

$$TC = \frac{1}{0.10048}$$

$$TC = 9.95 \text{ seconds}$$

The inverse relationship between VOR phase and VOR time decay constant would suggest that, as phase increases for low-frequency head accelerations, the time decay constant decreases; and this would be true. Similarly, as VOR phase decreases for low frequency head accelerations, the time decay constant increases. For all practical purposes, the use of low-frequency SHA testing (for 0.01–0.04 Hz) and low velocity step testing are considered equivalent (Baloh & Honrubia, 2001);

however, use of low-velocity step testing (60°/second) is considered the preferred method for calculating the time constant of the VOR (Brey et al., 2008b; Shepard & Telian, 1996). This may be due to the fact that the velocity storage function of the central system may be best provoked with the use of a constant velocity stimulus as it likely incites a greater number of both irregular and regular afferent neural fibers, rather than a predominance of regular fibers incited during SHA testing.

Using the mathematical relationship between time constant and phase, it is possible to calculate the theoretical upper and lower limits of the VOR time decay constants. Let us apply the upper and lower limits of the normative data set for VOR phase presented in Chapter 6 to calculate the time constant limits. The upper and lower VOR phase leads presented in Chapter 6 at 0.01 Hz are 52.16° and 26.78°, respectively. Applying the lower VOR phase limit will estimate the upper limit for normal time decay constant (given its inverse relationship). Using the inverse equation, the upper time constant limit calculates to 31.55 seconds, which agrees well with upper published normative limit of 30 seconds. Conversely, applying the upper phase limit should estimate the lower limit of time decay. Using the inverse equation, the lower time constant limit calculates to 12.34 seconds. Although the 12.34 seconds is slightly higher than the generally agreed upon 10 second lower time decay limit, this estimation falls within normative reference ranges reported elsewhere

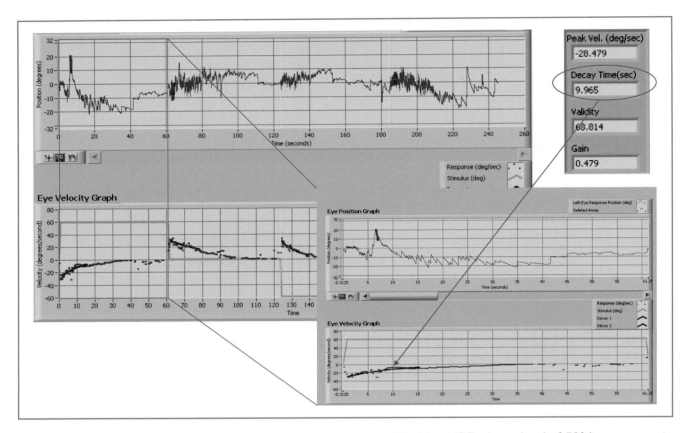

FIGURE 7–27. 60° step test for the same patient in Figure 7–26 with a VOR phase lead of 58° in response to a 0.01 Hz sinusoidal stimulus. VOR time decay constant using the rightward acceleration step stimulus is 9.965 seconds, which is precisely the time decay constant predicted using the VOR phase lead.

(Baloh & Honrubia, 1990; Baloh, Honrubia, Yee, Langhofer, & Minser, 1986; Cohen, Henn, Raphan, & Dennett, 1981; Goldberg et al., 2012; Goulson et al., 2016). One possible reason for a slightly higher predicted time constant lower limit when converting from VOR phase might be due to the difference in stimuli. The step stimulus is very different from the SHA stimulus. Consequently, the difference in time constants may be a subtle manifestation in how the neural integrator processes regular versus, regular *AND* irregular afferent signals generated during the SHA and step tests, respectively. Although this is only one idea, other nuances in stimuli and neural coding may contribute to the overall differences sometimes observed between time decay constants calculated from low frequency phase leads and low velocity step testing. Nonetheless, the time constant determined from VOR phase and the 60° step test

should be in near agreement when both tests are used clinically.

Time Decay Constant and Site-of-Lesion

Because the phase of the VOR during low-frequency SHA testing and time constant are (inversely) related, a measure of time constant is subsequently a reflection of the functional integrity of the central velocity storage mechanism (Brey et al., 2008b; Shepard & Telian, 1996). In fact, the general interpretation of time constants follows an interpretation similar to that of phase during SHA testing (Goulson et al., 2016). Thus, an abnormally short time constant (<10 seconds) suggests pathology of the peripheral vestibular end organ, the vestibular nerve, or the vestibular nuclei (Brey et al., 2008b;

Shepard & Telian, 1996). However, when no other central abnormalities are present, abnormally short time constants are usually associated with either a unilateral or bilateral peripheral pathology (Baloh & Honrubia, 1990; Brey et al., 2008b).

Similar to significantly reduced phase leads or phase lags, much less information is known regarding an abnormal *increase* in the VOR time constant (>30 seconds), but this finding may be related to central processing deficits such as those often associated with migraine or, specifically, from lesions in the nodulus region of the cerebellum (see Figure 3–3), as this region is highly influential on the regulation of the velocity storage mechanism (Shepard & Telian, 1996; Waespe, Cohen, & Raphan, 1985; Wearne, Raphan, Waespe, & Cohen, 1997).

The inverse relationship between low-frequency VOR phase and time decay is highly predictable. Performing both measures offers a significant clinical advantage, as concomitant results between step testing and SHA testing can often corroborate clinical pathology or even offer insight into possible technical, administrative, and/or tasking related problems that may occur in either SHA testing or step testing. Due to the strong relationship between VOR phase and time decay, it is rare that one parameter would be abnormal without the other. When the two outcome measures significantly differ, the results of one measure should be brought into question and the possible errors pertaining to the administration of either test should be carefully scrutinized, as there are numerous limitations and critical errors that can lower the reliability of either test.

General Limitations to 60°/Sec Step Testing

As during any test that evaluates the vestibular-ocular reflex, there are certain limitations that must be considered. Patient alertness can have a significant impact on the intensity of the vestibular nystagmus. Therefore, mental suppression of the induced vestibular nystagmus at the time of each acceleration impulse must be ameliorated with proper mental tasking. Although averaging multiple trials has been suggested as a possible way to improve low velocity step testing sensitivity and specificity, as it would lessen any chance of unintended suppression, this would add significant time to the test protocol and, most likely, fatigue and increased inattentiveness from the patient. In addition, symptoms of nausea can be a side effect of this test and extended time could create a significantly more noxious test. Static head position can also influence the VOR time decay constant insomuch as there occurs a proportional decrease in the time decay constant to the degree of forward head tilt (Leigh & Zee, 2006). This is likely due to contributions from the vertical canals, which may lead to a change in the axis of eye rotation and subsequently shorten the time constant (Leigh & Zee, 2006). Moreover, tilting of the head forward or laterally immediately following step acceleration (or deceleration) significantly reduces the duration of the time constant and nystagmus. This is likely secondary to a "dumping" activity of the velocity storage mechanisms with significant contributions from the otolith organs (Raphan & Cohen, 1979; Fetter et al., 1996; Fetter, Tweed, Hermann, Wohland-Braun & Koenig, 1992). Knowing this can actually be a useful clinical tool when forced to prematurely terminate a test session secondary to severe noxious symptoms, particularly if a patient is suffering from excessive nausea and impending emesis. Finally, similar to SHA testing, any CNS suppressants and/or stimulants are contraindicated during this test as significant effects on the VOR have been well reported (Shepard & Telian, 1996).

Sensitivity for Determining Laterality of a Peripheral Lesion Using 60°/Sec Step Testing

The ability to lateralize peripheral vestibular lesions with rotation is fundamentally dependent on one of two stimulus parameters, either a very quick acceleration of the head (i.e., quick head impulses) or a very high angular velocity. In fact, the identification of unilateral vestibular disease requires head accelerations that exceed 2000° per second squared, or head velocities that exceed 100° per second (Leigh & Zee, 2006). Unfortunately, the stimulus properties associated with low velocity step testing offer neither of these criteria. That being said, use of a low velocity step test (60°/sec) is *not* considered an effective stimulus for lateralizing peripheral vestibular pathology. As already alluded to, the primary reason for this lies in the relatively weak nature of the low velocity step stimulus. Despite the robust acceleration of 200°/sec², the low target velocity of 60°/sec severely governs the time each cupulae endure the force of angular acceleration (0.3 seconds). This, in turn, severely limits the degree of cupular deflection. Thus, the short acceleration time period fails to provide a sufficient sustained force to completely deflect the cupulae, which prevents the trailing cupula from experiencing complete inhibition (i.e., zero spikes per second). In light of this, the trailing (inhibitory) cupula contributes to the VOR output during low velocity step testing. As such, the overall neural output (the VOR) fails to reflect a pure (isolated) *excitatory* afferent drive from a single cupula, which would theoretically allow for a comparison between labyrinths and subsequent detection of unilateral pathology (but more to come on that in the next section on high velocity step testing). Therefore, due to the weak nature of the 60°/sec target velocity stimulus, the output represents a contribution from both an excitatory AND inhibitory afferent cupular contribution. Consequently, a lesioned periphery from either the trailing ear (inhibitory) or the leading ear (excitatory) may cause an abnormally reduced time decay constant, regardless of whether an acceleration or deceleration stimuli is applied. As such, general comparisons of right versus left time constants should not be compared, or used to suggest laterality of peripheral pathology. An exception to this interpretation, however, can be applied if supplemental or corroborating clinical evidence clearly lateralizes a peripheral lesion. That is, if concomitant vestibular results (e.g., caloric, VEMP) lateralize a vestibular lesion, and the low velocity step test data corroborate an abnormal time constant ipsiversive to the lesion, then the step data could offer additional evidence that would support the specific unilateral lesion.

Given what was previously stated—that identifying unilateral vestibular disease during step testing requires head accelerations exceeding 2000° per second squared, or head velocities ex-

ceeding 100° per second—it would stand to reason that increasing the target velocity stimulus above 100°/second would provide greater sensitivity for lateralizing unilateral vestibular disease. This is essentially true. If lateralization of a unilateral lesion is routinely desired (and generally, when is it not?), the velocity step stimulus must be increased to a level that saturates the trailing ear's cupular response. This is the premise for performing high-velocity step testing, which we will now discuss.

HIGH VELOCITY STEP TESTING

Premise for Performing High Velocity Step Testing

High velocity step testing directly attempts to address the primary limitation of rotational testing, by providing evidence to accurately identify the laterality of a unilateral vestibular lesion. Administration procedures for high velocity step testing are equivalent to the 60° step test with the exception of selecting a higher target step velocity. As opposed to the low velocity step stimulus, use of a high target velocity stimulus can now effectively saturate the inhibitory response of the trailing ear while maximizing the excitatory response of the leading ear. Acceleration is the same as that employed during a low velocity step test (200°/sec²), however, because the target velocity is now much greater at 240 to 300° per second, the cupulae experience the acceleration (or deceleration) force for a longer period of time. Specifically, during a target velocity of 240°/sec, the cupulae are subjected to an angular acceleration for 1.2 seconds as opposed to 0.3 seconds during a low velocity step stimulus of 60°/sec (Baloh & Honrubia, 2001). Figure 7–28 illustrates the stimulus characteristics of a high velocity step stimulus. Note that the stimulus paradigm of acceleration followed by deceleration in both clockwise and counterclockwise directions is identical to the 60° step rotational paradigm, only now with a higher target velocity of 240° per second.

Such high velocity step stimuli subsequently create a saturation effect in the first order ves-

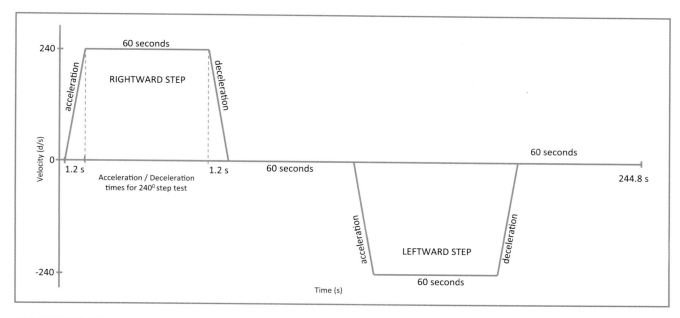

FIGURE 7–28. A 240°/second step velocity paradigm showing each 60-second per and post, rightward and leftward step stimuli. Time (in seconds) is plotted on the x-axis and velocity (in degrees/second) is on the y-axis. Acceleration and deceleration stimuli are held constant at 200°/second^2, which produce an acceleration and deceleration period equal to 1.2 seconds. Total test time including the acceleration, deceleration, and constant velocity stimuli periods of 60 seconds each, equals 244.8 seconds.

tibular afferent neurons in the trailing ear (Wall, 1990). Because the dynamic range for excitation is approximately four times that of inhibition, (Chapter 3) and cupular mechanics respond preferentially to excitatory stimuli (Ewald's second law), such longer periods of acceleration cause a near complete ("hard") saturation of the inhibitory neural response from the trailing ear and an incomplete ("soft") saturation of the excitation neural response from the leading ear (Wall, 1990). As a result, the trailing inhibitory ear's spontaneous firing rate of 90 spikes per second is driven to, or near, zero spikes per second (saturation), while the leading excitatory ear's spontaneous neural firing rate is elevated to a higher tonic level up to a theoretical maximum of 350 to 400 spikes per second (Baloh & Honrubia, 2001). As a consequence of inhibitory saturation, the resultant VOR response is, theoretically, entirely a reflection of the excitatory response from the leading ear (although keep in mind that the trailing ear provides the excitatory response during abrupt decelerations). In theory, such high velocity step stimuli allow for identification and quantification of the excitatory response from a

single labyrinth, much like that of the caloric stimulus. Similarly, the high velocity step stimulus can be repeated in the opposite direction, from which the opposing excitatory VOR peak response can be used for the determination of labyrinthine symmetry, again, much like the caloric response. In a perfectly calibrated and/or equally opposed vestibular system, the clockwise and counterclockwise high velocity step stimuli would produce an equal or symmetrical VOR response. It is important to keep in mind that the above discussion regarding excitation from the *leading* ear applies only to *acceleration* stimuli. During deceleration stimuli, the opposite is true. Overall, the intensity (or degree) of the VOR response principally reflects the labyrinthine response from a single ear (the excitatory ear or the leading ear during accelerations and/or the trailing ear during decelerations).

Physiologic Response Characteristics

Cupular deflections during a high velocity step test are similar to that experienced during a low velocity step test, insomuch that the principles of the cupular pendulum model still apply. That being said, because the pendulum model predicts cupular deflection that is commensurate with the degree and duration of angular acceleration, during high velocity step testing, the degree of cupular deflection approaches maximum displacement. Figure 7–29 graphically illustrates the difference in the cupular deflection of a 60° step stimulus versus a 240° step stimulus. This maximal displacement creates a hyperexcitable afferent environment in the leading ear and a near-to-complete inhibitory afferent environment in the trailing ear (for acceleration stimuli). These opposing neural environments create a proportionate central asymmetry and results in a significant and robust VOR nystagmus (with often a concomitant robust subjective vertigo).

High Velocity Step Parameters

High velocity step testing generates a nystagmus response that is precisely the same as the low velocity step test, with one exception; the VOR peak eye velocity response is much greater follow-ing high velocity step acceleration and deceleration. Figure 7–30 provides an example of a 240°/second step response and compares it against a 60°/second step response. A robust peak eye slow-phase velocity response (VOR) can clearly be seen in response to a rightward acceleration step stimulus that is significantly greater follow-ing the 240° stimulus than the 60° stimulus. This is true for all acceleration and deceleration step intervals. Figure 7–31 provides an example of the total raw nystagmus response and the slow phase peak eye velocity data plots for each of the step intervals. The significantly robust slow phase peak eye velocity response can clearly be seen. It is critical to recall that the greater peak eye slow phase velocity response is due to the more robust acceleration (or deceleration) stimulus that occurs in response to the extended period of angular acceleration required for the chair to obtain the higher target rotational velocity of 240° per second (1.2 seconds). Again, this concept is supported by the pendulum model of cupular mechanics, which states that the slow component velocity of rotation-induced nystagmus is proportional to the deviation of the cupula, and that the deviation of

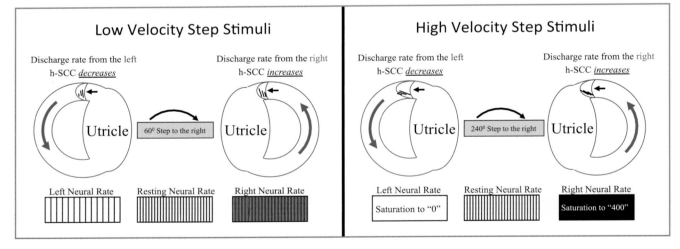

FIGURE 7–29. Cartoon comparing the cupular mechanics and subsequent afferent neural firing rate of a low velocity step paradigm (e.g., 60°/sec) versus a high velocity step paradigm (240°/sec). Green arrows and small black arrows represent direction of endolymph force against the cupulae during a rightward angular rotation like a step stimuli. Degree of cupular deflection is commensurate with the velocity of angular rotation, such that the high velocity stimuli depict the displacement of the cupular stereocilia near maximum displacement. Relative (or hypothetical) neural firing rates are depicted beneath each image for both the inhibitory and excitatory labyrinth.

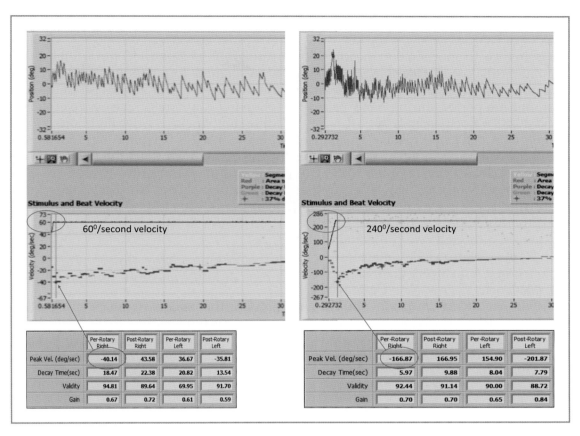

FIGURE 7–30. Normal 60°/second velocity step test and 240°/second velocity step test (after correcting/deleting for noise) depicting the difference in peak slow phase eye velocity in response to a similar rightward (clockwise) acceleration of 200°/second^2. Solid black line represents chair velocity.

FIGURE 7–31. Example of a 240°/second step stimulus response for all rightward and leftward acceleration and deceleration stimuli. Similar to the 60°/second, the acceleration stimulus is held constant at 200°/sec^2. Peak slow phase eye velocity peaks are identified similar to a 60°/second step stimulus. Each peak eye velocity response is identified in the insert chart.

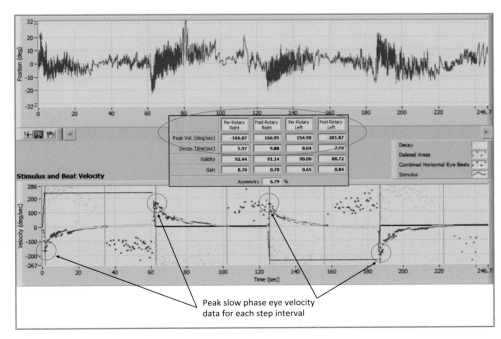

the cupula is, in turn, proportional to the intensity of the stimulation (Baloh & Honrubia, 1990). Figure 7–32 graphically reminds us of the difference in acceleration time period during a 60° velocity step test and a 240° velocity step test.

Following the peak eye velocity response, there is a similar natural non-linear decay of the slow phase eye velocity (nystagmus) to that of low 60° velocity step testing. However, unlike low velocity step testing, we are no longer concerned with the time decay constant of the nystagmus response (although one can certainly be calculated). Rather, high velocity step testing is primarily concerned with a very distinct response parameter: *the single greatest slow-phase peak eye velocity response immediately following acceleration and deceleration in both the clockwise and counterclockwise rotations*. That is, for each 60 seconds of per- and postrotary nystagmus, one *single beat* of

nystagmus is identified for a total of four beats of nystagmus (one following clockwise acceleration, one following clockwise deceleration, one following counterclockwise acceleration, and one following clockwise deceleration). If this seems remarkable, it is. To put things into a broader perspective, for a total test time of a little more than four minutes, the critical response parameters needed for analysis consists of only four beats of nystagmus, each lasting no more than a few hundred milliseconds each!

High Velocity Step Response: Peak Slow-Phase Eye Velocity

Because the peak slow phase eye velocity of the response is fundamental to the analysis, identification of the peak eye velocity during each per- and post rotation is imperative during high veloc-

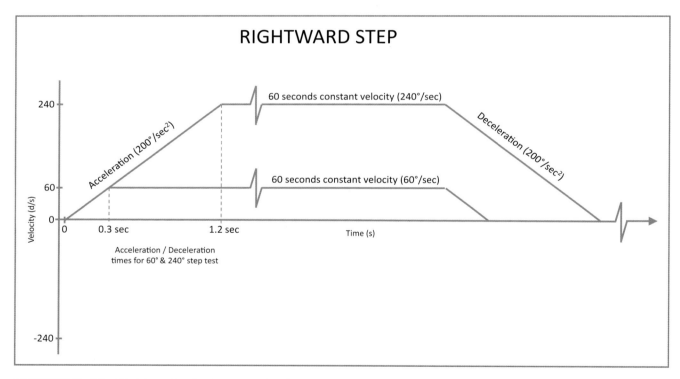

FIGURE 7–32. Rightward velocity step stimulus highlighting the difference in acceleration time between a high velocity and low velocity step stimulus. The acceleration stimulus is held constant at 200°/sec^2, and the duration of the acceleration stimulus is dependent upon the target angular velocity. For a target velocity stimulus of 60°/sec, the acceleration stimulus will occur for a duration of 0.3 seconds, whereas for a higher target velocity stimulus of 240°/sec, the duration of the acceleration stimulus persists for 1.2 seconds. The duration of the deceleration stimulus is similar to that of the acceleration stimulus. Rightward step stimulus is only shown for this illustration but the acceleration stimulus for the leftward step stimulus is the same.

With Only Four Beats of Nystagmus Needed, Can the High Velocity Step Test Be Shortened?

Many students often ask if the test can be shortened if only a *single* beat of peak nystagmus is all the data that is required for analysis. They often ask if the 60-second period of constant velocity rotation per and post clockwise and counterclockwise acceleration (and deceleration) can be shortened to only 10 seconds (or less). Unfortunately, to incite an appropriate and, more importantly, an equivalent response for each velocity period post acceleration and deceleration, the entire nystagmus response must fully extinguish itself (a complete discharge of velocity storage). For most normal physiological systems, this takes approximately three time constants, or nearly the entire 60 seconds for the nystagmus response to fully extinguish and any lingering effects from velocity storage to be negated. So the short answer is no, the test cannot (and likely should not) be shortened. The only caveat to this is when the test is significantly abnormal and the peak VOR slow-phase eye velocity response is severely reduced with little to no nystagmus to undergo decay. During such abnormal responses, completion of the full 60 seconds of constant velocity rotations per- and post-clockwise and counterclockwise acceleration could be potentially shortened. This is *only* true if there is no evidence of any nystagmus response, thus suggesting no evidence for any needed extinction of an intact velocity storage mechanism. Under these circumstances, where velocity storage does not require diminution or extinction, the 60-second constant velocity stimulus period may be shortened and the test advanced to the next stimulus period (whether it is deceleration or acceleration in the opposite direction). Of course, it goes without saying that if any test stimulus period is to be shortened, it should be done with good reason and without concern for contamination or loss of data.

ity step testing. Figure 7–33 (inset box) depicts only the initial period of nystagmus decay in response to leftward acceleration. The slow phase eye velocity plot is depicted, and the *single* peak eye velocity response is identified. The remaining slow-phase eye velocity responses from the decaying nystagmus are plotted precisely the same way as low velocity step testing, with even a time decay constant appropriately calculated (best fit yellow line). Although it is not unreasonable to analyze the high velocity time decay constant and apply it to clinical populations (many software algorithms will actually plot a time decay of the nystagmus response), one must remember that if such clinical application of the data is to be done, it is critical that site-specific normative data ranges for high velocity time decay constants are established, as the lower cutoff of 10 seconds is only applicable to *low velocity* step testing. In fact, time decay constants normally *decrease* as the

intensity of the step velocity increases (Shepard, Goulson, & McPherson, 2016), and may actually approach or even fall below the 10-second cutoff limit applied during low velocity step testing. A primary reason for such a rapid decay during high velocity step testing is that the peak response is so intense that the stored neural input cannot effectively be maintained and is rapidly "dumped" by the neural integrator. In this light, if time decay data for high velocity step testing are reported and applied during clinical use, it is imperative the provider highlight their normative data and not simply apply the lower cutoff of 10 seconds.

High Velocity Gain

In addition to identifying the peak eye velocity response, a high velocity step *gain* can also be calculated. This is done simply by dividing the peak slow phase eye velocity response by the target

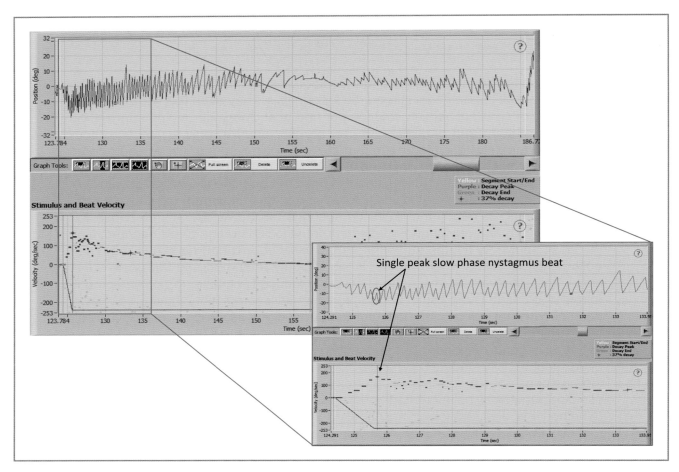

FIGURE 7–33. Corrected 240°/sec step test response data. Initial 10 seconds of data have been expanded to illustrate the peak slow phase eye velocity selection.

step velocity (240°/second in this case). As with all other rotational analysis measures, reduced VOR gain can significantly decrease the spectral purity from which most analyses are derived, particularly when the gain falls below 0.15. Furthermore, there are no established normative data regarding VOR step gain. Baloh and Honrubia report lower limits for normal high velocity step gain to be approximately 0.27, whereas others report lower VOR gain limits of 0.40 (Shepard et al., 2016). Because of such a wide discrepancy of normative limits, it is highly recommended that site-specific step gain values be established if such values are to be used for clinical interpretation. Although high velocity gain is not traditionally a response parameter that has received a great

deal of clinical attention, Shepard and colleagues (2016) have reported a possible clinical value for comparing high velocity step gain against low velocity step gain to infer compensated versus uncompensated vestibular status. They suggest that a directionally similar abnormal gain asymmetry for *both* low velocity step stimuli and high velocity stimuli suggest an uncompensated vestibular status with hypofunction assigned to the weaker labyrinthine response. Conversely, they suggest that when VOR symmetry for low velocity stimuli is within normal limits, and a significant VOR asymmetry persists for high velocity step stimuli, that a centrally compensated vestibular status is likely, with hypofunction assigned according to the high velocity asymmetry.

They summarize by indicating that the low velocity data assist in assigning compensation, whereas the high velocity data assist in segregating asymmetries. However, it is important to realize that establishing VOR gain normative reference ranges is absolutely vital when applying this interpretive strategy, as even slight changes in test protocols can change VOR gain data.

High Velocity Step Response: Peak Slow-Phase Eye Velocity Symmetry

Use of high velocity step data is analyzed to assist in the identification of labyrinthine asymmetry. Similar to caloric analysis, peak slow-phase nystagmus velocities from the right and left labyrinthine responses are compared and a symmetry ratio is calculated. However, unlike the caloric analysis where warm (excitation) and cool (inhibition) responses are totaled for each ear and compared, right and left labyrinthine responses are determined from the two step stimuli conditions that incite excitation. Specifically, an excitatory right labyrinthine response is elicited from per-rotational acceleration to the right and post-rotational deceleration from the left. Conversely, an excitatory left labyrinthine response is elicited from per-rotational acceleration to the left and post-rotational deceleration from the right. A response symmetry ratio is then calculated much like how the Jongkees formula is applied during caloric irrigations.

$$\frac{Right\ Response - Left\ Response}{Right\ Response + Left\ Response} \times 100$$

Specifically, the equation for high velocity step testing is written as such:

$$\frac{(per\ rotation\ right + post\ rotation\ left) - (per\ rotation\ left + rotation\ right)}{(per\ rotation\ right + post\ rotation\ left) + (per\ rotation\ left + rotation\ right)} \times 100$$

Once the symmetry ratio is determined, labyrinthine asymmetry (or labyrinthine hypofunction) can be determined. Although an asymmetry ratio as high as 30% has been reported to be significant for unilateral dysfunction (Shepard et al., 2016), an asymmetry greater than 20% (similar to a caloric asymmetry) is generally agreed upon as

significant for unilateral dysfunction (Baloh & Honrubia, 2001). As always, it may be useful to establish site-specific normative cutoff limits for the identification of unilateral asymmetry as site-specific test protocols, specifically the intensity of the high velocity stimulus, can often vary from one clinic to another. Figure 7–34 shows an example of a normal high velocity step test. Figure 7–35 shows an example of a high velocity step test demonstrating a significant asymmetry. The difference in peak slow phase eye velocity is clear in this example and can easily be visualized by comparing the positive slow-phase peak VOR responses (left acceleration and right deceleration) against the negative slow-phase peak VOR responses (right acceleration and left deceleration).

Interpreting the High Velocity Step Test

Like many physiological stimuli, the more robust the velocity step stimuli, the greater the ability to segregate asymmetries, and, subsequently, potential pathology. When compared to the low velocity step stimuli of 60° per second, an increase in the peak chair velocity over 200°/second can often expose a peripheral vestibular asymmetry that would otherwise be masked by less robust velocities (Paige, 1989). This was previously alluded to, insomuch that higher target velocity stimuli are more effective in driving the periphery into saturation on the lesion side when compared to the 60°/second step stimuli (Baloh & Honrubia, 1990; Brey et al., 2008a). This is further elaborated by Tusa, Grant, Buettner, Herdman, and Zee (1996) insomuch that "high-velocity step rotations toward the intact ear generate higher gain values than when rotating toward the ear with a unilateral lesion because the lagging ear in unable to drive the firing rate below zero" (p. 294). The sensitivity of this measure, however, is dependent on the severity of the vestibular lesion. In general, Baloh, Sills and Honrubia (1979) found that asymmetries were more commonly associated with patients exhibiting more severe unilateral lesions, even when higher velocity step frequencies were administered. They reported an 87% sensitivity for 240° step testing when caloric responses were

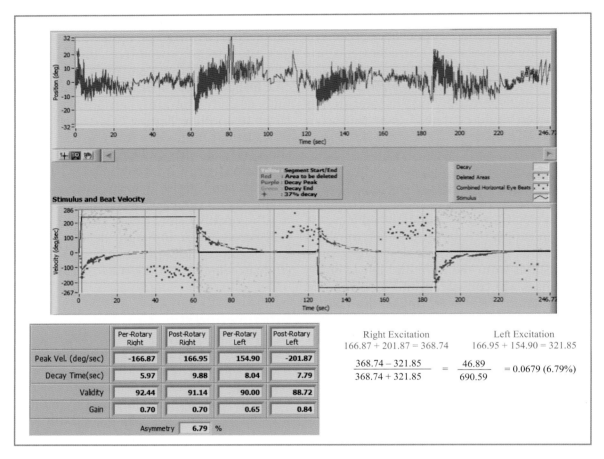

FIGURE 7–34. Normal 240°/second velocity step test (after correcting/deleting for noise). Asymmetry calculation is shown.

absent, but only a 67% sensitivity when caloric responses were reduced (but not absent). Therefore, despite increasing the target step stimuli above 200°/second, the greater the unilateral damage, the greater the likelihood of an observed physiologic high velocity step asymmetry. That being said, it is likely true that if an abnormal high velocity step asymmetry exists, that a significant labyrinthine asymmetry is almost always present, regardless of the frequency being tested. However, when a high velocity asymmetry is within normal limits, a borderline to marginal asymmetry *may* still actually be present, especially for lower frequency stimuli (i.e., caloric stimuli). The reason for this is likely secondary to the preferential loss of labyrinthine function for lower frequency stimuli, similar to

a preferential loss of SHA gain for the lower frequencies when vestibular pathology is present.

Before finishing our discussion on the significance of identifying labyrinthine asymmetries using 240° step testing, it is important to also highlight the usefulness of 240° step data for identifying residual bilateral labyrinthine hypofunction. We have determined that the intensity of the high velocity 240° step stimulus is essentially the strongest (or at least one of the most robust) stimuli that we clinically present to the vestibular system. That being said, it is conceivable that, if a 240° step stimuli failed to provoke a labyrinthine response, then the plausibility that the vestibular system was severely (if not entirely) damaged is greater than if caloric, SHA, or 60° step stimuli were

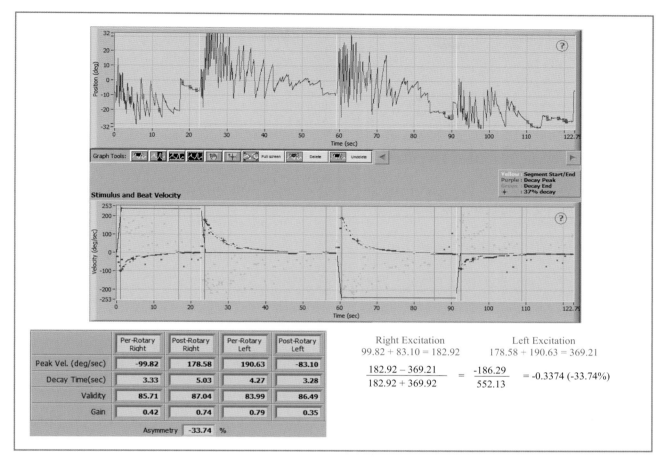

FIGURE 7–35. Abnormal 240°/second velocity step test (after correcting/deleting for noise). Asymmetry calculation is shown. The VOR gain is greater than 20%. Labyrinthine hypo-function is assigned to the weaker excitation conditions (right ear).

used alone. Therefore, the complete lack of VOR response to a 240° step stimulus provides strong evidence to suggest profound labyrinthine hypofunction. However, if a minimal response were obtained, does this provide evidence to suggest a minimal degree of labyrinthine reactivity is present? To help illustrate this point, consider Figure 7–36, which depicts the VOR 240° step response from an individual with significant bilateral peripheral vestibular disease. In this example, an appropriately beating VOR response is clearly identified in response to each step stimuli. These data suggest that, if given an appropriate amount of stimuli, this patient's labyrinth (or at least the horizontal semicircular canals) retain some residual function and provide some evidence to refute complete

labyrinthine areflexia. The data not shown in this example were the absence of any detectable VOR to standard caloric stimuli, SHA stimuli, and 60° step stimuli. Therefore, the only data that provides some salient evidence to refute complete labyrinthine areflexia were the 240° step stimuli. This, however, does not speak to the functional "usability" or rehabilitation of such labyrinthine reactivity; only that minimal residual response exists.

Late "Reversal" Nystagmus During High Velocity Step Testing

At times, the presence of a reversing nystagmus may occur toward the end of a high velocity stimulus period, either per or post acceleration. In fact,

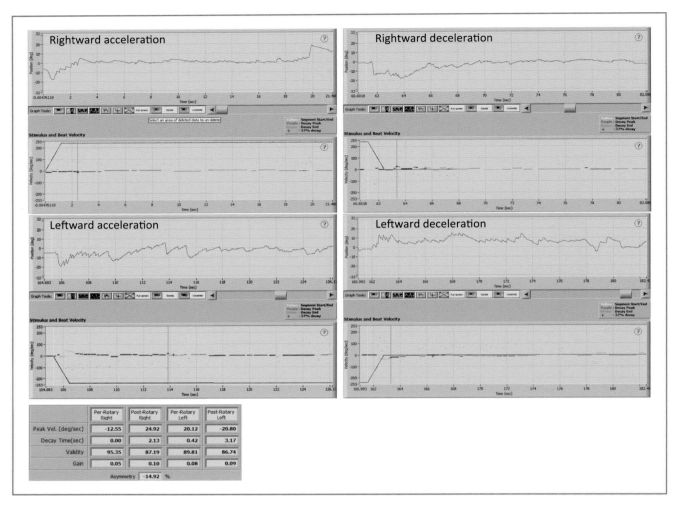

	Per-Rotary Right	Post-Rotary Right	Per-Rotary Left	Post-Rotary Left
Peak Vel. (deg/sec)	-12.55	24.92	20.12	-20.80
Decay Time(sec)	0.00	2.13	0.42	3.17
Validity	95.35	87.19	89.81	86.74
Gain	0.05	0.10	0.08	0.09
Asymmetry	-14.92 %			

FIGURE 7–36. The VOR and slow phase eye velocity plots for rightward and leftward, acceleration and deceleration stimuli during a 240° step test. Despite the incredibly weak VOR response, these data confirm very limited labyrinthine activity (VOR response is appropriately beating to all stimuli conditions) that would otherwise have gone undetected by traditional caloric or even SHA stimuli.

it is actually quite common for a burst of opposite beating nystagmus to occur following complete decay of the nystagmus response. Figure 7–37 shows a nystagmus reversal in a healthy individual following a 240° rightward step stimuli. Reversal of nystagmus is generally more prominent following acceleration than deceleration stimuli. Furthermore, reversal of nystagmus most often occur when cupulae are subjected to constant acceleration of a moderate-to-high velocity, such as step stimuli greater than 100°/second (Baloh & Honrubia, 2011; Baloh et al., 1979). Although

nearly all nystagmus during rotational testing can effectively be explained by the *pendulum model* and cupular mechanics, the primary explanation for this reversal is known as the *adaptation phenomenon* (Baloh et al., 2011).

To explain the adaptation phenomenon, we must first summarize the fundamental principles of the pendulum model of cupular mechanics we have previously discussed. The pendulum model states two fundamental properties of cupular dynamics. First, the degree of cupular deflection is in direct relationship to the degree of the accel-

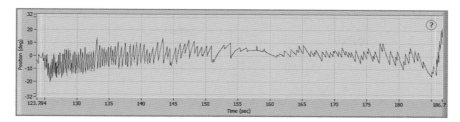

FIGURE 7–37. Example illustrating a robust "reversal nystagmus" following a 240°/second step test on a healthy individual.

eration stimulus. Second, the time it takes the cupulae to reach maximum deviation is directly proportional to the viscosity of the endolymph and inversely proportional to the elasticity properties of the cupulae (Baloh et al., 2011). What is implied, however, but not directly stated, is that the pendulum model is constrained to explaining *cupular* dynamics and fails to take into consideration the regular and irregular *afferent firing properties* of the vestibular nerve. Following sustained accelerations, a substantial portion of afferent nerve fibers exhibit adaptation properties that are not explained by the pendulum model. When exposed to a sustained velocity of approximately 100°/second, or greater, these adaptation neurons experience a biphasic response that demonstrate a secondary prolonged decrease in firing rate that return to baseline at a much slower rate than the monotonic phasic excitatory neurons. It is this slower return of biphasic neurons that is most likely responsible for the emergence of the reversal nystagmus observed during high velocity step testing. Although the exact origins of this response is not know (anatomic versus synaptic), this adaptation phenomenon is a more pronounced behavior from irregular neurons than regular neurons (Baloh et al., 2011). Recall, that properties of irregular afferent nerve fibers also respond best to stimuli with more robust onset characteristics such as those experienced during (high velocity) step testing, whereas regular afferent nerve fibers respond best to more sustained angular stimuli such as those experienced during SHA testing. Clinically speaking, however, the absence of a reversal nystagmus in an otherwise healthy and intact vestibular system has not received any prognostic attention and should

not be interpreted as abnormal until identified as such.

Limitations to 240° Step Testing

There are a couple of critical limitations to the high velocity step test. First, it is absolutely critical that appropriate mental tasking and sharpened mental alertness occur during administration of all step stimuli, and especially during high velocity step testing. Although this is true of all measures that assess the VOR, such mental tasking during step testing is essential, particularly during the initial burst of acceleration and deceleration to ensure equivalent and maximum peak responses are produced and recorded. Because the high velocity step test is primarily concerned with only four discrete beats of nystagmus, it is imperative that the signal to noise ratio during these precise (and extremely brief) periods of data collection be extremely high. Keep in mind that the peak slow-phase eye velocity responses should occur immediately post the acceleration and deceleration stimulus periods. It is not uncommon for patients to experience significant vertigo and even a "jolt of suspense" or "surprise" immediately following such high velocity stimuli. Consequently, their physiological "knee jerk" (or more precisely "ocular jerk") response may be to close their eyes, tense their ocular muscles, or even roll their eyes up into the orbits. Figure 7–38 depicts an example of a patient for whom reliable data was not obtained during the critical recording period secondary to increased ocular tension. All of these physiological responses will contribute to lower peak eye velocities and subsequently create a

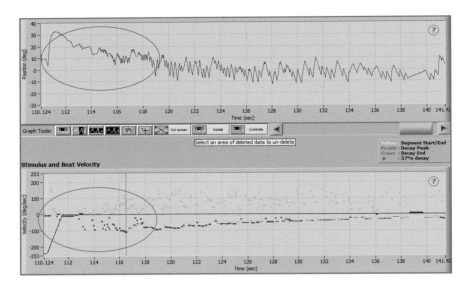

FIGURE 7–38. Example illustrating the difficulty with obtaining the *single* peak slow phase eye velocity response during a 240°/sec step test due to ocular tightening. This example shows the absence of any eye velocity data in response to decelerating from a leftward 240°/sec step velocity. As a result of an abrupt onset of vertigo often experienced secondary to the abrupt deceleration from the chair rotation, the peak slow phase eye velocity was missed for the first 6 seconds following deceleration (from 110 seconds to 116 seconds). Subsequently, the slow phase peak eye velocity response of −107.24°/sec is considered inaccurate and the test must be either repeated or negated. This example again highlights the importance of capturing "clean" data at the critical periods of acceleration and deceleration—as the entire four-minute test must be repeated due to the single loss of one slow phase eye velocity data point.

diminished response. When you're only collecting a single beat of nystagmus, a significant (although transient) decrease in signal to noise ratio during this critical "first second" time period immediately post the acceleration or deceleration stimulus, will often cause peak responses to be missed, or recorded a few seconds *after* the acceleration or deceleration period (only after the "knee jerk" ocular reflex has abated and the patient re-opens their eyes). By this time, the peak response may have declined by a significant percentage. Unfortunately, there is not a great deal of flexibility in the administration protocols during step testing that would allow a clinician the tractability to stop the test in order to quickly repeat a single step acceleration or deceleration period (i.e., *portions* of a step test cannot be repeated; the *entire* test must be repeated). Figure 7–39 depicts an example of a

patient who experienced a difficult time keeping their eyes open during and immediately after the onset of the acceleration and deceleration stimulus. In this example, the test was performed a second time with a significant degree of cajoling by the clinician to maintain eye opening throughout the entire test, and particularly during the critical recording periods. As can be seen in the example, an increase in peak slow phase eye velocity by 157% would potentially have been missed if the test had not been performed another time. Such a difference can create significant problems with your data analysis, particularly when a single data point constitutes 25% of your entire data! In light of this, it is critical for the clinician to know precisely when the step of acceleration and/or deceleration is going to occur so as to appropriately prepare and task the patient just prior to, during,

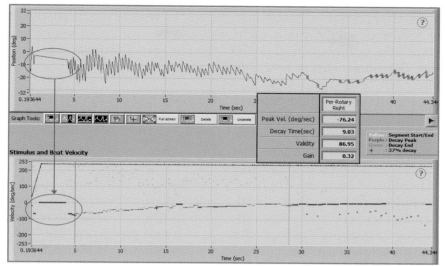

A

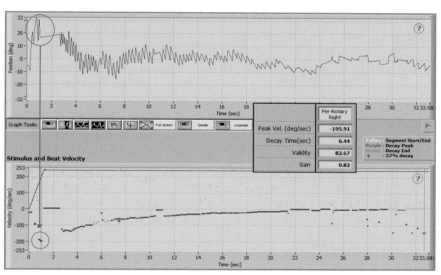

B

FIGURE 7–39. Example illustrating the occasional difficulty with obtaining the peak slow phase eye velocity response during a 240°/sec step test. **A.** Shows the absence of any eye velocity data immediately following a rightward 240°/sec step acceleration due to eye closure. As a result, the peak slow phase eye velocity was subsequently identified as −76.24°/sec at 5 seconds. The 240° step test was repeated while the patient was encouraged to keep their eyes open. These data are shown in **B**. Despite the patient's eyes being closed for a brief period of time between 1 and 3 seconds, the slow phase peak eye velocity response was nevertheless cleanly obtained within the first second of the test. The peak slow phase velocity response was −195.91°/sec (an increase in the slow phase peak velocity response from the previous test by 157%). This example clearly illustrates the importance of data collection during the critical time period during and immediately post acceleration (or deceleration).

and a few seconds post the onset of each stimulus. Of course, another foolproof method to combat missing these discrete time periods is to task the entire 4-plus minutes of testing. This is generally good clinical practice.

A second critical limitation to high velocity step testing is the physiological contamination of the peak slow phase eye velocity response. Because of the intense step velocity stimulus, the slow phase eye response data (and subjective response) can often be similarly intense. This may cause spurious physiological noise in the individual slow phase components of the nystagmus, such as noisy beats due to tracking inadequacies or, worse, unwanted physiologic noise (such as blink artifact) that can often be misinterpreted as actual data. The problem with these spurious data points is that the beat detection algorithms employed in many software programs often identify and may include these aberrant data points within your analysis (i.e., the algorithms cannot distinguish between noise and real nystagmus data). Moreover, these data points can often be significantly greater in their velocity than the actual surrounding "true" data points. Unfortunately, unless the clinician recognizes this error, and either deletes the spurious "noise" or adjusts the peak velocity response to the "correct" data point, the symmetry calculation will erroneously include a possibly inflated peak slow phase velocity response, and inaccurately reflect the true labyrinthine symmetry. Figure 7–40 illustrates such an example of blink artifact inappropriately identified as the peak slow phase eye velocity response. This example constitutes a single data point that, if taken to be true, would have elevated the peak slow phase response by 335%. Therefore, it is vital that the response data be carefully scrutinized. Fortunately, the analysis is fairly simple, as you only need to confine your data analysis to four discrete "true" beats of nystagmus that should occur within the first 1 to 2 seconds after completion of the acceleration or deceleration stimulus. Figure 7–41 is another example of both an incorrect identification of the peak velocity response as well as the corrected response. Although this example is less extreme, it is just as common and just as easy to identify. Finally, similar to the low velocity step test, contraindicated medications that could deleteriously suppress or stimulate the CNS, as well as significantly alter the VOR gain, should be avoided unless otherwise instructed by the patient's administering physician.

ALTERNATIVE STIMULUS VELOCITIES AND VELOCITY STEP PROTOCOLS

Certainly a variety of target velocities can be selected when performing low and high velocity step testing; however, there is no clear knee-point as to what constitutes "low" versus "high" velocity step stimuli. Although a 60°/second velocity is almost universally chosen for performing the low velocity step test, from which the VOR time decay constant is calculated, the choice of high velocity step stimuli is less "unanimous." One could argue that the velocity at which reversal nystagmus occurs may be sufficient evidence to suggest that the knee-point exists at approximately 100°/second. Regardless of what velocity is designated for the low versus the high velocity step target stimuli, it is critical that site-specific normative values for VOR gain and/or time decay constants be obtained given slight variations in protocol administration. Remember though, the higher the velocity stimuli, the better the chance of segregating and identifying unilateral pathology.

Velocity Storage "Cancellation" Protocol

For patients who have a suspected uncompensated vestibular pathology, it is often useful to determine the functional integrity of the velocity storage mechanism, or the lack thereof. As we have already discussed, the velocity storage mechanism is uniquely responsible for both the initiation and maintenance of central compensation, as well as the preservation of the VOR beyond that of simple cupular mechanics. We have already discussed various outcome measures that infer velocity storage function, specifically the VOR decay time constant during 60° step testing. However, there is an additional outcome measure that can provide insight into velocity storage function. The velocity storage "cancellation" protocol (also

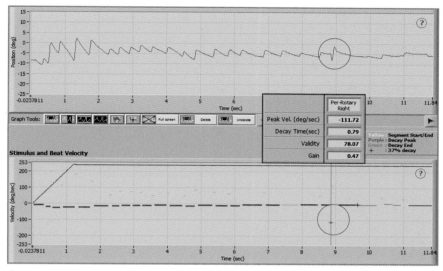

A

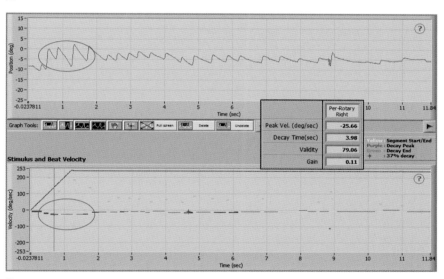

B

FIGURE 7–40. Example illustrating the effects of noise offsetting peak detection during a 240°/sec rightward step acceleration. **A.** Shows an inappropriate selection of the −111.72°/sec peak response just prior to 9 seconds. The raw tracing clearly shows this response to be noise (likely a blink response). **B.** Shows the correct selection of the -25.66°/sec peak response during the rightward step acceleration just prior to 1 second. Proper inspection of the data has significantly changed the interpretation of this response from a robust peak VOR response (47% gain) to a significantly weak VOR response (11% gain)—all due to a single introduction of blink artifact misinterpreted by the response algorithm as actual data.

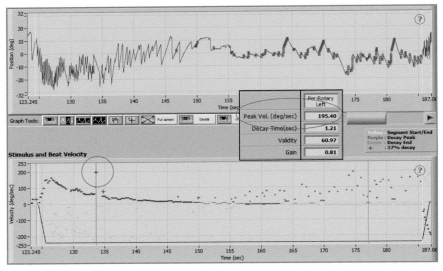

A

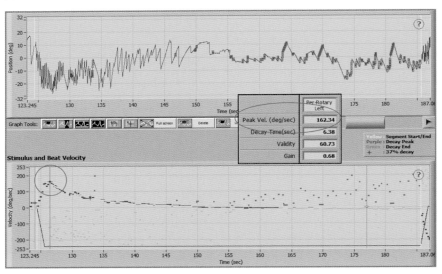

B

FIGURE 7–41. A–B. Example illustrating an incorrect identification of the peak slow phase velocity response following a leftward 240°/sec step acceleration. Peak slow phase velocity response (*circled*) changed from 195.40°/sec to 162.34°/sec. It is imperative that such peak identification be meticulously inspected as these individual slow phase peak data points from each step acceleration and deceleration interval (leftward acceleration only shown here) are the only four points of data analyzed during the 240°/sec step test.

referred to as the tilt suppression protocol; velocity storage "dumping" protocol; or velocity storage "short circuit" protocol) can be performed to determine the effectiveness of cancelling (or "short circuiting") the velocity storage mechanism. Following initiation of the velocity storage mechanism, such as that during 60° velocity step testing, the stored neural response can be rapidly "cancelled" ("short circuited" or "dumped") simply by lowering one's chin toward their sternum post cessation of step rotation. The abrupt re-orienting of one's head is thought to "dump" the stored neural response due to otolith-semicircular canal interaction (Benson & Bodin, 1966; Shepard et al., 2016). Specifically, reduction of the stored angular VOR by head tilt is hypothesized to represent a nodulo-uvular mechanism by which the discordant central conflict between neural signals from the otoliths (stationary head) and the semicircular canals (rotating head) is resolved (Wiest, Deecke, Trattnig & Mueller, 1999). The resultant VOR time decay constant following reorientation (tilting) of the head has been shown to be effectively reduced the time constant to that of cupular mechanics (Benson & Bodin, 1966, Waespe et al., 1985).

Determination of velocity storage cancellation is often made while performing 60° velocity step testing. Specifically, the VOR time constant is measured after lowering the patient's chin to their sternum *post cessation* of the 60° velocity step stimulus (it is important to avoid reorientation of the head during the ongoing step stimulus, as such movement can initiate tremendous vertigo and nausea, similar to OVAR testing discussed in Chapter 8). The "head tilted" VOR time constant is then compared against the time constant acquired during standard 60° velocity step testing. A reduction of the time constant by at least 40% should be recorded during the velocity storage cancellation protocol (Lockette, Shepard, Lyos, Boismier, & Mers, 1991). In patients for whom such "velocity cancellation" fails to occur, a central pathology impacting the nodulus and the ventral uvula of the cerebellum has been implicated (Hain, Zee & Maria, 1988; Lee et al., 2016; Moon et al., 2009; Waespe et al., 1985; Wiest, Deecke, Trattnig, & Mueller, 1999), as have lesions of the posterior cerebellar vermis (Waespe et al., 1985). Unfortunately, other pathologies have also been implicated (essential hypertension) so the diagnostic sensitivity for localizing pathology exclusively to the neural integrator or velocity storage mechanism should be interpreted with caution (Lockette, Shepard, Lyos, Boismier, & Mers, 1991). However, when collective data does suggest a potential lesion impacting the neural integrator, velocity storage cancellation can be useful for further strengthening or corroborating a potential (midline) cerebellar lesion.

Of particular note regarding velocity storage cancellation testing, however, is that reorientation of the patient's head following step rotation requires the absence of head restraints. This clearly requires particular concern for the patient's safety during step acceleration and constant velocity rotation. In addition, the lack of any head restraints requires particular care to ensure the patient maintains a steady head position during the step test to maximize the VOR step response and minimize the onset of acute vertigo due to the Coriolis effect. Finally, because the investigation of velocity storage "cancellation" is often performed post cessation of velocity step stimuli, this requires the addition of another velocity step test. Unfortunately, if the patient in question suffers from uncompensated dizziness or vertigo, the addition of another velocity step rotation may be problematic if the patient finds such stimuli adverse or noxious.

CHAPTER SUMMARY

Like any other vestibular test, interpreting results from velocity step testing should be performed in association with other vestibular test results (SHA, ocular motor, VNG, VEMP, etc.). Low and high velocity step testing can concurrently confirm and provide novel aspects to the diagnosis of vestibular pathology, as well as increase the ability to better identify the potential site-of-lesion. Table 7–1 summarizes the more common abnormal findings and respective interpretations associated with both low and high velocity step testing.

Overall, velocity step testing offers two valuable insights into vestibular physiology. First, low

Table 7–1. Common Abnormalities from 60⁰/Second and 240⁰/Second Velocity Step Testing

	Velocity Step Testing		
	Abnormality	*Possible Interpretation*	*Rule Out*
60°/sec	Low time constant (<10 sec)	1. Peripheral unilateral vestibular lesion if ocularmotor testing is normal, likely labyrinth or VIII Nerve 2. At 60° or 100°/sec, information is from both labyrinths 3. Non-localizing cupular time constants plus velocity storage—gains should be >0.3; if not, consider migraine	Inattention; too much blinking; bilateral loss; fixation
	If 3 of 4 time constants are abnormal	1. Abnormal study; nonlocalizing	Inattention; too much blinking
240°/sec	Consider peak slow phase velocity; >20% difference between CW and CCW directions?	1. Significant asymmetric results in peak SPV indicate peripheral unilateral vestibular lesion and side of loss	Eye closure (eyes must be open when chair starts and stops)

velocity step testing provides a significant contribution to the evaluation of central vestibular function. Velocity step testing offers the ability to gain a greater perception of central velocity storage. In addition, when VOR gain is compared between low and high velocity step stimuli, step testing offers the ability to gain a better insight into central compensation mechanisms. These two advantages alone support the inclusion of step testing as a critical component to the standard rotational test battery. Although there are those who argue that, because of the inverse relationship between low frequency VOR phase and VOR time decay constant, the use of low-frequency SHA testing (for 0.01 to 0.04 Hz) and low velocity step testing are considered equivalent and, therefore, redundant (Baloh & Honrubia, 2001). Although this point is not without merit, many agree that the use of low-velocity step testing is considered the preferred method for calculating the time decay constant of the VOR (Brey et al., 2008b; Shepard & Telian, 1996). This is primarily because the velocity storage function of the central system is best provoked with the use of a constant velocity stimulus, as it likely incites a greater number of both irregular and regular afferent neural fibers (rather than a predominance of regular fibers incited during SHA testing).

The second valuable insight velocity step testing provides is that it addresses the primary limitation of SHA testing; that is, the inability to lateralize peripheral vestibular pathology. The use of high velocity step testing currently offers a moderate sensitivity for the detection of unilateral peripheral vestibular pathology. It is uncertain whether high velocity step testing will ever take the place of caloric testing for the identification of labyrinthine asymmetry. However, newly developed rotational stimulus protocols, such as high acceleration chair thrust testing, may hold promise (Chapter 8). In addition, as advancements in hardware and software continue to be developed, more precise recording techniques and stimulus paradigms will undoubtedly emerge and contribute to a greater ability to detect unilateral vestibular lesions.

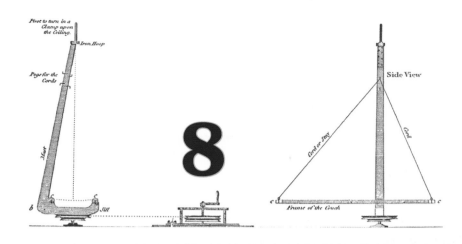

8

Supplemental and Specialized Rotational Tests

INTRODUCTION

A basic rotational evaluation consists of sinusoidal harmonic acceleration testing (SHA) and velocity step testing (VST), perhaps even using both a low and high velocity stimulus. Both of these tests have been discussed at length in Chapters 6 and 7, respectively. The capabilities of the rotational assessment, however, do not end there. There are additional rotational tests that may be routinely used in some facilities as part of a regular assessment, whereas other facilities may reserve their use only when clinically indicated. The more widely used ancillary rotational tests are those that investigate the complex interaction between the visual and vestibular systems. There are two primary tests of visual-vestibular interaction: VOR suppression and visual-vestibular enhancement. Clinically, these tests offer added insight into central [vestibular] pathology that often expand our understanding of vestibular disease and non-specific dizziness beyond that offered by VST and SHA testing.

Rotational tests have also been developed in an attempt to evaluate otolith function. Unilateral centrifugation testing, or UCF testing, was developed to evaluate utricular function, and involves yaw rotations along an eccentric path. Such eccentric rotations generate a centripetal linear force over the outwardly displaced utricle that produces a subsequent subjective tilt, much like that experienced during circular amusement park rides. During such rotations, the subjective tilt can usually be quantified in the clinical setting by having the patient self-adjust a target line to what they believe to be vertical. Although this test had been receiving some clinical attention over the past decade, it has seemingly been migrating out of the clinic and fading back into the research literature. In addition, off-vertical axis rotational testing, (OVAR) was developed to explore otolith function. This test involves yaw rotations that are performed while the chair is slightly tilted off its earth-vertical axis. The integration of OVAR testing into standard clinical use, however, has experienced a great deal of resistance for a variety of reasons. One of the likely reasons that OVAR testing has failed to achieve routine clinical use is its added expense above the standard rotational chair apparatus, which already has a relatively high cost, in relation to its limited increase in diagnostic power. Moreover, its poor widespread clinical use has limited its expansion into mainstream diagnostic discussions and clinical comparisons to other vestibular tests. Unfortunately, due to such limited diagnostic power, and current normative clinical data, OVAR testing has been strictly limited to research use by the Federal Drug Administration (FDA) at the time of this publication.

Finally, as technology continues to advance, the capabilities of rotational testing will concomitantly advance. There are a number of emerging tests that may have clinical applications in the future, but are not yet fully developed or characterized across various populations. I refer to these tests as more research-driven tests. Such research tests, given enough development, efficacy studies, and clinical application studies to patient populations, will generally become more recognized as routine clinical tests. These tests include vertical canal assessment using yaw rotations, whole-body "en-bloc" head thrust testing (chair head impulse testing or crHIT), and psychophysiological measures of vestibular (acceleration) threshold detection.

Prior to discussing some of the more research-driven tests, as well as some of the future advancements in rotational testing, let us first discuss the two most common tests of visual-vestibular interaction, (i.e., VOR suppression testing, visual-vestibular enhancement testing), as well as eccentric rotation testing.

VISUAL-VESTIBULAR INTERACTION TESTING

We have thoroughly reviewed how two rotational tests, SHA and VST, can provide a tremendous amount of clinical insight into peripheral and, at times, central function. We have seen how known lesions of the peripheral system can significantly impair the VOR, and we have seen how known lesions of the central nervous system can cause subtle abnormalities that have little to no effect on VOR sensitivity (i.e., gain). We have also seen how both peripheral and central lesions can negatively impact the efficiency of the VOR, as with the processing of the phase, symmetry, and time decay constants. Therefore, when analyzing rotational results, it is sometimes difficult to specifically localize lesions to the central nervous system or to the peripheral vestibular system. This is why it is often critical to incorporate a comprehensive vestibular assessment in order to identify particular patterns within your vestibular test results. Often it is far easier to identify a peripheral vestibular lesion than a central lesion. However, there are two rotational tests that are able to provide direct insight into central nervous system function. Such tests tap into the complex neurophysiological interaction between the visual and the vestibular systems. These tests are referred to as visual-vestibular interaction tests.

Visual-vestibular interaction tests (VVI) are specialized rotational tests that target central vestibular processing, and are able to highlight central pathology that impacts the efficiency of the VOR, even when VOR gain is within normal limits (Baloh, Honrubia, & Kerber, 2011). Confining a rotational assessment solely to SHA and velocity step testing can, therefore, potentially limit the diagnostic power of a "comprehensive" *rotational* assessment, specifically when attempting to identify possible central lesions that can often cause generalized (non-specific) dizziness in patients. For example, cerebellar floccular lesions have little-to-no impact on the production (gain) of the VOR (Goldberg et al., 2012); however, such lesions can significantly impact the ability to suppress the VOR. Such processing is critical for canceling the VOR during combined head-eye tracking and, when dysfunctional, can cause non-specific dizziness symptoms in patients, particularly in the aging population. Lesions impacting this central processing can often be confirmed or further elucidated through tests of visual-vestibular interaction, which can increase the diagnostic power of your clinical assessment and potentially help to reduce the number of nebulous diagnoses that occur far too often with age-related or non-specific dizziness phenotypes.

Although abnormalities in ocular motor assessment can often suggest central pathology, such abnormalities are too often underappreciated or dismissed as inattentiveness, age-related, or too subtle to classify as meaningful or pathologic. In light of this, the contribution of visual-vestibular interaction testing on the VOR deserves a greater degree of clinical consideration when assessing our patients for neurotological disorders (Demer, 1996). Therefore, let us consider the two visual-vestibular interaction tests: VOR suppression testing, and visual-vestibular enhancement testing.

VOR Suppression Testing

Vestibular Ocular Reflex (VOR) suppression testing has also been referred to as VOR cancellation, VOR fixation testing, or Visual-Vestibular Fixation (VVI-FX). The principal concept of VOR suppression testing is not new. In fact, vestibular clinicians typically perform VOR fixation testing at least twice during the caloric irrigation test. Following each warm (or cool) caloric irrigation, we instruct our patients to visually fixate, or suppress, their VOR response. The only difference between rotational and caloric VOR fixation is that during caloric testing, the patient is attempting to suppress an induced-vestibular response from an extremely low frequency stimulus (0.003 Hz), whereas during rotational assessment, the patient is asked to suppress the VOR to much more robust stimuli, generally frequencies greater than 0.04 Hz.

The principal components of VOR suppression testing have already been well examined during our discussion of sinusoidal acceleration testing. In fact, the VOR suppression test is nothing more than the same sinusoidal accelerations we discussed in Chapter 6, only now these angular rotations are performed in the presence of a visual fixation target. In fact, this test is often performed at the exact same harmonic frequencies conducted during SHA testing, but this is not required. However, prior to discussing the exact details of the rotational VOR suppression clinical protocol, let us first review the different stimuli that can be used to suppress the VOR, as well as the neurophysiological substrate that is being evaluated during VOR suppression testing.

Rotational VOR Suppression Stimuli and Neurophysiology

Rotational VOR suppression testing is most often performed with fixation upon a *visual* target. This is because a visual stimulus is approximately two to three times more effective in suppressing the gain (sensitivity or response) of the VOR than an auditory or somatosensory target (Jacobson, Piker, Do, McCaslin, & Hood, 2012). The VOR suppression test can also be performed to imagined targets; however, the effectiveness is essentially equivocal to somatosensory and auditory targets (Jacobson et al., 2012). Therefore, it is possible to suppress the VOR response to nearly any target, imagined or otherwise; however, visual targets are the most effective. The differences in the suppressive nature of each target would subsequently suggest different underlying neural pathways governing each one. This is, in fact, true. There is significant evidence that the underlying neurophysiological substrates involved in the suppression (or cancellation) of the VOR are different whether the suppressive target is a visual one, versus an auditory or somatosensory one, versus an imagined one. Before we discuss the various attributes of each suppressive target, let us review the neurophysiological substrates associated with each target stimuli used during VOR suppression testing.

Neurophysiological Substrate of VOR Suppression Associated with Non-Visual Fixation Targets. Use of non-visual fixation targets is not routinely performed during clinical assessment of VOR suppression. This is primarily due to the statistically greater suppressive effects provided by visual targets. Nevertheless, research has been conducted to investigate the effects of such non-visual fixation targets. The most common non-visual targets include somatosensory and auditory fixation stimuli. For these stimuli, there is good evidence to suggest that there exist supplementary neurocortical pathways that are specific to these modalities, in lieu of the primary direct pathways associated with visual target suppression. It has been shown that corticofugal fibers originating from the premotor cortex, the cingulate cortex, the intraparietal sulcus, the insula, the retroinsular cortex, and the posterior region of the superior temporal cortex, all have primary projections to the vestibular nuclei. All of these projections have been shown to activate VOR suppression to non-visual stimuli in primates (Akbarian, Grusser, & Guldin, 1992; Faugier-Grimaud, & Ventre, 1989; Guldin, Akbarian, & Grussehave, 1992; Kawano, Sasaki, & Yamashita, 1980; Leinonen, Hyvarinen, & Sovijarvi, 1980; Nishiike, Guldin, & Baurle,

2000, in Jacobson et al., 2012). Data provided by Jacobson and colleagues (2012) have shown that such efferent inhibitory pathways, mediated by auditory and somatosensory feedback, offer modest suppressive effects on the VOR by as much as 28% to 44%, but that such effects are significantly less than that provided by the more direct visual motor pathways (84% to 87%).

Alternatively, there is evidence to show that *imagined* targets also have suppressive effects on the VOR. If visual targets are imagined and move with the head, evidence has shown that the resultant suppressive effects can reduce the gain (sensitivity) of the VOR to nearly 0.1 (Leigh & Zee, 2006). Jacobson and colleagues (2012) reported only a modest suppression of the VOR (44%) in a group of individuals who imagined a patient-fixed simple visual target during angular rotations. In addition, they showed that the suppressive effect of the imaginary target was not significantly different than the suppressive effects of an auditory or somatosensory target. However, the suppressive effects of an imagined target were significantly less than a patient-fixed visual target. Interestingly, Leigh and Zee (2006) reported that if the imagined target is an *earth-fixed* visual scene, (i.e., one that is stationary like a picturesque horizon), the VOR is not suppressed at all, but actually augmented to a near perfect gain of 1.0 (Leigh & Zee, 2006). This is similar to visual-vestibular enhancement (albeit with an imagined visual target), which is discussed after VOR suppression.

Neurophysiological Substrates of VOR Suppression Associated With a Visual Fixation Target. Most evidence has identified that the neurophysiological substrates for visual suppression of the VOR follows the direct smooth pursuit and optokinetic pathways, which heavily involve the accessory optic system, the nucleus of the optic tract, and the flocculonodular lobe in the vestibulocerebellum (Baloh, Honrubia & Kerber, 2011; Leigh & Zee, 2006). Although evidence suggests that this *direct* pathway is the *primary* contributor to the efficiency of VOR suppression, there exists some evidence to suggest that an *indirect* pathway also exists. This indirect pathway is mediated by the vestibulocerebellum, which includes the nodulus

and uvula (Baloh, Honrubia, & Kerber, 2011; Leigh & Zee, 2006; Shepard & Telian, 1996). This neuroanatomical substrate is the essential component of the velocity storage mechanism, which we have discussed at length throughout this text. Evidence has shown that this indirect pathway may, in fact, modify the direct pathway through a distributed network of neural projections between vestibulocerebellar and vestibular dedicated neurons within the vestibular nuclei, (known as vestibular-only neurons) (Goldberg et al., 2012). Some of the evidence supporting this distributed network involving brainstem and cerebellar neural projections comes from data showing that stimulation of the nodulus and ventral uvula reduces the VOR time constant, similar to the effects of visual suppression (Goldberg et al., 2012). However, despite this evidence suggesting a network distribution, it is clear that concomitant abnormalities of smooth pursuit, optokinetic reflexes, and VOR suppression occur as a result of cerebellar lesions involving the flocculi and ventral paraflocculi (Goldberg et al., 2012). Overall, it is almost universally agreed that VOR suppression is *heavily* mediated by the direct smooth pursuit and optokinetic ocular motor pathways, with only a minor influence of the indirect flocculonodular pathway.

VOR Suppression Protocol

Conducting rotational VOR suppression testing is as straightforward as performing SHA testing, with the exception that the patient is instructed to fixate their gaze on a head-fixed (i.e., rotation-fixed) target. Rotational frequencies are usually greater than 0.04 Hz, and most often occur between 0.08 and 1.0 Hz. Given the simplicity of introducing a visual target during sinusoidal rotations, as well as the two- to three-fold increase of VOR suppression by a visual target over a non-visual target (Jacobson et al., 2012), it is understandable that a *visual* target is most often used during VOR suppression protocols. Furthermore, one could argue that, given the complex nexus of corticoneural pathways and neural centers that are associated with non-visual stimuli, compared to the (essentially singular) heavily mediated direct neural pathway that is associated with visual stimuli, the localizing power of VOR suppression is much greater with the use of a visual target than a non-visual target.

There exists one more potential reason to perform VOR suppression testing with the use of a visual target rather than a non-visual target. In light of the (minor) indirect contributions of the flocculonodular lobe to VOR suppression, the assessment of this neurophysiological response may be of some importance, as the nodulus, along with the ventral uvula, is heavily involved in the down-regulation and clamping of the commissural processes that occur during central compensation. Therefore, performing rotational VOR suppression testing could potentially provide invaluable insight into the efficiency and effectiveness of the central compensation mechanism. This can be of significant prominence in the rotational test battery, particularly if the efficiency of the central compensation mechanism needs to be examined prior to a planned unilateral labyrinthectomy that will depend on (and demand) such mechanisms postsurgically. Moreover, VOR suppression testing can and should be assessed if a lack of central compensation is suspected. Figure 8–1 illustrates such an example in a patient with Cryptococcal meningitis. These data depict a severe lack of VOR suppression for all octave frequencies tested from 0.08 through 0.64 Hz. These data (along with abnormal smooth pursuit testing and optokinetic testing data, which are not shown here) were instrumental in providing evidence to suggest a lack of cerebellar control over this patient's VOR, as well as their complaint of unremitting dizziness.

Clinical Indicators for Rotational VOR Suppression

Rotational VOR suppression testing should be considered for nearly all patients undergoing rotational testing, just as all patients receiving caloric irrigations receive caloric-fixation testing. In fact, one could argue that rotational VOR suppression testing should be adopted as a routine component to a standard rotational test battery for three reasons. First, it produces little (if any) nausea, emesis, or patient discomfort. Second, it extends the overall test time less than a few minutes. Finally,

the clinical yield for the identification of central pathology that rotational VOR suppression testing can offer is far greater than the clinical sensitivity of the caloric fixation test. This is primarily because fixation of the VOR becomes increasingly more difficult as the stimuli become more intense (Demer, 1996). In fact, suppression of the caloric response requires significantly less physiological "effort" when compared to suppression of high frequency rotational responses, which are inherently more robust.

Because VOR suppression relies heavily upon the direct smooth pursuit pathway, effective suppression can be expected through approximately 1.0 Hz (Goldberg et al., 2012). Above this frequency, suppression of the VOR becomes less efficient with a concomitant decrease in efficiency of the smooth pursuit pathway (Baloh, Honrubia, & Kerber, 2011). Moreover, because the efficiency of the smooth pursuit pathway has been shown to be age-dependent, VOR suppression performance may also be influenced by age. Although, this does not imply that rotational VOR suppression cannot be performed above 0.1 Hz, one just needs to be cognizant that the previously cited 84 to 96% suppression observed at frequencies less than or equal to 0.1 Hz (Furst et al., 1987; Jacobson et al., 2012; Moller et al., 1990) will likely not be commensurate for frequencies >0.1 Hz (Baloh, Honrubia & Kerber, 2011). Overall, it is strongly suggested that site-specific normative reference ranges be obtained for any and all frequencies performed on a routine basis, and particularly if the target population includes aging patients. This recommendation is similar to SHA and velocity step testing, as slight changes in methodology, peak chair velocity, and age distribution can influence the variance of the data.

Clinical Advantages of Rotational VOR Suppression Over Caloric VOR Suppression. We know that VOR suppression can be performed during both caloric testing and rotational testing, however, rotational VOR suppression is considered to be superior to caloric-induced VOR suppression for a number of reasons. First, the rate of VOR suppression is significantly greater for rotational stimuli than caloric stimuli. Brey, McPherson, and Lynch (2008) reported visual suppression of the VOR to be

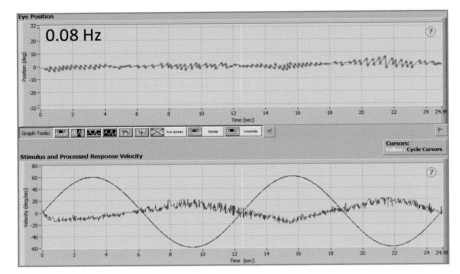

A

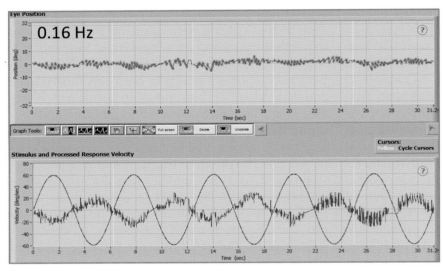

B

FIGURE 8–1. Failure of fixation suppression in a patient with Cryptococcal meningitis. Individual cycle data and raw nystagmus tracings are shown for 0.08 to 0.64 Hz (**A–D**). Overall gain for each frequency is plotted in **E**..
continues

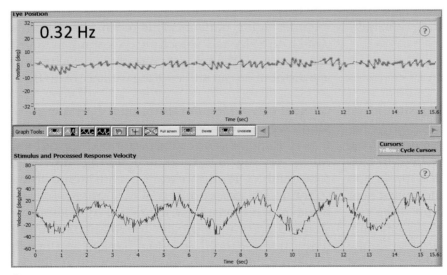

C

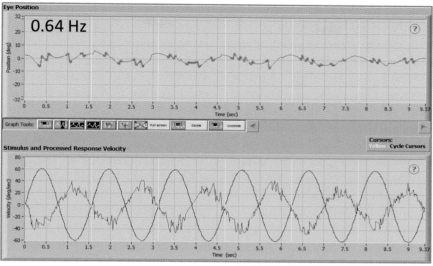

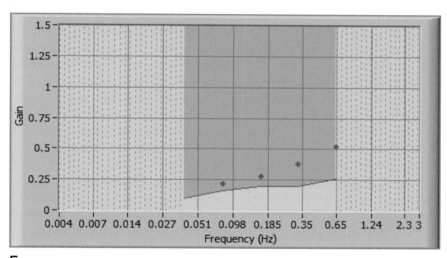

FIGURE 8–1. *continued*

as great as 75 to 90% for rotational stimuli, whereas Barber and Stockwell (1980) were cited as reporting a marginally lower suppression of the VOR by only 40 to 70% for caloric stimuli (Brey, McPherson, & Lynch, 2008). Consequently, these data would suggest a greater opportunity for segregation and identification of central pathology. Second, suppression of the VOR via rotational testing not only allows for evaluation across a more natural stimulus frequency range, but also allows for more precisely administered stimuli (Goulson, McPherson, & Shepard, 2016). Third, unlike the fixation of a caloric response, suppression of a rotationally induced VOR remains consistent across patients and time, as the applied sinusoidal stimulus is always constant (both across and within test sessions). Conversely, suppression of a *caloric*-induced VOR is highly dependent upon the intensity of the slow phase response, which significantly changes over time post stimulus delivery. That is, suppression of a caloric-induced VOR can be conducted immediately following the crescendo and onset of the peak slow phase response, or much later after the slow phase response has significantly dissipated. This variability of the timing with respect to the presentation of the fixation visual target is often clinician dependent. Therefore, suppression of a caloric-induced VOR is, by default, highly variable, and is inherently associated with greater inconsistency as to when suppression of the VOR was measured (at a relatively high or relatively low period of the peak caloric nystagmus). Finally, rotational testing allows for investigation of VOR suppression at multiple frequencies in lieu of just a single frequency (i.e., the caloric frequency). Although conducting VOR suppression at multiple frequencies is preferred, others have suggested that a single frequency is, in fact, sufficient. If a single frequency is performed due to clinical or time limitations, a target frequency of 0.8 Hz has been suggested (Goulson, McPherson, & Shepard, 2016).

VOR Suppression Summary

Overall, rotational VOR suppression testing is strongly recommended for all patients undergoing rotational testing, and particularly for those patients for whom a central lesion is suspected, as well as those for whom effective central compensation is questioned secondary to an anamnesis of chronic dizziness. Moreover, patients who generate ocular abnormalities during smooth pursuit and optokinetic testing should absolutely receive rotational VOR suppression testing because of the shared neurosubstrate. This is particularly true when smooth pursuit and optokinetic abnormalities are subtle, or when such subtle abnormalities are questioned because of a perceived lack of attention, anxiety, or fatigue. All things considered, rotational VOR suppression offers a precise, repeatable, reliable, and robust measure for detecting CNS pathology. Rotational VOR suppression is minimally impacted by patient performance/cooperation, and is probably the simplest rotational test to administer with minimal added time commitment. Above all, the clinical yield can be quite significant when VOR suppression is abnormal. Collectively, these conclusions would argue that VOR suppression is an excellent clinical test when weighing the time-to-benefit ratio.

Visual-Vestibular Enhancement Testing

As the name implies, visual-vestibular enhancement, testing (often abbreviated VVI-enhancement, or VVOR for visual-vestibular ocular reflex) investigates how the visual and vestibular system interact with one another in order to augment, or improve, the neurophysiological VOR response. We have previously discussed the relatively weak nature of the VOR in the absence of any visual cues (i.e., lack of VOR gain unity during SHA testing in darkness). Specifically, we have seen how the sensitivity (gain) of the vestibular system, particularly for frequencies below 1 Hz, is inherently weak, with gain values often [well] below 1.0 (see Figure 6–18). Unfortunately, if such a weak VOR gain were to persist in the presence of visual cues (i.e., anything less than 1.0) the functional outcomes would be catastrophic during head movement, as even minor retinal slips of the visual target off the fovea can cause significant blurring in visual acuity, which would subsequently be reported as "dizziness" in most patients. We are reminded that the fovea represents a viewing area of only 1° (approximately 1 mm) in a field of vision as large as 200°, and any deviation of the target from the fovea severely compromises visual clarity. In fact, the required precision of the visual system is so demanding that, even if the visual-vestibular system produced a VOR gain of 0.90 with a peak head velocity (movement) of 90°/sec (such as that experienced during running), an unassisted vestibular response would cause a retinal image velocity of 8°/sec. This would produce more than enough retinal slip to reduce visual acuity by a factor of 2 (Demer, 1996). If such retinal slip occurred during every active head movement, the resultant effects during daily activities would not only be devastating, they would be life limiting. In fact, if the VOR were *solely* responsible for providing compensatory eye responses to every head movement, the vestibular system's inadequacies would be highly detrimental to the maintenance of visual acuity during nearly every natural head movement. Fortunately, the inadequate VOR is effectively modified and *enhanced* by the visual system to near perfect sensitivity (gain), so such visual blurring is rarely a problem during routine daily activities. This visual-vestibular relationship, or enhancement, is heavily mediated through the central nervous system.

Prior to discussing the rotational protocol for visual-vestibular enhancement, let's first consider the various neurophysiological substrates associated with the complex interaction between the visual system and the vestibular system.

Neurophysiology of the Visual-Vestibular Enhancement

The visual system effectively supplements the imprecision of the vestibular system for processing certain accelerations, particularly those frequencies below 1 Hz where the vestibular system is inadequate to fully provide an accurate compensatory response by itself (Goldberg et al., 2012). By doing so, retinal slip is prevented and subsequent blurring of visual acuity if averted. In fact, the interaction between the visual system and the vestibular system is so precise that compensatory eye movements are almost always produced within a few percentages of near perfect gain for both horizontal and vertical head movements (Demer et al., 1990; Baloh, Honrubia, Yee, & Jacobson, 1986; Ferman, Collewijn, Jansen, & van den Berg, 1987). But what neurophysiology structures coordinate such a perfect visual and vestibular interaction to produce near perfect compensatory responses? Visual-vestibular enhancement is exclusively mediated by the central nervous system. Specifically, this highly coordinated and precise effort is heavily regulated by the optokinetic and, to a lesser degree, the smooth pursuit neural pathways. Because of the dependence on these neural pathways, visual-vestibular enhancement relies upon the cortical eye fields, the nucleus optic tract, the accessory optic system, and the flocculus and paraflocculus (Leigh & Zee, 2006). Therefore, central lesions that influence optokinetic performance (and to a lesser extent smooth pursuit performance) are likely to also exhibit deficits in visual-vestibular enhancement.

Alternative Neurophysiological Inputs to Visual-Vestibular Enhancement

There is also evidence that supports subordinate neurological inputs to the visual-vestibular interaction process. Evidence has shown that VOR gain is higher during active head movements that involve trunk and neck movements rather than passive head movements like those experienced during "en-bloc" whole body rotations (i.e., rotational chair testing) (Demer, 1996). The underlying hypothesis for this increase in VOR gain has been suggested to be secondary to efference copy signaling from skeletal muscle commands that allow the brain to predict head movement while simultaneously driving the needed compensatory eye movements (Demer, 1996). That being said, because rotational testing is performed "en-bloc" and does not incorporate active neck and skeletal muscle movements, a discussion regarding such neural contributions will not be addressed. However, the reader is nevertheless alerted to the potential contributions of larger visual-vestibular enhancement under conditions of dynamic head and neck movement due to such efference copy commands (i.e., vHIT).

Visual-Vestibular Enhancement Protocol

Conducting visual-vestibular enhancement testing is as straightforward as rotational VOR suppression testing, inasmuch as the testing consists of performing SHA rotations in the presence of a stationary optokinetic stimulus. Because the optokinetic stimulus field is not rotation-fixed (as would be the case in VOR suppression testing), rotations of an individual with eyes open across a *stationary* optokinetic stimulus creates a strong retinal flow environment *while simultaneously stimulating the horizontal semicircular canal VOR response.* Such rotations are generally performed for precisely the same frequencies that are performed during SHA testing. As the name of the test would imply, the VOR gain reported for certain frequencies during SHA testing should improve (or be enhanced) by the retinal slip caused by the flow of the stationary optokinetic stimuli across the field of vision. Thus, the increased retinal flow causes a significant addition to the (inadequate) VOR elicited by the simple harmonic sinusoidal accelerations to near perfect unity. That is, the previously observed "sub-1.0 VOR" gain elicited during SHA testing now increases to a near perfect gain of 1.0. Similar to VOR suppression, visual-vestibular enhancement above 1.0 Hz is subject to deterioration, as the underlying smooth pursuit system begins to break down above this frequency. This is corroborated by the fact that the smooth pursuit sys-tem has also been shown to have a substantial age-dependent effect by the sixth decade of life (Kanayama, Nakamura, Sano, Ohki, Okuyama,

Kimura, & Koike, 1994). Given the fact that visual-vestibular enhancement shares the same neural substrate as optokinetic and smooth pursuit pathways, visual-vestibular enhancement is, then by default, also age-dependent. Overall, the improvement of the inadequate VOR response to near perfect sensitivity (gain) confirms the relative importance of the visual system's enhancement of the imprecise VOR for ensuring functional integrity of the ocular fixation system during active head movements.

Lesions Impacting Visual-Vestibular Enhancement

In light of the underlying neurophysiological pathways shared by the optokinetic system and the smooth pursuit system, lesions will often be comorbid for these ocular motor tests and visual-vestibular enhancement. However, rotational induced visual-vestibular enhancement testing likely provides a more stable and accurate response. This is because the increase in VOR gain to near perfect unity during visual-vestibular enhancement testing is driven by an autonomic reflex pathway. That is, the increase in VOR gain to near 1.0 is not dependent on a subjective response by the person being rotated. This is in direct opposition to smooth pursuit testing, and to a lesser extent optokinetic testing, which requires active participation from the individual. Any time a test is dependent upon a subjective response from an individual, a number of performance variables could deleteriously impact the ocular motor response (e.g., lower gain or abnormal phase). As such, abnormalities associated with smooth pursuit testing and optokinetic testing may, in fact, be secondary to poor attention, anxiety, or fatigue rather than true pathology. Because enhancement of the VOR is provided by the (autonomic) optokinetic reflex, the sensitivity of visual-vestibular testing is likely far greater than any ocular motor test, which are often heavily dependent on patient performance and attention. This is particularly true of younger patients who do not always understand the test, and for patients with attention deficits, chronic fatigue, or those patients for whom optokinetic testing is problematic.

Specifically, lesions that impact the cortical eye fields, the nucleus optic tract, the accessory optic system, and the flocculus and paraflocculus all have been reported to have deleterious effects on the direct smooth pursuit and optokinetic pathways (Leigh & Zee, 2006). Therefore, by extension, these lesions will likely have a concomitant impact on visual-vestibular enhancement testing. Such lesions are therefore exclusive to the central system and, as such, are limited to pathologies that impact central function. For example, migraine has been shown to have significant central pathway inhibitors. In a report by Arriaga and colleagues (2006), an astounding 71% of their migrainous patients exhibited elevated visual-vestibular enhancement responses, compared to only 5% (one single patient) of control subjects. They concluded that, in light of the heavily mediated central pathways examined during visual-vestibular enhancement, this test might provide diagnostic power for patients with migraines manifesting disequilibrium and motion sensitivity. Figure 8–2 illustrates an example of a patient exhibiting a significant (uncontrolled) increase in visual-vestibular enhancement. She also displayed deficits in her smooth pursuit tracking and optokinetic testing. This patient has an autoimmune disease and began reporting chronic difficulty with recurrent (nonpositionally provoked) vertigo and dizziness for 6 to12 months. Additional vestibular testing provided ancillary evidence to support a unilateral left ear peripheral weakness, however, these VVOR and ocular motor data also provided evidence to support a concomitant central lesion that may involve the vestibulo cerebellum (flocculi and paraflocculi). Although this patient's VOR suppression testing was within normal limits, these data may offer some evidence to suggest a slowed compensation process that may be mediated by the autoimmune disease.

Summary of Visual-Vestibular Interaction Testing

Conducting rotational visual-vestibular interaction testing offers the clinician with a direct insight into the central neurophysiological function of the smooth pursuit, optokinetic, and the flocculonodular pathways. These direct and indirect pathways are essential to enable contributions provided by the visual system to either augment the deficient VOR, or cancel it during

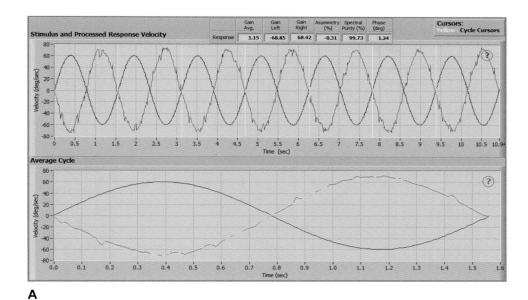

A

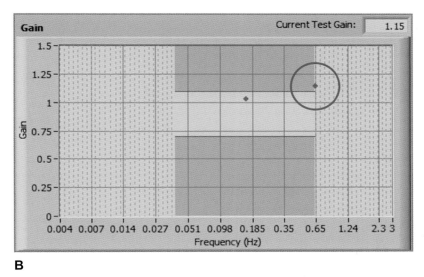

B

FIGURE 8–2. Abnormally high visual-vestibular enhancement in a patient with an autoimmune disease. **A.** Individual and average cycle data shows the high VOR gain in relation to the chair (head) velocity of 60°/second. **B.** Average visual-vestibular enhancement gain of 1.15 is plotted and circled in green.

eye-head tracking. Although these pathways can be assessed during ocular motor testing, the confounding factors of patient performance and subjective variability during ocular motor testing provides evidence for visual-vestibular interaction testing to be the preferred method for assessment of these central pathways. Rotational visual-vestibular testing offers a precisely controlled stimulus, and the ability to record an autonomic reflex response that essentially negates the confound-

ing effects of poor ocular motor performance or attention issues. Figure 8–3 illustrates an example of a patient with a rare cerebellar degenerative disease. The degenerative nature of the disorder has severely reduced the cerebellum's control over the VOR, which is documented in this patient's failure of fixation suppression, as well as the significant reduction in the enhancement of the visual system to the VOR. Concomitant abnormalities are also identified in saccadic

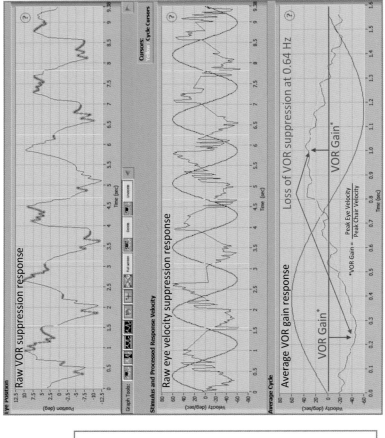

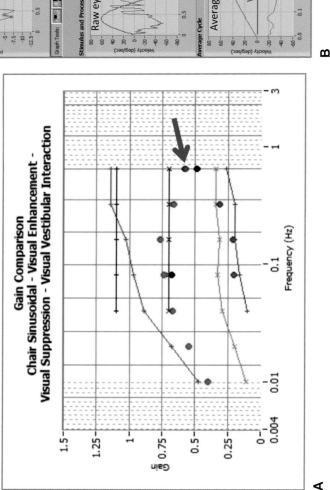

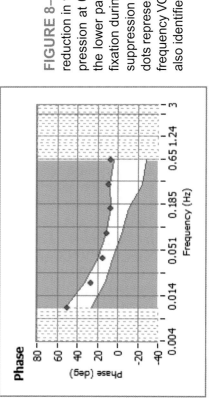

FIGURE 8–3. Patient with a rare cerebellar degenerative disorder. Data reveal a significant reduction in visual fixation (suppression) of VOR (**A**), and a near complete loss of VOR suppression at 0.64 Hz (**B**) where the abnormal VOR gain during visual fixation (identified in the lower panel in image **B**) is essentially identical to the VOR gain exhibited without visual fixation during SHA testing (*green arrow on image* **A**). **A.** Blue dots represent abnormal VOR suppression (*above blue line*). Red dots represent normal VOR gain (*between black lines*). Black dots represent abnormal visual-vestibular enhancement (*below black lines*). Concomitant high frequency VOR phase leads (**C**) and saccadic horizontal and vertical smooth pursuit (**D**) were also identified. *continues*

272

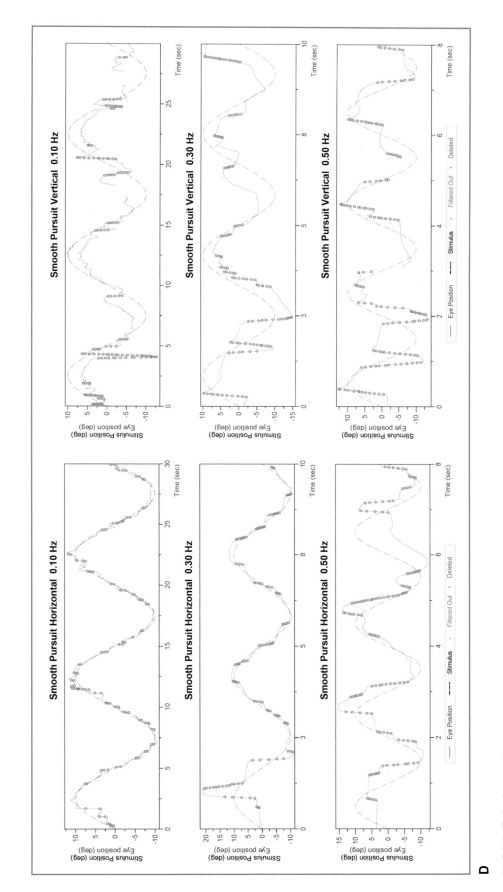

FIGURE 8–3. *continued*

273

smooth pursuit, increased high frequency VOR phase, and reduced performance on optokinetic testing (optokinetic data not shown). As one would expect, this patient has significant difficulty with ambulation, image stabilization, as well as any control over smooth motor movements.

ECCENTRIC ROTATIONAL TESTING

Eccentric rotation testing is also known as dynamic unilateral centrifugation testing (DUC), or simply unilateral centrifugation testing (UCF). Fundamentally, eccentric rotation testing is a test of utricular function that imparts a linear acceleration force (centripetal force) on an outwardly displaced utricle. Wetzig and colleagues (1990) were the first to describe the value of eccentric rotational testing in the identification of bilateral otolith asymmetries in man. Eccentric rotation consists of off-center rotations whereby the center point (z-axis) of rotation is located through the vertical plane of either utricle while the other utricle is displaced outward. Figures 8–4 and 8–5 illustrate the differences in linear forces experienced between on-center rotation and off-center rotation as they relate each respective utricle. During such lateral linear acceleration, the laterally displaced utricle experiences a centrifugation (lateral-linear) force as it endures *off-center* (eccentric) vertical

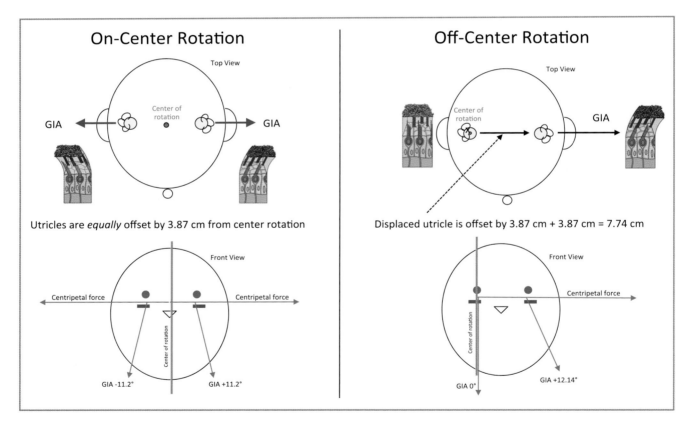

FIGURE 8–4. Diagram illustrating the differences in applied GIA force across the utricular epithelium (blue rectangles) for each ear during on-center rotation versus off-center (eccentric) rotation. During on-center rotation, a theoretical equal GIA (11.2°) is applied across opposing utricular epithelia. During eccentric rotation, a single utricle identifies the center point of rotation and, therefore, perceives zero GIA as no lateral force is applied across the epithelium. However, the opposing (eccentric) utricular epithelium receives a theoretical maximum GIA of 12.14° (using a 300°/sec velocity stimulus and an offset of 7.74 cm, which is the average interaural utricular distance) (Brey et al., 2008a).

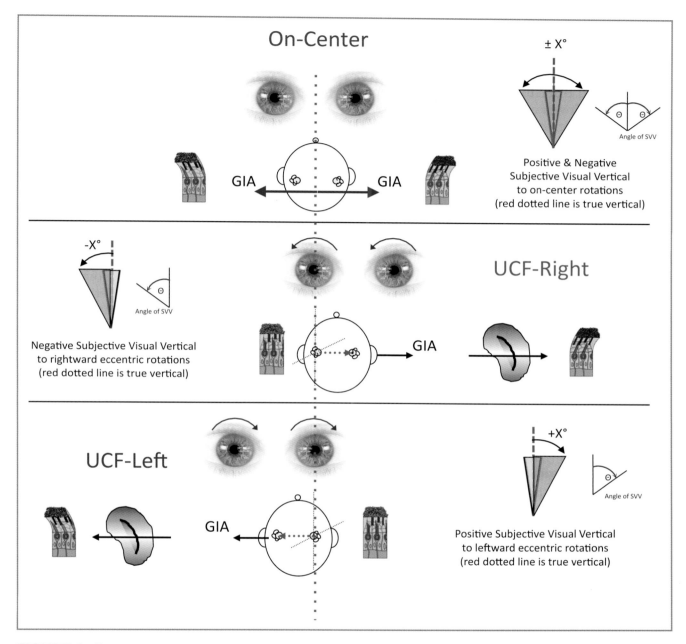

FIGURE 8–5. Images illustrating utricluar displacement, the GIA linear force, the physiologic ocular counterroll, and the expected SVV given the indicated rotational paradigm. Red center dotted line indicates the theoretical axis of rotation for all three rotational paradigms.

axis rotation while the contralateral utricle experiences *on-center* rotation rendering it free of any centrifugal stimulating force. As Ödkvist (2001) indicates, eccentric rotation at a constant velocity will provoke centrifugal force acting upon the outwardly displaced utricular maculae. Gresty

and Lempert (2001) suggest that such a lateral-linear acceleration will provoke a "pure otolithic" response that is essentially uncontaminated by the SCCs. There is little-to-no contribution from the semicircular canals to the VOR response, secondary to the habituation of the cupular response during constant velocity rotation (post acceleration stimulus period). This is similar to the habituation of the semicircular reactivity post velocity step acceleration with the exception that the acceleration period prior to eccentric displacement is considerably slower at 5°/sec². As a result of such slow acceleration, the degree of cupular displacement is significantly less (in accordance with the cupular pendular model) than during VST. Consequently, the VOR response is subsequently less and habituates more quickly once the target velocity stimulus is achieved. Thus, the contributions from the horizontal semicircular canals are considerably less and extinguish rapidly following the acceleration period. The exact methods for eccentric testing will be discussed shortly. First, let us consider the anatomical substrate and normal physiological response that occurs during eccentric rotational testing.

Anatomical and Physiological Response During Eccentric Rotation

Anatomically speaking, a centrifugal force will be imparted on the eccentrically (laterally) driven utricle causing an excitatory response from the medial hemimacula as well as a cross-striolar inhibitory response from the lateral hemimacula (Figure 8–6) (Leigh & Zee, 2006).

Subsequent to this translation force (t), a primary ocular counterroll (c-VOR) and a slight, contralaterally directed slow-phase horizontal nystagmus (t-VOR) occur. The induced ocular counterroll (c-VOR) and horizontal nystagmus (t-VOR) under such dynamic conditions is attributed to the asymmetric neural tonus created from the laterally driven utricular macula under centrifugal force and the quiescent utricular macula receiving on-center rotation (see Figure 8–5). In such cir-

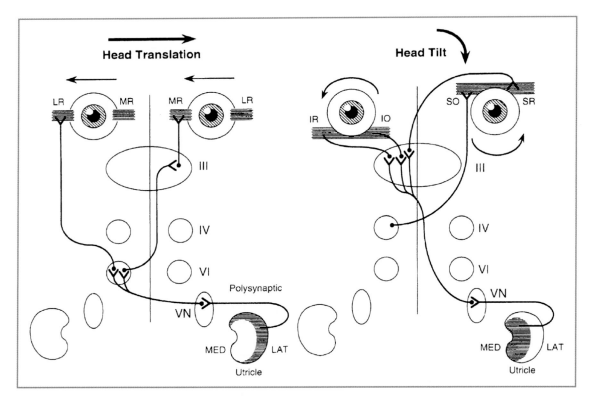

FIGURE 8–6. Utricular pathways for tilt and translation. The medial hemimacula contributes to counterrolling of the eyes by innervating the vertical torsional muscles. The lateral hemimacula contributes to a contraversive horizontal slow phase by innervating the horizontal muscles. From *The Neurology of Eye Movements* (5th ed., p. 75) by R. J. Leigh and D. S. Zee, 2015, New York, NY: Oxford University Press. Reprinted with permission.

Centrifugal Force Versus Centripetal Force: Which Is Correct?

Actually, the force present during eccentric testing is one of centripetal force. All forces applied during angular velocity from a center point are referred to as centripetal forces. However, centrifugal force is often used synonymously, so much so, that the idea of centripetal force is seldom referenced. The actual concept of centrifugal force is a fictitious, or imaginary, one, and often inappropriately applied—as it is in this case. This text will continue to use the term centrifugal to reference the applied force to the outwardly displaced utricle, as it is most commonly reported elsewhere (and even applied to the test's name). However, the reader is encouraged to review the differences between a centripetal and centrifugal force, as well as understand the theoretical reference of using centrifugal force to describe the dynamics of eccentric testing.

cumstances, where an abrupt acceleration is imparted eccentrically with a constant level of *acceleration*, the *initial* ocular response would be that of a horizontal compensatory eye movement contraversive to the direction of applied lateral force. This would occur at a relatively short latency (15–60 msec) secondary to excitation of the lateral hemimacula of the laterally driven utricle, and subsequent firing of afferent neurons in the superior branch of the vestibular nerve. If the centrifugal force is sustained, similar to that of the sustained tilting of the head, a slow ocular counterroll (cyclotorsion) occurs. The latency of this response is slower (than the t-VOR) at approximately 300 msec (Gresty & Lempert, 2001). As previously stated, an ocular counterroll occurs secondary to excitation of the medial hemimacula of the laterally driven utricle and subsequent firing of afferent neurons in the superior branch of the vestibular nerve.

Gravitational Inertial Acceleration (GIA) and the OCR-GIA Slope

In the presence of the induced ocular cyclotorsion (during eccentric constant velocity), a healthy patient often reports a consequent perception of subjective tilt. The degree of ocular cyclotorsion and subsequent subjective tilt is determined by a number of factors, specifically, the velocity of the eccentric rotation, the constant gravitational force, and the distance of otolith displacement from the center of axis rotation. Collectively, these factors produce a new "inertial force vertical" (g), also known as the gravitational inertial acceleration (GIA), with a mathematical relationship determined by the equation:

$$g = \frac{r\omega^2}{G}$$

Where: (g) equals the degrees relative to true vertical (GIA);

(r) equals the radial displacement from center axis of rotation;

(ω) equals the angular velocity of rotation; and

(G) equals the earth's gravitational acceleration constant (980.7 cm/sec^2)

The combined forces of eccentric angular acceleration ($r\omega^2$), and the earth's gravitational (vertical) acceleration (G), determine the degrees of subjective tilt (g) relative to the earth's true vertical. The resultant force is known as the gravitational inertial acceleration, or GIA and is represented by (g). In short, the GIA (g) is a function of the rotary chair angular velocity multiplied by the radial offset distance from the center of rotation to the eccentrically located utricle divided by the gravitational constant (G) (Brey, McPherson & Lynch, 2008a). Let us consider an example. Using a rotational velocity (ω) of 300°/sec, a radius of 7.74 cm, and where G is the gravitation constant of

981.7 cm/s^2, the resultant GIA (g) can be expressed by the following example equation:

$$GIA = arcTAN \left[\frac{r\left(\frac{\omega}{180°}\pi\right)^2}{G} \right] \frac{180°}{\pi}$$

$$GIA = arcTAN \left[\frac{0.0774m\left(\frac{300\,d/_s}{180°}\pi\right)^2}{9.81\,m/_{s^2}} \right] \frac{180°}{\pi}$$

$$GIA = arcTAN \left[\frac{2.108799}{9.81\,m/_{s^2}} \right] \frac{180°}{\pi}$$

$$GIA = arcTAN\,[0.21496]\frac{180°}{\pi}$$

$$GIA = 0.21174\,radian\frac{180°}{\pi}$$

$$GIA = 12.41°$$

The resulting GIA during the maximal point of chair displacement used in this example (0.0774 m or 7.74 cm) is therefore ±12.14° relative to true vertical (see Figure 8–4). This is, essentially, the new perceived subjective vertical tilt felt by an individual undergoing such eccentric rotation.

During eccentric rotation, a new "inertial force vertical" is integrated by the laterally displaced healthy utricle, and the resultant c-VOR and t-VOR ensues. Perceived postural tilt in the healthy individual is in the direction of lateral dis-

placement. However, the primary ocular counterroll in the upright-seated healthy individual will create a subjective visual vertical perception opposite that of the subjective tilt, as the ocular counterroll attempts to maintain the vertical meridians of the retinae in relation to the earth's true vertical (see Figure 8–5). For example, during eccentric rotation with the right utricle projected laterally, an upright healthy individual will perceive a subjective postural tilt to the right. To compensate for this perceived postural tilt, the right utricle produces a compensatory ocular counterroll to the left in order to maintain "vertical uprightness" in relation to the earth's true vertical (see Figure 8–5). Ultimately, the perception of "vertical" during eccentric rotation is the sum of the two forces (gravity and centripetal acceleration), which gives a new perceived force (angle) that is tilted toward the center of axis rotation (Raphan & Cohen, 1996; Wuyts et al., 2003). However, in reality, the actual ocular counterroll and subsequent subjective visual vertical is only a proportion of the sum of the forces, secondary to the influence of cognitive factors.

The rate of OCR change produced during the eccentric displacement of the chair can be determined once the GIA is known. Using the calculated GIA value (12.14° in this example), an OCR-GIA slope can be calculated by dividing the rise (change is OCR) by the run (±12.14° tilt as a result of dynamic displacement) for each eye during each eccentric position (UCF-Right and UCF-Left). The OCR-GIA slope is always negative

---

Why is the GIA Zero Degrees During On-Center Rotations?

As a point of clarification, the OCR-GIA slope during on-center rotation is theoretically null (equal) as the radial offset distance from the center of rotation to each utricle is equal, which negates the opposing radial g-force accelerations and produces no consequential OCR (see Figure 8–5). During such on-center (centric) rotations, an equal lateral GIA force of 11.2° is applied to each utricle leaving only the upward acceleration applied by the downward pull of gravity (Wuyts, Hoppenbrouwers, Pauwels, & Van de Heyning, 2003) (see Figure 8–4). This on-center rotational condition applies a theoretical equal and opposite afferent utricular response (i.e., equal utricular sensitivity) causing an absence of any observed ocular cyclotorsion in either direction, as well as an upright perception of earth-vertical as measured by SVV (Böhmer & Mast, 1999).

secondary to the counterroll nature of the ocular response (Figure 8–7).

GIA/OCR Linear Regression Model

Research in eccentric rotational testing has identified a *linear* relationship between the degree of ocular counterroll (OCR) and gravitational inertial acceleration (GIA). This linear relationship is known as the OCR-GIA slope. Wetzig et al. (1990), and later Wuyts and colleagues (2003) identified this linear relationship between the distance of lateral displacement during eccentric rotations and degree of ocular counterroll. Moreover, Wetzig, Hofstetter-Degen, Maurer, and von Baumgarter (1992) identified, and Wuyts and colleagues (2003) later confirmed, that the slope of this linear relationship is dependent on (or reflective of) utricular

reactivity. Although a linear relationship persists in patients with unilateral or bilateral utricular dysfunction, the slope of this relationship varies with utricular reactivity. This is significant because this predictable linear relationship could be used to lateralize utricular dysfunction based on a linear regression model.

The neurophysiological substrate of the utricular VOR dictates that a lateral translation to the right (positive GIA) during sustained rotation will induce an ocular counterroll to the left (negative OCR), whereas a lateral translation to the left (negative GIA) induces an ocular counterroll to the right (positive OCR) (Wuyts et al., 2003) (see Figure 8–5). The degree of OCR in relation to the lateral displacement of the eccentric utricle uniquely reflects the sensitivity of only the laterally displaced utricle. The more laterally displaced the eccentric rotation is to the left, the greater the

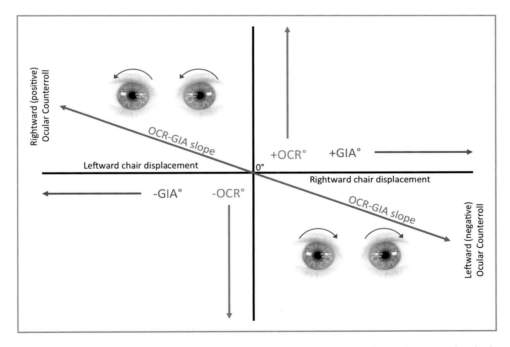

FIGURE 8–7. Theoretical OCR-GIA slope. With dynamic leftward eccentric chair displacement (negative GIA), the cVOR produces an increasing rightward (positive) ocular counterroll. Conversely, with dynamic rightward eccentric chair displacement (positive GIA), the cVOR produces an increasing leftward (negative) ocular counterroll. The relationship between OCR to GIA has been shown to be linear (Wuyts et al., 2003). That is, in a healthy and symmetrical vestibular system, the amount of change in OCR (degrees) is the same for every degree of GIA produced by lateral displacement of the chair (to a theoretical limit). The slope of the OCR-GIA function will always be negative due to the physiologic counterroll inherent to the cVOR.

theoretical OCR will be to the right (more positive). Conversely, the more laterally displaced the eccentric rotation is to the right, the greater the theoretical OCR will be to the left (more negative). The linear regression model predicts that all data points between the eccentric extremes will fall in a straight line, whereby the slope of the regression line directly reflects the sensitivity of a utricular system. Given two equally sensitivity and functional utricles, the preponderance of positive and negative degree of OCR should be equal when the GIA equals zero. Therefore, by applying the linear regression model to the GIA/OCR data, two response parameters can be used to describe utricular sensitivity and symmetry; slope of the linear regression line and the and the intercept of the regression line at 0° GIA, respectively.

Slope of the GIA/OCR Linear Regression Model

The slope of the linear regression model reflects the sensitivity of a utricular system. Identification of a steeper slope indicates a more robust OCR with respect to a greater lateral displacement of eccentric rotation, thus reflecting greater utricular sensitivity to the applied centrifugal acceleration. Wuyts et al. (2003) reported a mean GIA/OCR slope (sensitivity) of −0.232 (SD 0.054) for healthy participants. Conversely, a decreased slope reflects a decrease in the induced OCR and a subsequent decrease in the sensitivity of one or both utricles (Wuyts et al., 2003). If, in fact, the relationship of GIA to OCR is linear and independent of utricular status, one would predict that the slope of the regression line for an individual with a complete loss of unilateral utricular function to be half of the physiologic gain of a normal utricular system. This is, indeed, the case as presented by Wuyts and colleagues (2003). These authors documented a 50% reduction of the GIA/OCR slope (sensitivity) in a group of patients with unilateral vestibular dysfunction (UVD) when compared to the GIA/OCR slope in a group of healthy participants (-0.104, SD 0.036 right UVD patients; −0.107, SD 0.026 left UVD patients). For patients with bilateral vestibular loss, the GIA/OCR slope is at or near 0° indicating little to no utricular sensitivity.

Intercept of the GIA/OCR Linear Regression Model

The intercept of the GIA/OCR linear regression model at 0° GIA reflects the physiologic preponderance of a utricular system. In short, the intercept indicates the balance of utricular physiology. In a healthy individual with near balanced utricular gain (sensitivity), the intercept of the regression line would be expected to be at, or near, zero degrees. In the case of equal utricular sensitivity during on-center rotation, both utricles are subjected to equal and opposite centrifugal forces, which essentially cancel opposing right and left afferent signals leading to no measurable OCR and earth-upright vertical sensation (Böhmer & Mast, 1999; Clarke, Schönfeld & Helling, 2003). That is, the observed prevalence of positive OCR with lateral displacements of eccentric rotation to the left (negative GIA), and the observed prevalence of negative OCR with lateral displacements of eccentric rotation to the right (positive GIA) would be similar, only in opposite directions. Consequently, the slope of the linear regression line in this case would inevitably intersect 0° GIA, at or near, 0° OCR. However, in the case of unilateral asymmetry, or complete utricular loss, a preponderance of either negative or positive OCR is elicited by the stronger (more intact) utricular end organ, even during on-center rotation. The relative balance between utricular sensitivity will dictate a more positive or negative OCR with respect to the GIA. Although this OCR preponderance will be most evident during eccentric rotations in each direction, a slight bias will also exist during *centric* (on center) rotations identified by the positive or negative intercept of the regression line from 0° GIA. This occurs as a result of an unbalanced utricular tonus (secondary to a UVD) that produces a measureable OCR during on-center rotations because the asymmetric utricles no longer interpret the opposing centrifugal force equally. A resultant ocular counterroll is subsequently produced by the utricle with greater sensitivity. A positive OCR at 0° GIA reflects a greater bias or preponderance from the left utricle, whereas a negative OCR at 0° GIA reflects a great bias or preponderance from the right utricle (Wuyts et al., 2003). Figure 8–8 illustrates the theoretical bias and OCR-GIA slope for a unilateral utricular loss for each ear.

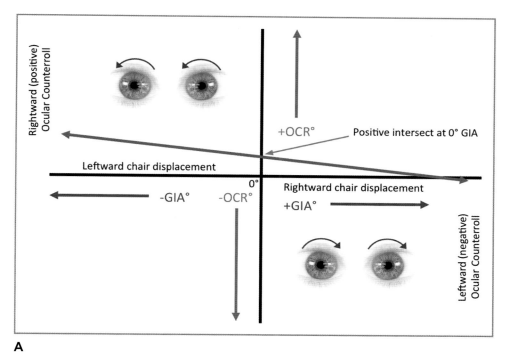

A

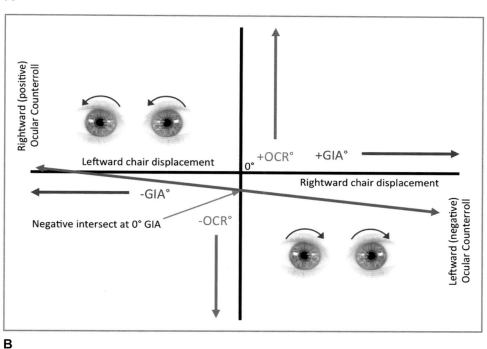

B

FIGURE 8–8. Theoretical OCR-GIA slope for a right unilateral utricular loss (**A**), and a left unilateral utricular loss (**B**). For a left unilateral utricular loss (**A**), on-center rotations (0° GIA) produces a positive ocular counterroll due to the stronger intact left utricular reactivity. This is evident by a positive-intersect of the OCR-GIA slope at 0° GIA. Conversely, for a right unilateral utricular loss (**B**), on-center rotations (0° GIA) produces a negative ocular counterroll due to the stronger intact right utricular reactivity. This is evident by a negative-intersect of the OCR-GIA slope at 0° GIA. The utricular asymmetry will produce an on-center rotation bias that should (theoretically) consistently produce an ocular counterroll toward the lesion ear. The slope of the OCR-GIA function will continue to be negative due to the physiologic counterroll inherent to the cVOR; however, the slope will be theoretically half that of the normal bilaterally intact system (Wuyts et al., 2003).

The intercept data would also suggest that dynamic SVV testing during on-center rotation could have significant clinical relevance. Böhmer & Mast (1999) specifically indicated that during *on-center* rotations, unilateral vestibular disordered patients would perceive a lateral tilt provoked by the intact ear (unilateral GIA) and should, consequently, align an SVV that was tilted toward the lesioned side. This measure is significant as these data provide evidence to support a key clinical concept; that the use of dynamic SVV testing during on-center rotation may be useful in lateralizing compensated utricular UVD simply by comparing the direction of SVV tilt to that of the static SVV measure. In the case of a UVD, on-center rotation could effectively produce a utricular afferent asymmetry, similar to a lateral GIA force that is capable of inducing an OCR and SVV tilt similar to that during UCF testing, although *without* the need for enhanced eccentric rotation protocols. Although this method may only be effective for complete unilateral utricular loss, any degree of asymmetry in bilateral utricular dysfunction, or partial unilateral utricular dysfunction, may require more robust stimuli and enhanced methods of eccentric rotational testing to produce reliable data. The research supporting this premise, however, is currently lacking.

Finally, it is important that the slope and intercept be interpreted in conjunction with one another. The slope will assist in the identification of utricular sensitivity, whereas the intercept will reveal a potential lateral bias (or weakness) in utricular function. A shallow slope with a concomitant positive intercept would indicate right utricular dysfunction. Whereas, a shallow slope with a concomitant negative intercept would suggest left utricular dysfunction. A shallow slope with an intercept near or at zero would be consistent with bilateral utricular dysfunction.

Eccentric Rotational Test Methods

Now that we have a good understanding of the complex neurophysiological response that occurs during eccentric rotation testing, let us now consider the clinical methods by which patients are tested. Prior to rotations, care should be taken to ensure the patient is positioned as near the center of rotation as possible, both in the nasion-occipital axis position, as well as the interaural axis. Although this is important for *all* rotational tests, it is even more imperative during eccentric rotational testing. Positioning the patient over the precise center of rotation will help to ensure the right and left vestibular systems are receiving equal GIA during on-center rotations, as well as pure unilateral GIA during eccentric rotations. A plumb bob can easily be used to help position the patient near the exact center of rotation prior to securing them in place with the various head and shoulder belt restraints.

Prior to performing eccentric rotations, patients first undergo an on-center rotational paradigm using the same stimuli protocol as the eccentric rotation protocol. That being said, the basic eccentric test protocol is designed to measure patient's SVV and OCR during on-center rotation followed by both right and left eccentric rotations.

Eccentric Rotational Stimuli

During eccentric (and on-center) rotational testing, secured patients are subjected to a slow, on-center acceleration (~5°/sec²) until the predetermined target velocity is reached (if using a target velocity of 300°/sec, the acceleration period will be 60 seconds at 5°/sec²). The direction of rotation is generally nasioncentric (i.e., clockwise rotations during left eccentric displacements and counterclockwise rotations during right eccentric displacements). The reason for nasioncentric rotations is discussed below under "Factors Impacting Eccentric Rotational Testing." The target velocity stimulus can vary but is generally quite robust.

The target velocity is also largely dependent by the degree of lateral inertia force (GIA) desired across the outwardly displaced utricle, which is, in turn, dependent on the amount of lateral displacement. Ultimately, the stronger the lateral force (GIA) applied across the utricle, the stronger the physiologic response. Therefore, given the often-diminutive physiological cyclotorsion response elicited from eccentric rotational studies, the best outcomes usually come from either a robust angular velocity or a large lateral displacement (or both). Recall from our discussion above regarding the inverse relationship of the inertial force vertical that produces the OCR; the further the displacement from center, the less velocity required to achieve the same GIA and, subsequently, similar ocular cyclotorsion and subjective vertical tilt. In light of this relationship, eccentric paradigms of 100 cm displacement may require only a rotational velocity of 120° per second whereas a 4 cm displacement may require up to 300° to 400° per second (or more), for an equivocal physiologic response. Figure 8–9 depicts the comparative GIA with respect to two lateral displacements for a variety of angular velocity stimuli. It can clearly be seen from Figure 8–9 that the degree of lateral displacement from the center of rotation has a significant impact on the GIA. Unfortunately, no standard test paradigms currently exist. However, the variable of displacement versus angular velocity is of (relatively) minor significance because the resultant subjective vertical tilt (GIA) can easily be predicted given the equation $g = (r\omega^2) + G$. That being said, there are advantages and disadvantages for choosing the

appropriate angular velocity and degree of lateral displacement, both of which will be discussed below when review factors that impact eccentric rotation testing.

Once the target constant velocity stimulus has been achieved, the chair is then dynamically displaced off-center (i.e., laterally moves off-center after completing acceleration and *during* constant high velocity rotation). Similar to determining the target angular velocity, the distance of chair displacement is entirely dependent upon the degree of lateral force desired and the target angular velocity.

Eccentric Response Measures

Universal to most testing paradigms is a period of sustained eccentric rotation at a constant target angular velocity (e.g., 300°/sec). Once the sustained eccentric angular velocity has been achieved and the angular SCC response has completely dissipated in accordance with the cupular pendular model (i.e., approximately 3 time decay constants

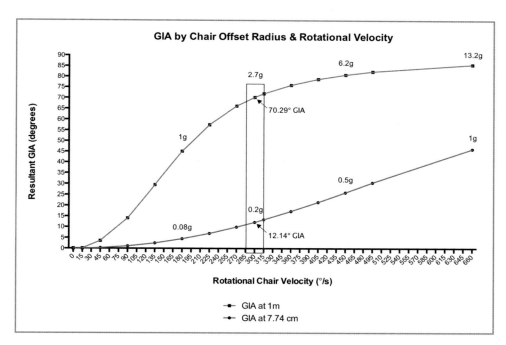

FIGURE 8–9. Graph depicting the degree of GIA (measured in degrees) as a function of chair displacement (radial offset) and angular velocity. The rectangle highlights the difference in the amount of GIA produced during a 300° angular velocity stimulus between a radial offset of the chair by 1 m (*red line*) versus 7.74 cm (*green line*). The respective g-force accelerations are shown for various angular velocity stimuli.

Non-Dynamic Eccentric Rotation Paradigms

At times, eccentric rotational testing is also conducted without "dynamic" displacement. Some rotational paradigms actually begin accelerating to the target velocity with the chair already displaced in the eccentric position. Historically, this method was routinely performed as a "dynamic" displacement of the chair required specialized lateral drive components within the torque motor. Even today, non-dynamic methods of eccentric rotations continue to be performed, particularly when eccentric rotations involve large displacements from the center of rotation. Such rotations involving large eccentric radii (e.g., ≥ 1 m) have a distinct advantage of producing a significant increase in lateral force that requires a relatively low angular velocity stimulus. This can also be explained by the mathematical inverse relationship between velocity and displacement, given the equation $g = (r\omega^2)/G$, and is further illustrated in Figure 8–9. Incredibly large g-force accelerations, up to 40 g's, have been generated using extreme centrifuges that have an exceptionally long radial displacement and high angular velocity, such as the Johnsville Centrifuge (see Figure 1–17).

or 30 seconds), a series of subjective visual vertical measures are presented during eccentric rotation. Although not discussed at length here, subjective visual horizontal (SVH) testing can also be performed in the same manner as SVV testing is conducted. The goal of SVV testing is to capture and quantify the degree of cyclotorsion generated by the c-VOR during eccentric rotation and applied lateral inertial force (GIA). This is performed by having the patient adjust a diode LED bar or laser target (usually a vertical line) to what is perceived by the patient to best represent true vertical (or horizontal). Multiple independent SVV measures (6–10 trials) should be obtained in each rotational condition (on-center as well as right and left eccentric rotations), from which a mean subjective tilt is calculated. Sufficient time should be given to the patient to complete each SVV trial (approximately 10–15 seconds). Concomitant to the SVV measures, an independent measure of the degree of ocular cyclotorsion, or OCR, can also be recorded. Although this measure is best acquired through sclera coils, modern videographic recording techniques are able to capture and calculate the degree of ocular torsion (provided that the manufacturer's software is capable of ocular torsion tracking). Again, for on-center rotations (prior to conducting eccentric rotations), displacement of the chair is not performed and measures of SVV and OCR are

conducted during on-center constant velocity rotation prior to the chair decelerating back to 0°/sec.

Following sustained eccentric rotation and SVV testing, the chair is once again returned to the center of rotation before decelerating back to 0°/sec velocity. The opposing utricle is then examined using essentially the same rotational protocol; only that rotation is performed in the opposite direction while maintaining nasioncentric rotation. Subjective visual vertical and OCR measures are recorded and the chair is once again returned to center and decelerated back to 0°/sec velocity. Figure 8–10 depicts a rotation and data collection paradigm for both on-center and eccentric rotations. The presentation of right versus left eccentric displacements should be delivered with a sufficient inter-stimulus interval in order to ensure quiescence of the physiological response. Inter-stimulus intervals of at least 5 minutes have been proposed (Akin, Murnane, Pearson, Byrd, & Kelly, 2011).

Factors Impacting Eccentric Rotational Testing

In light of the complexities of eccentric rotational testing, many factors can impact the validity, reliability, and overall significance of data collected. Such factors would include the degree of lateral displacement from the center of rotation, nasion-

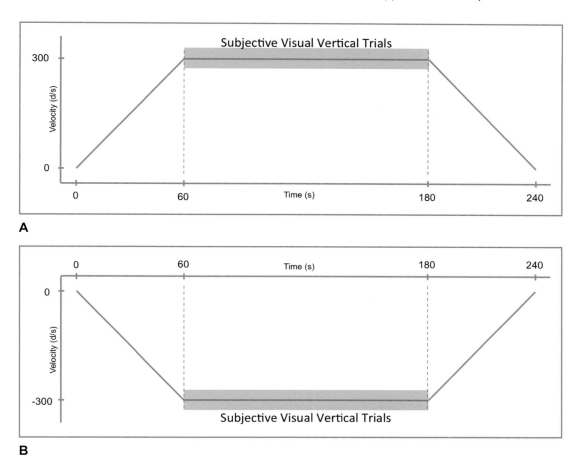

FIGURE 8–10. Four different rotational paradigms. **A.** On-Center (On-Axis) Clockwise Rotational SVV Paradigm. **B.** On-Center (On-Axis) Counterclockwise Rotational SVV Paradigm. *continues*

centric versus occipitalcentric rotation, starting angle and direction of the visual stimulus, and any ocular abnormalities such as astigmatism, pre-existing ocular torsion, or visual/somatosensory memory. Let us briefly review each here.

Degree of Lateral Displacement. Most current eccentric rotation paradigms laterally displace the utricle of interest to a point where the contralateral utricle is over the center of axis rotation. This paradigm attempts to isolate and lateralize a single utricular response by attempting to "silence" the neural response of the utricle receiving on-center axis rotation. The degree of off-axis displacement, however, seems to be one of loose academic agreement. Some paradigms reports lateral displacement by as little as 3.87 cm (Brey et al.,

2008a), whereas others report as great as 100 cm (Ödkvist, 2001). The mean distance between utricles has been reported to be 7.22 (±0.06) (Nowé et al., 2003), to as much as 7.74 cm (Brey et al., 2008a). Determining the distance from the center of the head to the individual utricles calculates to a distance of 3.61 to 3.87 cm. In light of these data, a value of ±4 cm of lateral displacement is sometimes used in order to approximate one utricle directly over the axis of rotation. In doing so, the off-axis utricle will be approximately 8 cm from the center of rotation (given idiosyncrasies between patient head size, etc). Although on-axis utricular rotation appears to conform to sound scientific methods, the degree of lateral displacement, and the consequential effects on ocular cyclotorsion, have yet to be fully determined.

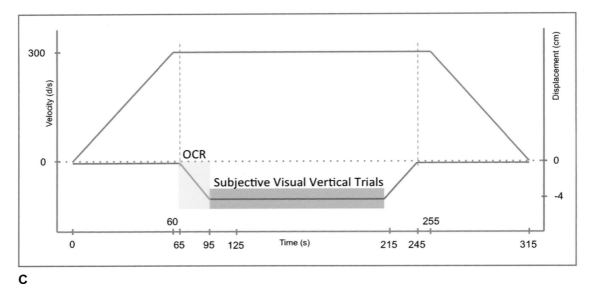

C

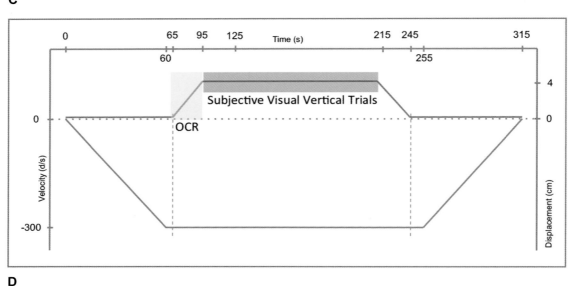

D

FIGURE 8–10. *continued* **C.** UCF-Left Eccentric Rotational SVV Paradigm [using rightward (clockwise) yaw rotation]. **D.** UCF-Right Eccentric Rotational SVV Paradigm [using leftward (counterclockwise) yaw rotation]. For all rotational paradigms, blue line represents yaw rotational velocity; red line represents chair displacement (4 cm); green shaded area represents time period for SVV measures; and yellow shaded area represents dynamic chair displacement and time period of active ocular counterroll (OCR) measures.

Direction of Rotation. The direction of eccentric rotation is likely critical to the degree of cyclotorsion as well as the perceived subjective visual vertical. In light of the anatomical orientation and morphology of the utricle, it would not be surprising if the centripetal force applied to the utricle would be different during nasion-centric versus occipital-centric rotations. Most test paradigms have stressed the importance of maintaining nasion-centric rotations, as angular rotations in the occipital-centric direction are not only functionally less relevant, but are presumed to have a significant difference in excitation pattern of the elliptically shaped utricle (Ödkvist, 2001). Although data regarding these comparisons (nasioncentric versus occipitalcentric) have yet to be published, it would stand to reason that, unless testing was conducted in the same direction of rotation, results between utricles could potentially be unequivocal. In fact, Ödkvist (2001) has argued that eccentric rotation protocols dictate that the patient should be seated some distance from the center of rotation and *facing* the direction of rotation. However, to date there are no reliable data indicating the difference between directions of rotation on the utricular response.

Starting Tilt Angle and Direction. A variable that has received little, if any, attention is the starting skew angle of the misaligned vertical (or horizontal) stimulus during subjective visual vertical (horizontal) testing. It is unclear as to whether or not the degree of initial skewness would have a significant impact on the final judgment of subjective visual vertical. Visual and vestibular memories have been shown to impart a significant impact on the SVV (Berthoz & Rousié, 2001; Van Nechel, Toupet, & Bodson, 2001). Moreover, it is even less clear whether or not the initial skew angle in relation to the patient's altered subjective vertical would have a significant impact on subjective vertical testing. These variables have yet to be fully vetted in the normal population.

Monocular Versus Binocular Testing. Extraocular muscle innervation from a single utricle will differ depending upon the ipsilateral versus the contralateral eye. Because of the different extraocular muscle innervation, there exists a slight asymmetry in the degree of ocular torsion exhibited from each eye, depending on which utricle is stimulated (Van Nechel et al., 2001 Vibert, Häusler, & Safran, 1999). Evidence has also shown a smaller standard deviation of subjective vertical alignment using binocular rather than monocular vision (Van Nechel et al., 2001). It was postulated that this is due to the fusion of the binocular cues that effectively 'corrects' any idiopathic cyclodeviations between the two eyes often found in the normal population. Van Nechel and colleagues (2001) determined that, if testing were conducted under monocular conditions, such idiopathic monocular cyclodeviations would contribute to a greater deviation in subjective visual vertical measures. Vibert, Häusler, and Safran (1999) investigated the degree of subjective vertical tilt in patients with vestibular disease using both monocular and binocular measurement techniques. In

their study, they identified a greater sensitivity for detecting SVV tilt using a monocular recording method over a binocular method. Moreover, they identified a more robust deviation of the ipsilateral eye to the affected ear. To supplement these findings, Van Nechel and colleagues (2001) measured the degree of monocular versus binocular counterroll in healthy subjects while the head was tilted bidirectionally in the roll plane. They also confirmed an asymmetrical ocular counterroll (although this time in healthy subjects) using the monocular method with a most robust ocular torsion in the ipsilateral eye to head tilt. These data not only support a slightly more robust ipsiversive ocular counterroll both in healthy as well as pathologic patients, but also support a preference for using a monocular method, of measurement when identifying the ocular counterroll response over a binocular method (Dieterich & Brandt, 1992; Van Nechel et al., 2001; Vibert, Häusler, & Safran, 1999).

Conversely, test-retest studies investigating monocular versus binocular recordings of ocular counterroll have revealed no significant differences in OCR between recording methods (Ödkvist, 2001). Ödkvist (2001) reported equivalent ocular measures even if the test is performed with one eye open while the other is closed. These data may have significant relevance during testing, particularly if a study participant, or patient, is noted to have an ocular abnormality, such as that observed in myasthenia gravis, and may require testing with one eye patched. It light of such conflicting reports, further research on the effects of monocular versus binocular recordings is warranted.

Pre-existing Ocular Dysfunction. Any image must first be filtered through the retina and various structures of the eye. It is here where deviations of the visual scene can first be introduced and, at times, even be unfiltered or uncompensated by the cortical eye fields. Such deviations of visual imagery can be altered by frank pathologies like astigmatism, as well as a congenital or acquired ocular cyclotorsion. In fact, an uncorrected oblique astigmatism can alter the perception of visual vertical by as much as 3.8° (Van Nechel et al., 2001). This could spuriously introduce significant artifact in many normative studies of otolith function because patients are rarely screened for any visual myopia or astigmatism. Moreover, ocular motor testing does not effectively identify such visual pathologies and would, consequently, not be identified during routine assessment. Because most rotational testing utilizes some form of goggle or mask, which does not allow for corrective lenses, any significant effect of astigmatism could potentially be unaccounted for. Therefore, it is imperative to determine any ocular abnormalities prior to otolith assessment involving subjective visual vertical/horizontal measures. This determination quickly becomes apparent when collecting normative data during both static and dynamic (eccentric) visual vertical testing. Furthermore, the potential additive effect of an ocular cyclotorsion and/or any astigmatism in a patient with a latent otolith disease could be significant when analyzing and interpreting clinical results.

Presence of Somatosensory Cues. During eccentric rotation, many somatosensory cues can contribute to the subjective sensation of true vertical. Such cues likely occur from the cutaneous pressure receptors, the tendon and muscle receptors, as well as the proprioceptive cervical receptors activated during rotation (Van Nechel et al., 2001). This may have some implications during eccentric rotational testing, as head restraints and straps are often used to ensure cephalic verticality and stability. Although Van Nechel and colleagues (2001) have shown that this constraint does not appear to be relevant when otolithic cues are present, they did show that when otolithic cues were unavailable, secondary to disease, the head restraints and straps could provide an orthogonal reference that could possibly mask a subjective visual vertical deviation. Although testing of the subjective visual vertical in water submersion would likely neutralize such somatosensory cues, such testing is fraught with complexities and may be more representative of a measure of subjective postural vertical rather than subjective visual vertical.

Normative Eccentric Rotational Data

Published data regarding eccentric rotational testing are not only sparse, but many of the reports are difficult to compare secondary to the varying paradigms under which the data were collected. To date, there exist no published reports characterizing the normal effects of various factors affecting utricular function during eccentric rotational testing. Reports have identified subjective visual tilts varying by as much as 20° from true vertical during eccentric rotational testing (Ödkvist, 2001; Tran Ba Huy, & Toupet, 2001).

Work performed at the NIH vestibular lab has established normative reference ranges for both SVV and OCR in response to eccentric and on-center rotations. These data are presented in Figure 8–11 and Appendix B. Testing paradigm for these reference ranges were established using a clockwise rotation for on-center rotations and nasioncentric rotations during eccentric rotations (as depicted in Figure 8–10).

Identifying and Recognizing Otolith Disease

Prior to discussing the clinical applications of SVV, OCR, and OCR-GIA slope data, it is first important to briefly review the symptoms and pathophysiology accompanying otolith disease. Otolith dysfunction in the absence of any damage to the SCCs is likely rare (Van Nechel et al., 2001). In general, the pathophysiology of an otolithic disorder is poorly understood, however, as Gresty, Bronstein, Brandt, and Dieterich (1992) suggest, an otolith disorder should be suspected if a patient describes sensations of linear motion or tilt, or reports specific instabilities of ocular motor, postural orienting, or general imbalance with falls. In light of the biomechanical and morphological complexities of the otolith system, it is not surprising that diagnosing isolated macular dysfunction can be difficult, and is often a process of exclusionary diagnoses (Schönfeld, Helling, & Clarke, 2010).

Symptoms of Otolith Disease

In general, otolith dysfunction will result in three primary symptoms. First, acute otolith disease will often impart visual disturbances, often in the form of vertical or horizontal diplopia, oscillopsia, or subjective skew deviation. Second, acute postural

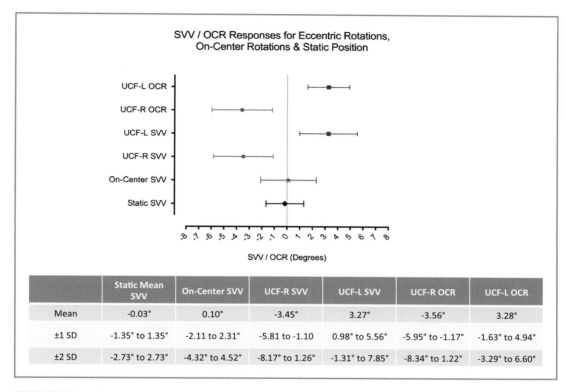

SVV / OCR Responses for Eccentric Rotations, On-Center Rotations & Static Position

	Static Mean SVV	On-Center SVV	UCF-R SVV	UCF-L SVV	UCF-R OCR	UCF-L OCR
Mean	-0.03°	0.10°	-3.45°	3.27°	-3.56°	3.28°
±1 SD	-1.35° to 1.35°	-2.11 to 2.31°	-5.81 to -1.10	0.98° to 5.56°	-5.95° to -1.17°	-1.63° to 4.94°
±2 SD	-2.73° to 2.73°	-4.32° to 4.52°	-8.17° to 1.26°	-1.31° to 7.85°	-8.34° to 1.22°	-3.29° to 6.60°

FIGURE 8–11. Normative reference ranges for subjective visual vertical (SVV) and ocular counterroll (OCR) for the static seated position, on-center rotation, as well as both right and left eccentric rotation conditions. Graph depicts ±1 standard deviation (SD). Also referenced in Appendix B.

changes will occur. These postural changes are often manifested by a postural tilt in the direction of the lesioned otolith. Finally, perceptual changes will be noted in the patient's self-orientation with respect to that of the surrounding environment. Such reports of mismatched self-perception to that of the surrounding environment may include abnormal sensations of levitation, translation, or tilting; inappropriate sensations of moving up or down, similar to that of standing on a floating dock; sensations of lateropulsion, or being pulled to the ground; severe sensations of disorientation, dissociation, or illusory self-propulsion; and even hallucinations. Other mismatched self-perceptions of otolith origin have been specifically labeled as discrete disorders such as mal de débarquement, orthostatic hypotension, and motion sickness (Gresty et al., 1992).

Most otolithic disorders will also share common presenting or historical reports by the patient. First, most are triggered by translational or static movements. Second, most patients will report an exacerbation of symptoms when the visual and/or proprioceptive surroundings are altered. Finally, there is a highly variable pattern of reported intensity and duration of symptoms, often within the same patient. This is likely secondary to the otoliths multisystemic connections and autonomic reflexes, the mirrored redundancy of bilateral maculae, the rate of central compensation, and the degree/location of macula damage.

Pathophysiology of Otolith Disease

The pathophysiology of otolith dysfunction is as complex as the morphology and physiology of maculae reflexes themselves. As a result, the pathophysiology of otolith dysfunction is poorly understood (Brandt, 2001). Any dysfunction of the otoliths will invariably cause a change in the way linear acceleration, gravity perception, and head tilt perception are integrated. In a diseased or damaged state, any linear or static tilt force will be aberrantly perceived by the damaged maculae. Symptoms of otolith disease are likely caused by incorrect signaling from the maculae for the correct control of upright posture, self-motion, and spatial orientation and awareness. These symptoms are likely exacerbated during movement, which can often provoke strange reports of disorientation, detachment, or postural instability that can even contribute to feelings of generalized psychological disturbances, anxiety, or panic (Tran Ba Huy, & Toupet, 2001).

However, it is important to consider that the pathophysiology of otolith dysfunction is dependent on the specific region(s) of the macula(e) affected. Given the morphologic segregation of the hair cell bundles and afferentation structure, as well as the physiological differences governing the t-VOR and the c-VOR, localized damage to a small area of the macula would likely fail to impact all aspects of otolith function. If this were to occur, it is likely that only minor and discrete symptoms would be reported. This occurs, in part, because a single macula contains a population of sensory cells that is capable of sensing and signaling movement in any linear direction. Furthermore, in light of the omni-orientation of hair cells and stereocilla bundles within each macula and the redundancy provided by the homologous maculae on the contralateral side, any localized destruction of hair cells within a specific region on a single macula would likely be compensated by the opposing, undamaged macula in the contralesional ear within a few weeks (Tran Ba Huy, & Toupet, 2001). Ultimately, it is this mirrored anatomical symmetry and neurophysiology between opposing maculae that offers a highly efficient compensation process that quickly occurs in response to unilateral impairment (Tran Ba Huy, & Toupet, 2001).

Otolith Function Following Unilateral Vestibular Damage

In the presence of a unilateral otolith disorder, or significant asymmetry, the clinical manifestations are a primary postural tilt toward the hypotonic side, as well as cyclotorsion of the eyes toward the lesioned side. This cyclotorsional response in the static upright-seated position can be attributed to an unopposed tonus of the medial portion of the surviving (contralesional) utricle (Gresty & Lempert, 2001). Such a skew of the ocular system would undoubtedly result in the aberrant perception of subjective visual vertical. This indeed, is, the case, as was initially exploited first in 1970 by Friedman in the form of the visual vertical test of unilateral otolith dysfunction.

Under dynamic conditions, the ocular manifestations of unilateral otolith disease are more complex. In the case of a unilateral utricular disorder under dynamic conditions, there is a distinct reduction in linear compensatory amplitude when accelerating to the side of the lesion. This is due to the fact that the sole excitatory response when accelerating toward the lesioned side is provided by the medial hemimacula of the contralesional utricle, which is primarily responsible for the isolated cyclotorsional compensatory VOR. Hence, an absence of t-VOR is noted due to the damaged ipsilesional lateral hemimacula. This is, however, quickly compensated in a period of several months, whereby bi-directional sensitivity is once again regained (Gresty & Lempert, 2001). It is important to note that a robust c-VOR is not produced by excitation of the surviving contralesional medial hemimacula, because the abrupt and transient linear acceleration is insufficient for the longer latency needed to trigger the c-VOR (300 ms). Similarly, when static head tilts are delivered toward the lesioned side, a clear absence of c-VOR is noted. However, when the head is tilted toward the healthy side, a robust c-VOR is observed. Such ocular manifestations are clearly observed during an acute unilateral otolith lesion or significant asymmetry. Although these physical manifestations are generally apparent in the acute phase of an otolith disorder, the presence of a subjective tilt is not always a clear indicator of otolith disease, insomuch that a potential asymmetry of the vertical SCCs can also produce similar symptoms.

Central compensation of a utricular or saccular asymmetry is complex but rapid given the omni-directional orientation of the maculae sensory epithelium. In most cases, the abnormal c-VOR and t-VOR is quickly compensated and no longer observed under static conditions, even within a few weeks following otolith insult (Tran Ba Huy, & Toupet, 2001). However, under dynamic conditions the ocular manifestations secondary to the underlying asymmetric otolithic tonus can often be enhanced or exposed. In fact, it is possible to provoke the abnormal c-VOR or t-VOR response from a statically compensated otolithic disorder if a patient is subjected to linear (translational) acceleration or lateral linear acceleration (e.g., off axis rotational testing or eccentric rotational testing). This is, however, difficult in routine clinical testing, as it requires specific and often expensive and elaborate instrumentation. Fortunately, a major achievement in recent years has been the development of more reliable and precise tests capable of investigating otolith dysfunction. Such tests would include more precise static and dynamic tests of visual vertical and horizontal perception, eccentric and off-axis rotational testing, and cervical/ocular VEMP testing. Although many of these tests (excluding VEMP testing) continue to remain extremely expensive, scarce in their availability, often restricted to research settings, labor intensive, and/or require a high degree of sophistication to administer, progress toward a better evaluation and understanding of otolith disorders is burgeoning.

Clinical Application of SVV Data to Identify Otolith Disease

The clinical usefulness of the SVV has been shown to be integral in the diagnosis of otolith disease (Schönfeld & Clarke, 2011; Valko, Hegemann, Weber, Straumann, & Bockish, 2011). However, the ±2 standard deviation (*SD*) normative reference ranges for the absolute SVV measures for each rotational condition collected at the NIH suggest that eccentric rotational SVV testing may be clinically insensitive to the identification of utricular disease (see Figure 8–11). This is largely due to the fact that the eccentric conditions are meant to provoke a distinctively larger utricular-induced ocular counterroll (and subsequent SVV offset) than that observed during on-center rotation. For example, if the on-center SVV mean response occurs between −4.32° and +4.52°, then the eccen-

tric rotation should elicit an SVV response that is larger than the SVV reported during the on-center rotation with essentially no overlap, (that is, less than and greater than −4.32° and 4.52°, respectively). However, this was not observed in the normative reference data collected at the NIH. In fact, the eccentric SVV response ±2SD normative reference range for the UCF-R condition is between −8.17° and +1.26°, and the SVV response ±2SD normative reference range for the UCF-L condition is between −1.31° and +7.85°. Not only do both ranges clearly extend within the range of on-center rotation, but, both the UCF-R and UCF-L ±2SD normative reference ranges also encompass SVV responses that include zero degrees. These normative reference ranges pose a significant diagnostic dilemma, insomuch that an individual could present with an on-center SVV of 0° (exactly vertical), a UCF-R SVV of −4.0°, and a UCF-L SVV of +3.0°. The inherent problem with this example is that, although both eccentric SVV responses are within the normative range for the UCF-R and UCF-L conditions, they also fail to extend beyond the normative range for *on-center* rotation, which creates suspicion for whether or not the eccentric rotations actually elicited a c-VOR utricular response. This clearly creates a diagnostic quandary when attempting to differentiate a healthy from a diseased utricular system. In short, these data suggest this test offers neither adequate sensitivity nor specificity for utricular disease.

A previously reported alternative for determining what constitutes a normal SVV response is to calculate the *difference* in the eccentric SVV skew from the on-center response, rather than use the absolute SVV skew for each condition. Interpreting the change in eccentric SVV skew from the on-center SVV skew has been shown to represent a better indicator for utricular reactivity than the absolute SVV measures within each condition (Akin, Murnane, Pearson, Byrd, & Kelly, 2011). This is largely due to the fact that it accounts for any inherent asymmetric SVV response bias exhibited during on-center rotation. Overall, the resulting translation of chair to an eccentric rotational position further increases the SVV response data by approximately three and one-half degrees in either direction. Although this appears to be a good indicator for utricular reactivity, the variance of the response deleteriously contributes to an all too familiar large standard deviation. This, unfortunately, continues to limit the clinical application of these data and the subsequent usefulness of the SVV response. That is, if the normative reference range (±2 SD) was calculated for the change of SVV from the on-center condition to each eccentric condition, the lower limit would continue to suggest that no change in SVV during eccentric rotation (i.e., $0°$) is inclusive of a normal utricular response.

Reasons Supporting a Lack of Significant Skew (SVV) Deviation During Eccentric Rotations

One possible reason for the lack of skew deviation as a result of eccentric rotation is the difficulty with exclusively isolating a single utricle during eccentric rotation. The degree of chair displacement was based on the mean interaural utricular distance of 7.74 cm (Brey et al., 2008a). Therefore, the precise distance of chair translation for each participant should exactly be 3.87 cm (compared to our current discussion where chair translation is 4 cm). In light of these data, individual differences in the interaural utricular distance would undoubtedly have a deleterious impact on these measures. As a result of this methodological limitation, the observed mild-to-moderate variance in the change in SVV response data may not be surprising. One solution would be to individualize the testing procedures to accommodate each participant's interutricular distance (IUD). Determination of the IUD can be obtained through two methods. First, high-resolution magnetic resonance imaging techniques can be performed in order to more precisely measure each patient's IUD between the medial margins of the vestibules (Nowé et al., 2003). However, this method is costly and not likely adaptable to routine clinical assessment. The second method is to use external cranial landmarks such that the IUD can be estimated from the intermastoid distance (IMD). Nowé et al. (2003) identified the relationship between the IUD and the IMD was linear with an R^2 of 0.71, such that the IUD can be estimated by the equation:

$$IUD = 0.536 + 0.480 \,[(IMD \,(10^{-2}m)]$$

After accounting for sex differences, the authors were able to slightly improve the estimation of the IUD ($R^2 = 0.72$) by taking into account the nasion-inion distance (NID) and the height (H) of the individual, such that the IUD can be estimated by the equation:

$$IUD = 0.536 + 0.480 \,[(IMD \,(10^{-2}m)] - 6.80 \times 10^{-2} \,[(NID \,10^{-2}m)] + 0.884 \, H \,(m)$$

Although modifying the distance of chair translation according to each patient's IUD is technically possible through reprogramming of the test protocol, this is not a routine option and requires custom software and programming expertise. Consequently, this option is not easily adaptable in standard clinical assessment. Furthermore, the head restraint system currently in use for routine clinical assessment is not completely rigid, insomuch that slight head movement during testing (either in the pitch or yaw plane) is possible. Although random head movement within the restraint is likely less than 1 cm, even a 1 cm movement in one direction constitutes almost a 13% variance from "exact" center. This problem could be solved through a stricter head-restraint system, like a bite bar, self-centering head restraint system, or a whole-head moldable facemask restraint system. Although one of these systems is commercially available for use (self-centering head restraint), the use of such devices is likely to raise concern from human research protection policies and Institutional Review Boards.

Summary of SVV Data for Identifying Otolith Disease

Although a significant difference in right versus left eccentric SVV data has been identified, as well as a significant contraversive extension of the SVV beyond static or on-center rotation, the wide variances in the data makes it difficult to apply these data when ruling out utricular pathology. Theoretically speaking, a significant counterroll of the eyes should occur in response eccentric rotations, which should cause a clearly observable contraversive rotation of the SVV beyond the upper limits of the static or on-center rotation SVV data. Unfortunately, normative data collected at the NIH and other research facilities have found a wide data variance that includes 0° within the two-standard deviation reference range. This means that when eccentric rotations fail to produce a significant increase in contraversive SVV, utricular pathology cannot be assigned, as a response of 0° falls within two standard deviations of the mean. Therefore, these data support the conclusion that eccentric SVV and OCR data can only assist in the confirmation of *healthy* utricular reactivity (i.e., utricular integrity) but only when a significant SVV is recorded during eccentric rotations. Otherwise, because an eccentric rotation SVV response of 0° occurs in the normal reference range, failure of a significant contraversive SVV cannot be used to suggest utricular pathology.

Clinical Application of OCR and OCR-GIA Slope Data to Identify Otolith Disease

Wyuts and colleagues (2003) were the first to provide evidence suggesting that utricular sensitivity could be determined through eccentric rotational testing by determining rate of change in the ocular counterroll as a result of eccentric translation and gravitational inertial acceleration (GIA). It is often difficult to compare OCR, and OCR-GIA results across facilities due to significant (or even slight) differences in methodology and analysis methods. Moreover, ocular counterroll data is often technically difficult to measure, as even subtle amounts of ocular noise tend to have a significant deleterious impact on ocular torsion tracking. In addition, post-hoc analyses on OCR data tend to be difficult, and the unfortunate need for over- or under-sampling of the data (to stabilize subtle ocular noise) creates a situation where the data may become artificially clean and possibly unreliable. Such unreliability either reduces study sample sizes, or individual patient data are deemed unusable, and unfortunately, eliminated. Nevertheless, when the OCR data were found to be reliable, the mean OCR-GIA slope (and standard deviation) data collected at the NIH are similar to that observed by Wyuts et al. (2003), providing preliminary evidence suggesting that the OCR-GIA slope parameter is, in fact, reliable and repeatable.

Summary of OCR and OCR-GIA Data for Identifying Otolith Disease

The clinical usefulness of the OCR-GIA slope data is a significant advancement toward a better understanding of utricular physiology and the diagnosis of otolith disease. However, the relevance of the data is only as strong as it is available and reliable. The mean data collected at the NIH agree with that of Wyuts and colleague's (2003) healthy participants. However, secondary to technical challenges associated with the capturing of clean OCR data, the response rate is often poor. Interestingly, Wyuts et al. (2003) also reported a significantly reduced sample size with reliable OCR data (14 of 28 subjects with data judged to be reliable for analysis). Despite the similarity in the mean OCR-GIA slope data, most clinicians would likely argue against performing such a labor-intensive test in the presence of such a low usable response rate. As it stands now, the technical challenges underlying the measurement of the OCR reflex severely limit the overall success of this test and thereby limit its clinical relevance.

Despite the technical difficulties associated with eccentric rotational testing, unilateral centrifugation testing not only offers the opportunity to collect multiple outcome measures (SVV, OCR, OCR-GIA slope), but also has the potential to extend its analytical ability to capture even more subtle eye movements with better technology and more advanced analytical software. For example, the introduction of 250 Hz, high-speed infrared cameras may have the potential to capture previously unseen ocular movement or greater detail from torsional measures, which, to date, have only been possible through sclera search coil technology. In addition, the rotational chair's ability to consistently provide unequivocal stimuli with exquisite precision offers a unique ability to task the vestibular (utricular) system in ways not possible with acoustic stimuli. Gretsy and Lempert (2001) report a distinct advantage with using eccentric linear acceleration because it produces a pure-otolithic response (compared to the ocular VEMP response, which is elicited by an acoustic stimulus rather than an acceleration force). Ultimately, the final word on the clinical efficacy of such eccentric data will depend on its application to a disordered population and the ability for each measure to differentiate normal and abnormal function. Valko et al. (2011) offer an initial examination of this with good evidence to support the use of eccentric rotation testing in routine clinical practice. However, more research is needed to expand our understanding of the clinical implications of these measures in disordered populations.

OFF VERTICAL AXIS ROTATION (OVAR)

Off vertical axis rotation was first developed in the mid 1960s as an alternative method of introducing linear acceleration stimuli to the otolith system (Raphan & Cohen, 1996). Traditional methods prior to that time included linear sleds that required highly specialized equipment and a relatively large demand for lab space. Unfortunately over the past few decades, OVAR testing has not experienced a widespread acceptance and inclusion into routine (or even part-time) clinical use. In fact, recent to the time of this publication, the Federal Drug Administration has not approved the use of OVAR as a clinical measure. As a result, OVAR testing has remained exclusively under the auspices of research. Nevertheless, let us review certain aspects of OVAR testing in order to become familiar with the general nature of the test protocol, the general outcome measures, and the possible clinical applications of this test.

OVAR Test Protocol

Off vertical axis rotation involves the slow acceleration of a subject in the yaw plane to a constant velocity stimulus (generally 30°, 60°, or 90°/sec), much like the stimulus delivered during low-velocity step testing. During this time, the contribution of the horizontal canalicular response dissipates in a manner similar to that observed in the post stimulus period during step testing. Following decay of the canal reflex, the axis of rotation is tilted off earth-vertical by as much as 30°, all while constant velocity rotations are maintained.

Secondary to the fact that the angular velocity is kept constant, contribution from the semicircular canals is negated (Henn, 1996). However, as angular rotations are delivered about an axis that is tilted with respect to earth-vertical, the ever-present force of gravity now dictates a new downward vector that acts upon the otoliths as they dynamically reorient their position relative to earth-vertical during each "yaw" rotation (Gresty, 1996). In short, the constant force of gravity applies a varying sheer force across the otolith organs as each end organ rotates its position with respect to true vertical. The linear force of gravity creates opposing vectors across all planes of the striolar epithelium, which will vary depending on the position of the otolith, at any given time, in the rotation. Such dynamics of downward linear force across dynamically rotating otoliths can best be visualized in the extreme case where rotations are delivered to a laterally rotating subject, similar to a barbeque-spit rotation. Given the complex morphology of the maculae, the applied linear force causes ever-present dynamic neural responses that generate non-fatiguing (otolith-driven) ocular responses for as long as rotation of the chair continues.

VOR Response and Neural Substrate

During off vertical axis constant velocity rotations, a horizontal nystagmus is elicited that has both a steady-state and an oscillatory component. The continuous (steady-state) component is a horizontal slow phase velocity nystagmus that beats in the opposite direction of rotation, which can be easily identified. This is known as the bias component. The oscillatory component is the modulation of the steady-state bias component such that the nystagmus response actively records as a sinusoidal response. When the bias and modulated component are viewed together, the response assumes the characteristics of a steady-state right- or left-beating horizontal nystagmus (bias component) superimposed on a sinusoidal response (modulation component). An example of a normal OVAR response is depicted in Figure 8–12. The bias component is the more relevant of the two responses as it represents the ongoing constant eye velocity response in the presence of the constant velocity stimulus. This response likely represents the ongoing physiologi-

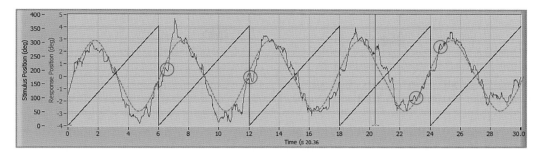

FIGURE 8–12. OVAR results showing the modulation (*red dashed line*) and the right-beating bias horizontal nystagmus component. The horizontal component has been periodically highlighted (*blue circles*) throughout the tracing for clarity. Image courtesy of Neuro Kinetics, Inc.

cal response of the maculae during constant velocity rotations, as the semicircular canal response is considered negligent or non-existent in the presence of a constant velocity stimulus (Furman, 2016). The modulation (oscillatory) component is less significant as it represents the unsuppressed horizontal eye response that occurs secondary to the misconception that the head is being oscillated linearly along the interaural axis (Furman, 2016). The horizontal nystagmus bias component of the response can be analyzed with respect to VOR gain, phase and symmetry. These analysis parameters are analyzed and interpreted precisely how the gain, phase, and symmetry parameters are analyzed and interpreted during SHA testing. That is, gain reflects the sensitivity of the vestibular response; phase reflects the central processing of the VOR; and symmetry reflects the inherent rightward of leftward bias or preponderance of the VOR.

Most evidence would suggest that the nystagmus elicited during OVAR testing is largely generated by the otolith maculae. However, data in primates have also shown that contributions from velocity storage mechanisms (nodulus and ventral uvula) have direct influences on production of the bias component of the nystagmus (Angelaki & Hess, 1995; Reisine & Raphan, 1992). Although the relative contributions of the saccule versus the utricle have yet to be systematically analyzed and elucidated (Raphan & Cohen, 1996), evidence shows that the neurophysiological substrate responsible for the VOR generated during OVAR testing is collectively mediated by the otoliths and velocity storage mechanisms.

Clinical Application and Limitations of OVAR Testing

Off vertical axis rotation testing has suffered from a significant lack of attention in clinical rotational assessments (whether routine or otherwise). Although it has received some attention in research, reports on OVAR testing in research have been scarce as well. The paucity of OVAR testing in clinical assessment is largely due to five factors.

First, OVAR testing suites are expensive or require a significant upgrade and cost to a current rotational test suite. For the minimal facilities that own rotational test suites, only a small percentage of those facilities have a rotational system capable of even performing OVAR testing. Moreover, only a portion of those facilities who own an OVAR chair actually conduct research on patient's (or healthy participants). Currently, this is solely due to the clinical non-approval status placed on conducting OVAR by the Federal Drug Administration, which exclusively limits its use to research.

The second reason for the lack of OVAR testing in clinical assessments (and research protocols) is that such rotations are highly provocative for nausea and potential emesis in most patients. Such a provocative response occurs secondary to the constant downward force applied to the otoliths as they are dynamically reoriented during rotations about the off-axis vertical rotation. Under such dynamic rotational conditions, the normal decay of the physiologic response to a constant velocity stimulus, similar to the canalicular decay response during VST, fails to occur. As a result of the omnipresent physiological response, an associated vertigo continues for as long as the stimulus is being delivered. That being said, the subsequent incitement of severe nausea in individuals significantly limits the application of such testing to vestibular patients who already report biliousness (nausea).

The third reason OVAR testing would offer a low clinical yield during vestibular assessments is that studies have shown OVAR to be relatively insensitive to unilateral peripheral vestibular pathology (Furman, 2016). This is likely secondary to the rapid compensation mechanisms that accompany unilateral otolith disorders, as well as the low velocity stimulus (albeit noxious) that is associated with OVAR testing. As discussed earlier, more robust stimuli are often required when segregating unilateral otolith disorders from healthy maculae. This point was also highlighted earlier when discussing GIA with respect to the degree of eccentric rotation and stimulus velocity.

The fourth reason OVAR testing has struggled gaining widespread acceptance (and, consequently, FDA approval) is that the clinical *application* of the data is not well understood. The reasons for this are multifactorial. The lack of understanding is most likely due to the paucity of its use and subsequent shortage of published reports. This has subsequently reduced its exposure and diagnostic significance for identifying vestibular pathology. As a result, the (clinical) applications of the test data, and by default, the (clinical) indications for performing the test, are not well understood. Off-vertical axis rotational testing is targeted primarily for the clinical assessment of otolith pathology. Unfortunately, the clinical indicators and patient triage process for otolith disease, combined with the lack of clinical reports and diagnostic sensitivity for unilateral otolith disease, have tremendously blunted the acceptance and expansion of OVAR testing in research studies and, subsequently, its approval in clinical-rotational assessments.

Finally, the clinical outcome data from OVAR testing is not well understood in large part because the data are highly complex. Angular "yaw" rotations performed on an off-vertical axis plane incite VOR responses that incorporate nearly every labyrinthine sensory end organ, as well as velocity storage mechanisms (Angelaki & Hess, 1995; Reisine & Raphan, 1992). Although the semicircular canal input quickly abates once achieving constant velocity rotation, the VOR response is believed to represent a complex neurophysiological response that incorporates both saccular and utricular reactivity (not to mention a *bilateral* contribution from both the right and left labyrinth). As such, the data are somewhat clinically nebulous with respect to localization of vestibular function and, more importantly, vestibular (otolith) disease. Consequently, such diagnostic implications are not accepted well by the clinical community insomuch that the effort spent performing OVAR testing offers little in the way of segregating vestibular disease.

Unfortunately, the combination of these shortcomings is somewhat self-limiting for the widespread acceptance for OVAR testing in routine rotational test protocols. Until additional research promotes significant increases in the diagnostic power of OVAR testing, its potential for clinical approval and subsequent use, will likely remain uncertain.

FUTURE ADVANCEMENTS IN ROTATIONAL TESTING

Advancements in technology will continue to promote the discovery, development, and use of new applications in clinical vestibular assessment. The introduction of video head impulse testing (vHIT) is a recent example of this. Such advancements often follow a course of "bench-to-bedside" development. Specialized assessment tools often spend years in research design (i.e., the "bench) concomitantly collecting enormous amounts of data on healthy and pathologic individuals prior to being introduced into routine clinical assessment (i.e., the "bedside"). Video HIT is an excellent example of a clinical measure that was able to quickly transition from research to clinical use.

There are a few tests that are receiving some attention for transitioning from the bench to the bedside. Two such tests include, whole body impulse testing and velocity/acceleration threshold detection measures. Let us briefly review each measure in order to become familiar with possible future advancements in rotational testing.

Chair Head Impulse Testing (crHIT)

Developments in impulse rotational testing have seen some recent attention. Although OVAR testing has struggled to make a clinical impact, other tests are being developed in an attempt to secure a more sensitive and specific clinical track record for the identification of vestibular disease. Similar to vHIT, quick thrusts of the chair can be delivered to the vestibular system in much the same fashion. In fact, such brisk accelerations ($1000°/sec^2$) can be delivered to the body "en-bloc" and produce a compensatory brisk VOR response similar to those seen during vHIT (Figure 8–13). Figure 8–14 depicts crHIT data from a series of chair thrusts (accerations) at $1000°/sec^2$ presented in the yaw plane to an individual with normal vestibular function. Figure 8–15 depicts data from a series of $1000°/sec^2$ accelerations presented to an individual with a normal vestibular system as well as an individual with a unilateral vestibular lesion. Not only can such "en-bloc" thrusts be delivered in all three orthogonal planes (horizontal, as well as the LARP, and RALP planes using a modified rotational chair), such testing is capable of delivering precisely controlled stimuli that can effectively be used to lateralize and compare VOR function between the right and the left "labyrinths". Recognizing the primary limitation for lateralization of peripheral pathology, crHIT provides a reasonable method for the detection of peripheral asymmetry. The sensitivity of such measures remains to be fully elucidated, although preliminary data look promising for segregating (and lateralizing) normal from abnormal vestibular function (Furman, Roxberg, Shirley, & Kiderman, 2016). Figure 8–15 depicts crHIT data that illustrates examples from an individual with unilateral vestibular disease.

There are some key advantages that crHIT can provide. First, it eliminates neck movement, such as those produced during vHIT, which can add to the potential contributions of larger visual-vestibular enhancement secondary to the presence of efferent copy commands under conditions involving dynamic head and neck movement (Demer, 1996). Second, it eliminates small positional errors within each orthogonal plane of excitation, such as those that may be experienced during vHIT. Third, it limits the unpleasant characteristics associated with head thrusts and neck rotation that accompany tests like vHIT. Fourth, given the precise delivery of the stimuli, it eliminates the need for a highly trained examiner (Furman, Roxberg, Shirley & Kiderman, 2016). Finally, because of the precise and *consistent* delivery of the stimuli (assuming an adequate head-to-chair velocity ratio), variability and repeatability of the results are less of a significant confounding variable from patient-to-patient, examiner-to-examiner, and from test-to-test.

One of the main challenges encountered during crHIT testing is maintaining a sufficient head-to-chair velocity ratio. As we previously discussed during high frequency SHA testing (i.e., frequencies >1.0 Hz), dermal slip and head lag become

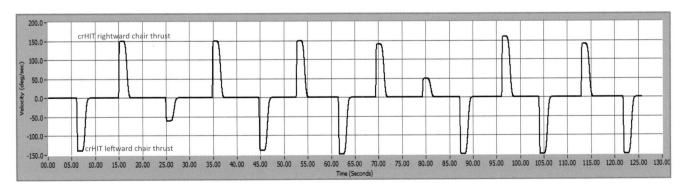

FIGURE 8–13. crHIT stimulus paradigm showing a series of chair thrusts delivered at $1000°/sec^2$ to a velocity of $150°/sec$. Image courtesy of Neuro Kinetics, Inc.

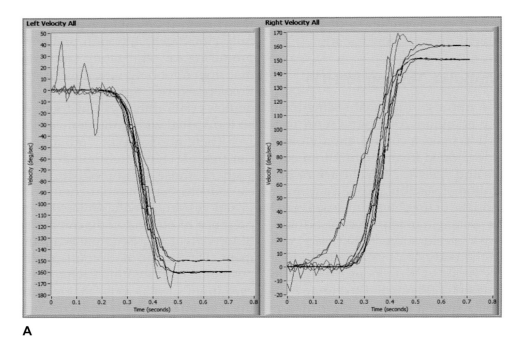

A

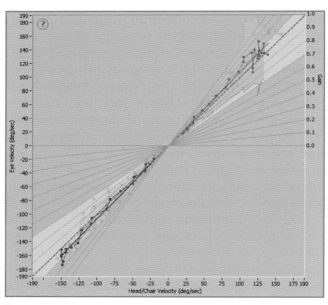

B

FIGURE 8–14. Individual crHIT results from a single individual with normal vestibular function using a 1000°/sec^2 acceleration between 25° and 150°/sec velocity chair thrust stimuli. **A.** Shows individual trial data of eye velocity to chair velocity. **B.** Shows eye velocity to chair velocity data for both right and left chair thrusts between 25° and 150°/sec stimuli. *continues*

an inherent problem, producing significant issues with phase lags that are secondary to poorly synchronized chair-to-head accelerations. Solutions to such phase problems can usually be remedied with the introduction of better head restraints. However, such restraints needed to limit dermal slip and head lag become more constraining and less comfortable for the patient. Straightforward

solutions, such as bite-blocks and moldable face-masks become increasingly intrusive, and safety becomes an increasing concern. Preliminary data suggest crHIT testing is possible with excellent repeatability (Furman et al., 2016), although significant attention to an excellent head-to-chair velocity ratio is vital. While the preliminary data look promising, more research is needed to deter-

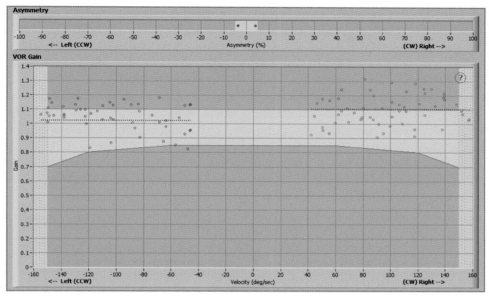

C

FIGURE 8–14. *continued* **C.** Shows individual trial gain data for the entire stimulus velocity range. Images courtesy of Walter Reed National Military Medical Center.

mine the reliability and validity of crHIT measures, if such a measure is to receive widespread acceptance in the routine rotational test battery.

Acceleration Threshold Detection

Similar to psychoacoustic measures of auditory threshold detection, previous research has investigated the psychophysiological measures of vestibular threshold detection using various frequency (acceleration) stimuli. Such measures are meant to exploit the just noticeable perception of acceleration (movement) by the vestibular system at various frequencies. Measures of acceleration detection (deg/sec^2) and/or velocity (deg/sec) threshold, in addition to directional awareness, can be determined, which is similar to an audiogram or, in this case, a vestibulogram. Very limited research has been performed in this area of psychophysiology for the vestibular system; however, Grabherr, Nicoucar, Mast, and Merfeld (2008) were able to describe such a vestibulogram for harmonic frequencies from 0.05 through 5 Hz. Their data reveal a precipitous increase in veloc-

ity detection thresholds at and below 0.2 Hz. For frequencies of 1 Hz and above, the thresholds for velocity detection plateaued around 1°/sec. Although this testing has largely been confined to research, with advancements in stimulus delivery, its introduction into clinical testing may have important applications in the future rotational assessment battery, particularly as a possible method to segregate a clinical aging vestibular phenotype, which has been, thus far, a significant challenge (Zalewski, 2015).

Summary of Future Advancements in Rotational Testing

The future of rotational testing is very promising. The advancements in technology in the last decade alone have allowed for significant improvement in the diagnosis of vestibular disease. Rotational testing offers an unparalleled clinical assessment platform for assessment of the vestibular system. In fact, no other test in our current comprehensive clinical test battery is capable of evaluating the vestibular system with a more appropriate stimu-

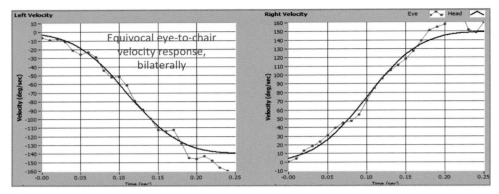

A

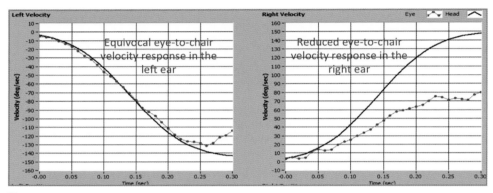

B

FIGURE 8–15. crHIT results from two individuals using a 1000°/sec² acceleration to a 150°/sec velocity chair thrust stimulus. **A.** Shows eye velocity to chair velocity data for an individual with normal vestibular results. **B.** Shows eye velocity to chair velocity data for an individual with a right unilateral vestibular lesion. Black lines represent chair velocity. Blue connected points represent eye velocity data. Images courtesy of Neuro Kinetics, Inc.

lus, one of motion. Rotational testing distinctively allows for the exacting delivery of a broad spectrum of motion stimuli to the vestibular system, while simultaneously having highly precise methods for capturing the subtlest of eye movements. In the ever-persistent search to improve the diagnostic sensitivity of current vestibular test methods, rotational testing offers perhaps the greatest potential for success. The need for increased diagnostic sensitivity has likely never been so great, as the prevalence of balanced-disordered patients, and particularly those with vestibular dysfunction, will likely see exponential increases over the next half century.

Appendices

Appendix A

*Sinusoidal Acceleration Normative Reference Ranges**

Response Parameter	0.01 Hz		0.02 Hz		0.04 Hz	
	Mean	2SD	Mean	2SD	Mean	2SD
VOR Gain	0.3951	0.15468	0.458	0.18274	0.5208	0.2174
VOR Phase	39.47	12.69	21.94	10.82	8.295	7.942
VOR Symmetry	4.238	16.348	3.457	17.442	5.603	18.246
Spectral Purity	92.82	6.394	93.87	7.896	96.67	3.89

Response Parameter	0.08 Hz		0.16 Hz		0.32 Hz	
	Mean	2SD	Mean	2SD	Mean	2SD
VOR Gain	0.508	0.2856	0.5108	0.2816	0.5376	0.302
VOR Phase	2.714	13.128	0.6483	13.428	0.2806	11.67
VOR Symmetry	3.777	16.868	−4.227	19.072	5.345	16.276
Spectral Purity	95.72	6.96	95.47	6.846	97.32	3.7

Response Parameter	0.64 Hz		1.28 Hz		2.0 Hz	
	Mean	2SD	Mean	2SD	Mean	2SD
VOR Gain	0.6018	0.2708	0.7925	0.216	0.7594	0.4214
VOR Phase	3.942	9.624	9.681	11.752	1.745	28.76
VOR Symmetry	2.883	14.538	0.5278	8.422	-2.675	48.52
Spectral Purity	98.46	3.672	99.12	1.1518	96.52	7.316

*Means and two standard deviations for sinusoidal acceleration testing (60° target velocity) for VOR Gain, VOR Phase, VOR Symmetry, and Spectral Purity from 0.01 to 2.0 Hz. Means and standard deviations based on a sample size of 47 healthy volunteers aged 18 to 62 years (*M*=27 years, *SD*=8).

Appendix B

Subjective Visual Vertical Normative Reference Ranges During Static, On-Center Rotation, and Eccentric Rotations[*]

	Static SVV	On-Center SVV	UCF-R SVV	UCF-L SVV	UCF-R OCR	UCF-L OCR
Mean	−0.03°	0.10°	−3.45°	3.27°	−3.56°	3.28°
±1 SD	−1.35 to 1.35°	−2.11 to 2.31°	−5.81 to 1.10°	0.98 to 5.56°	−5.95 to 1.17°	−1.63 to 4.94°
±2 SD	−2.73 to 2.73°	−4.32 to 4.52°	−8.17 to 1.26°	−1.31 to 7.85°	−8.34 to 1.22°	−3.29 to 6.60°

*Means and standard deviations based on a sample size of 47 healthy volunteers aged 18 to 62 years (M=27 years, SD=8).

References

Akbarian, S., Grusser, O. J., & Guldin, W. O. (1992). Thalamic connections of the vestibular cortical fields in the squirrel monkey (Saimiri sciureus). *Journal of Comparative Neurology, 3262(3)*, 423–441.

Akin, F. W., Murnane, O. D., Pearson, A., Byrd, S., & Kelly, J. K. (2011). Normative data for the subjective visual vertical test during configuration. *Journal of the American Academy of Audiology, 22(7)*, 460–468.

Anastasopoulos, D., Haslwanter, T., Fetter, M., & Dichgans, J. (1998). Smooth pursuit eye movements and otolith-ocular responses are differently impaired in cerebellar ataxia. *Brain, 121*, 1497–1505.

Angelaki, D. E., & Hess, B. J. (1995). Lesions of the nodulus and ventral uvula abolish steady-state off-vertical axis otolith response. *Neurophysiology, 73(4)*, 1716–1720.

Aoki, M., Ito, Y., & Burchill, P. (1999). Tilted perception of the subjective "upright" in unilateral loss of vestibular function. *American Journal of Otology, 20*, 741–747.

Arriaga, M. A., Chen, D. A., & Cenci, K. A. (2005). Rotational chair (ROTO) instead of electronystagmography (ENG) as the primary vestibular test. *Otolaryngology-Head and Neck Surgery, 133(3)*, 329–333.

Arriaga, M. A., Chen, D. A., Hillman, T. A., Kunschner, L., & Arriaga, R. Y. (2006). Visually enhanced vestibulo-ocular reflex: A diagnostic tool for migraine vestibulopathy. *Laryngoscope, 116(9)*, 1577–1579.

Arslan, O. (2001). *Neuroanatomical basis of clinical neurology*. New York, NY: Parthenon.

Baloh, R. W. (1998). *Dizziness, hearing loss, and tinnitus*. Philadelphia, PA: F. A. Davis.

Baloh, R. W., & Honrubia, V. (1990). *Clinical neurophysiology of the vestibular system* (2nd ed.). Philadelphia, PA: F. A. Davis.

Baloh, R. W., & Honrubia, V. (1998). Vestibular physiology. In C. W. Cummings, J. M. Fredrickson, L. A. Harker, C. J. Krause, M. A. Richardson, & D. E. Schuller (Eds.), *Otolaryngology head and neck surgery* (3rd ed., pp. 2584–2622). St. Louis, MO: Mosby.

Baloh, R. W., & Honrubia, V. (2001). *Clinical neurophysiology of the vestibular system* (3rd ed.). Philadelphia, PA: F. A. Davis.

Baloh, R. W., Honrubia, V., & Kerber, K. A. (2011). *Baloh and Honrubia's clinical neurophysiology of the vestibular system* (4th ed.). New York, NY: Oxford Press.

Baloh, R. W., Honrubia, V., Yee, R. D., & Hess, K. (1984). Changes in the human vestibulo-ocular reflex after loss of peripheral sensitivity. *Annals of Neurology, 16(2)*, 222–228.

Baloh, R. W., Honrubia, V., Yee, R. D., & Jacobson, G. P. (1986). Vertical visual-vestibular interaction in normal human subjects. *Experimental Brain Research, 64(3)*, 400–406.

Baloh, R. W., Honrubia, V., Yee, R. D., Langhofer, L., & Minser, K. (1986). Recovery from unilateral vestibular lesions. In R. J. Leigh & D. S. Zee (2006), *The neurology of eye movements* (4th ed.). New York, NY: Oxford University Press.

Baloh, R. W., Jacobson, K. M., & Socotch, T. M. (1993). The effect of aging on visual-vestibuloocular responses. *Experimental Brain Research, 95*, 509–516.

Baloh, R. W., Sills, A. W., & Honrubia, V. (1979). Impulsive and sinusoidal rotatory testing: A comparison with results of caloric testing. *Laryngoscope, 89*, 646–654.

Bárány, R. (1907). Physiologie und pathologie des bogengangsapparates [Physiology and pathology of the semicircular canal]. Wien, Austria: Deuticke.

Barber, H., & Stockwell, C. (1980). *Manual of electronystagmography* (2nd ed.). St. Louis, MO: C. V. Mosby.

Barber, H. O., & Wright, G. (1973). Positional nystagmus in normals. *Advancements in Oto-Rhino-Laryngology, 19*, 276–285.

Barin, K. (2006). Current state of static positional testing. *AudiologyOnline:* February 2, 2006. Retrieved August 4, 2010, from http://www.audiologyonline.com/articles/article_detail.asp?article_id=1540

Barin, K. (2009). Clinical neurophysiology of the vestibular system. In J. Katz, L. Medwetsky, R. Burkard & L. Hood (Eds.), Handbook of clinical audiology (pp. 431–466). Philadelphia, PA: Lippincott Williams & Wilkins.

Barin, K. (2013). *New tests for diagnoses of peripheral vestibular disorders*. Proceedings from the Illinois Academy of Audiology, January 30 to February 1, 2013.

Barin, K., & Durrant, J. D. (2000). Applied physiology of the vestibular System. In R. F. Canalis & P. R. Lempert (Eds.), *The Ear: Comprehensive otology* (pp. 113–140). Philadelphia, PA: Lippincott Williams & Wilkins.

Bartley, S. H. (1951). The physiology of vision. In S. S. Stevens (Ed.), *Handbook of experimental psychology* (p. 951). New York, NY: John Wiley & Sons.

Bear, M. F., Connors, B. W., & Paradiso, M. A. (2016). *Neuroscience: Exploring the brain* (4th ed.). Philadelphia, PA: Wolters Kluwer.

Belofsky, N. (2013). *Strange medicine: A shocking history of real medical practices through the ages.* New York, NY: TarcherPerigee, Penguin.

Benson, A. J., & Bodin, M. A. (1966). Effect of orientation to the gravitational vertical on nystagmus following rotation about a horizontal axis. *Acta Otolaryngologica, 61*, 517–526.

Berthoz, A., & Rousié, D. (2001). Physiopathology of otolith-dependent vertigo. In P. Tran Ba Huy & M. Toupet (Eds.), *Otolith function and disorders* (pp. 48–67). New York, NY: Karger.

Bhatnagar, S. C. (2013). *Neuroscience for the study of communicative disorders* (4th ed.). Baltimore, MD: Lippincott Williams & Wilkins.

Bischof, N. (1974). Optic-vestibular orientation to the vertical. In L.M. Beidler (Ed). *Handbook of sensory physiology, volume VI: Vestibular system* (pp. 155–190). Berlin, Germany: Springer.

Böhmer, A., & Mast, F. (1999). Chronic unilateral loss of otolith function revealed by the subjective visual vertical during off-center yaw rotation. *Journal of Vestibular Research, 9*, 413–422.

Brandt, T. (1999). *Vertigo: Its multisensory syndromes,* (2nd ed.). London, UK: Springer.

Brandt, T. (2001). Otolith vertigo. In P. Tran Ba Huy & M. Toupet (Eds.), *Otolith function and disorders* (pp. 34–47). New York, NY: Karger.

Breathnach, C. S. (2010). Hallaran's circulating swing. *History of Psychiatry, 21*(81 Pt. 1), 79–84.

Brey, R. H., McPherson, J. H., & Lynch, R. M. (2008a). Background and introduction to whole body rotational testing. In G. P. Jacobson & N. T. Shepard (Eds.), *Balance function assessment and management* (pp. 253–280). San Diego, CA: Plural.

Brey, R. H., McPherson, J. H., & Lynch, R. M. (2008b). Technique, interpretation, and usefulness of whole body rotational testing. In G. P. Jacobson & N. T. Shepard (Eds.) *Balance function assessment and management* (pp. 281–317). San Diego, CA: Plural.

Brödal, M. (1946). Three unpublished drawings of the anatomy of the human ear. Philadelphia, PA: W. B. Saunders. In C. W. Cummings, J. M. Fredrickson, L. A. Harker, C. J. Krause, M. A. Richardson, & D. E. Schuller (Eds.), *Otolaryngology head and neck surgery* (1998, 3rd ed.). St. Louis, MO: CV Mosby.

Brodal, P. (2004). *The central nervous system: Structure and function* (3rd ed.). New York, NY: Oxford University Press.

Bronstein, A., Gresty, M., & Rudge, P. (2004). Neuro-otologic assessment in the patient with balance and gait disorder. In A. Bronstein, T. Brandt, M. Woollacott & J. Nutt (Eds.), *Clinical disorders of balance, posture and gait* (2nd ed., pp. 99–129). London, UK: Arnold.

Cass, S. P., & Furman, J. M. (1993). Medications and their effects on vestibular function testing. *ENG Report, November 1993.* Chicago, IL: ICS Medical.

Clarke, A. H., Schönfeld, U., & Helling, K. (2003). Unilateral examination of utricle and saccule function. *Journal of Vestibular Research, 13*, 215–225.

Coats, A. C., & Smith, S. Y. (1967). Body position and the intensity of caloric nystagmus. *Acta Otolaryngologica, 63*(6), 515–532.

Cohen, B., Henn, V., Raphan, T., & Dennett, D. (1981). Velocity storage, nystagmus, and visual-vestibular interactions in humans. *Annals of the New York Academy of Sciences, 942*, 241–258.

Cohen, B., & Raphan, T. (2004). The physiology of the vestibuloocular reflex (VOR). In F. M. Highstein, R. R. Fay, & A. N. Popper (Eds.), *The vestibular system,* (pp. 235–285). New York, NY: Springer.

Colebatch, J. (2001). Vestibular evoked potentials. *Current Opinion in Neurology, 14*(1), 21–26.

Colebatch, J., & Halmagyi, (1992). Vestibular evoked potentials in human neck muscles before and after unilateral vestibular deafferentation. *Neurology, 42*, 1635–1636.

Colebatch, J., Halmagyi, G., & Skuse, N. (1994). Myogenic potentials generated by a click-evoked vestibulocollic reflex. *Journal of Neurology, Neurosurgery, and Psychiatry, 57*, 190–197.

Cumberworth, V., Patel, N., Rogers, W., & Kenyon, G. (2006). The maturation of balance in children. *Journal of Laryngology and Otology, 121*, 449–454.

Curthoys, I. S., & Halmagyi, G. M. (1996). How does the brain compensate for vestibular lesions? In R. W. Baloh & G. M. Halmagyi (Eds.), *Disorders of the vestibular system,* (pp. 145–154). New York, NY: Oxford University Press.

Curthoys, I. S., & Halmagyi, G. M. (2007). Vestibular compensation: Clinical changes in vestibular function with time after unilateral vestibular loss. In S. J. Herdman (Ed.), *Vestibular rehabilitation* (3rd ed., pp. 76–97). Philadelphia, PA: F. A. Davis.

Cyr, D. G. (1991). Vestibular assessment. In W. F. Rintelmann, *Perspectives in audiology series: Hearing assess-*

ment (2nd ed., pp. 739–803). Needham Heights, MA: Allyn & Bacon.

Cyr, D. G., Moore, G., & Möller, C. (1989). Clinical experience with the low-frequency rotary chair test. *Seminars in Hearing, 10,* 171–189.

Darwin, E. (1794). *Zoonomia; Or, the laws of organic life* (Vol. I). London, UK.

Darwin, E. (1796). *Zoonomia; Or, the laws of organic life* (Vol. II). London, UK.

Darwin, E. (1801). *Zoonomia; Or, the laws of organic life* (3rd ed., Vol. IV). London, UK.

Della Santina, C. C., Potyagaylo, V., Migliaccio, A., Minor, L. B., & Carey, J. P. (2005). Orientation of human semicircular canals measured by three-dimensional multiplanar CT reconstruction. *Journal of the Association for Research in Otolaryngology, 6*(3), 191–206.

Demer, J. L. (1996). How does the visual system interact with the vestibulo-ocular reflex? In R. W. Baloh & G. M. Halmagyi (Eds.), *Disorders of the vestibular system,* (pp. 73–84). New York, NY: Oxford University Press.

Demer, J. L., Goldberg, J., Porter, F. I., Jenkins, H. A., & Schmidt, K. (1990). Visual-vestibular interaction with telescopic spectacles. *Journal of Vestibular Research, 1*(3), 263–277.

Dieterich, M. & Brandt, T. (1992). Cyclorotation of the eyes and the subjective visual vertical. *Baillière's Clinical Neurology, 1*(2), 301–316.

Dix, M. R., Hallpike, C. S., & Hood, J. D. (1963). Electronystagmography and its uses in the study of spontaneous nystagmus. *Transactions of the Ophthalmological Societies of the United Kingdom, 83,* 531–557.

Ey, W., & Feldman, H. (1964). Der Heidelberger planeten-drehstuhl, eine neuartige mehrzweck-drehstuhlanlage fuer vestibularisreflexpruefungen. [The Heidelberg planet turning chair, a new type of multipurpose turning chair unit for vestibular reflex tests]. *Archives Ohren, Nasen- u. Kehlkopfheilkd, 184,* 73–80.

Faugier-Grimaud, S., & Ventre, J. (1989). Anatomic connections of inferior parietal cortex (area 7) with subcortical structures related to vestibulo-ocular function in a monkey (Macaca fascicularis). *Journal of Comparative Neurology, 280*(1), 1–14.

Ferman, L., Collewijn, H., Jansen, T. C., & van den Berg, A. V. (1987). Human gaze stability in the horizontal, vertical, and torsional direction during voluntary head movements, evaluated with a three-dimensional scleral induction coil technique. *Visual Research, 27,* 811–828.

Fetter, M., & Dichgans, J. (1996). Vestibular tests in evolution. II. Posturography. In R. W. Baloh & G. M. Halmagyi (Eds.), *Disorders of the vestibular system* (pp. 48–61). New York, NY: Oxford University Press.

Fetter, M., Hain, T. C., & Zee, D. S. (1986). Influence of eye and head position on the vestibulo-ocular reflex. *Experimental Brain Research, 64*(1), 208–216.

Fife, T, Tusa, R., Furman, J., Zee, D., Frohman, E., Baloh, R., . . . Eviatar, L. (2000). Assessment: Vestibular testing techniques in adults and children: Report of the therapeutics and technology assessment subcommittee of the American Academy of Neurology. *Neurology, 55,* 1431–1441.

Fluur, E. (1960). A novel rotary chair. *Acta Otolaryngologica, 52,* 210–214.

Fluur, E. (1970). The interaction between the utricle and the saccule. *Acta Otolaryngologica, 69,* 17–24.

Formby, C., Kuntz, L. A., Rivera-Taylor, I. M., Rivera-Mraz, N., Weesner, D. R., Butler-Young, N. E., & Ahlers, A. E. (1992). Measurement, analysis, and modeling of the caloric response. 2. Evaluation of mental alerting tasks for measurement of caloric-induced nystagmus. *Acta Otolaryngologica Supplemental, 498,* 19–29.

Frenckner, P., & Preber, L. (1956). Relationship between reactions and vegetative reflexes, studied in man by means of a revolving chair of new design. *Acta Otolarnygologica, 46*(3), 207–218; discussion, 219–220.

Furman, J. (2016). Rotational testing. In J. M. Furman & T. Lempert (Eds.), *Handbook of clinical neurology; Vol 137, Neuro-otology* (3rd series, pp. 177–186). Cambridge, MA: Elsevier.

Furman, J. M., Goebel, J. A., Hamid, M. A., Hanson, J., Honrubia, V., Peterka, R., . . . Wall, C. (1994). Interlaboratory variability of rotational chair test results. Interlaboratory rotational chair study group. *Otolaryngology-Head and Neck Surgery, 110*(4), 400–405.

Furman, J. M., Goebel, J. A., Hamid, M. A., Hanson, J., Honrubia, V., Peterka, R., . . . Wall, C. (2000). Interlaboratory variability of rotational chair test results II: Analysis of simulated data. *Otolaryngology-Head and Neck Surgery, 122*(1), 23–30.

Furman, J. M., Roxberg, J., Shirley, I., & Kiderman, A. (2016). *The Computerized Rotational Head Impulse Test (crHIT).* Poster presented at 2014 Bárány Society Meeting, Buenos Aires, Argentina.

Furman, J. M., Wall, C., & Kamerer, D. B. (1989). Earth axis rotational responses in patients with unilateral peripheral vestibular deficits. *Annals of Otology, Rhinology, and Laryngology, 98*(7 Pt. 1), 551–555.

Furst, E. J., Goldberg, J., & Jenkins, H. A. (1987). Voluntary modification of the rotary-induced vestibulo-ocular reflex by fixating imaginary targets. *Acta Otolaryngologica, 103*(5–6), 232–240.

Gacek, R. R. (2005). Anatomy of the central vestibular system. In R. K. Jackler & D. E. Brackman (Eds.), *Neurotology* (2nd ed., pp. 75–90). Philadelphia, PA: Elsevier Mosby.

Gianna, C., Heimbrand, S., & Gresty, M. A. (1996). Thresholds for detection of motion direction during passive lateral whole-body acceleration in normal subjects and patients with bilateral loss of labyrinthine function. *Brain Research Bulletin, 56,* 443–449.

Goebel, J. A., Stroud, M. H., Levine, L. A., & Muntz, H. R. (1983). Vertical eye deviation and nystagmus inhibition during mental tasking. *Laryngoscope, 93(9),* 1127–1132.

Goldberg, J (2000). Afferent diversity and the organization of central vestibular pathways. *Experimental Brain Research, 130,* 277–297.

Goldberg, J. M., & Fernandez, C. (1975). Vestibular mechanisms. *Annals Review of Physiology, 37,* 129.

Goldberg, J. M., & Fernandez, C. (1982). The vestibular system. In J. Brookhart & V. Mountastle (Eds.), *Handbook of physiology. The nervous system III* (pp. 977–1022). Washington, DC: American Physiologic Society. In L. Ödkvist (2001). Clinical and instrumental investigational otolith function. In P. Tran Ba Huy & M. Toupet (Eds.), *Otolith function and disorders* (pp. 68–76). New York, NY: Karger.

Goldberg, M. E., & Hudspeth, A. (2000). The vestibular system. In E. R. Kandel, J. H. Schwartz, & T. M. Jessell (Eds.), *Principles of Neuro Science* (4th ed., pp. 801–815). New York, NY: McGraw-Hill.

Goldberg, J. M., Wilson, V.J., Cullen, K. E., Angelaki, D. E., Broussard, D. M., Bütner-Ennever, J.A., . . . Minor, L. B. (2012). *The vestibular system: A sixth sense.* New York, NY: Oxford University Press.

Goulson, A. M., McPherson, J. H., & Shepard, N. T. (2016). Background and introduction to whole-body rotational testing. In G. P. Jacobson & N. T. Shepard (Eds.), *Balance function assessment and management* (pp. 347–364). San Diego, CA: Plural.

Grabherr, L., Nicoucar, K., Mast, F. W., & Merfeld, D. M. (2008). Vestibular thresholds for yaw rotation about an earth-vertical axis as a function of frequency. *Experimental Brain Research, 186(4),* 677–681.

Graybiel, A., & Hupp, D. (1946). The oculo-gyral illusion: A form of apparent motion which may be observed following stimulation of the semicircular canals. *Journal of Aviation Medicine, 17,* 3–27.

Graybiel, A., Niven, J., & Walsh, T. (1952). The differentiation between symptoms referable to the otolith organs and the semicircular canals in patients with nonsuppurative labyrinthitis. *Laryngoscope, 62,* 924–933.

Gresty, M. A. (1996). Vestibular tests in evolution. I. Otolith Testing. In R. W. Baloh & G. M. Halmagyi (Eds.), *Disorders of the vestibular system* (pp. 243–255). New York, NY: Oxford University Press.

Gresty, M. A., & Bronstein, A. M. (1992). Testing otolith function. *British Journal of Audiology, 26,* 125–136.

Gresty, M. A., Bronstein, A. M., Brandt, T., & Dieterich, M. (1992). Neurology of otolith function: Peripheral and central disorders. *Brain, 115,* 647–673.

Gresty, M. A., & Lempert, T. (2001). Pathophysiology and clinical testing of otolith dysfunction. In P. Tran Ba Huy & M. Toupet (Eds.), *Otolith function and disorders* (pp. 15–33). New York, NY: Karger.

Guedry, F. E., Jr., & Graybiel, A. (1961). *Rotation devices, other than centrifuges and motion simulators. A rationale for their special characteristics and use.* Washington, DC, National Academy of Sciences—National Research Council.

Guedry, F. E., Jr., Kennedy, R. S., Harris, C. S., & Graybiel, A. (1962). Human performance during two weeks in a room rotating at three rpm. *U.S. Naval School of Aviation Medical Research Report, 74,* 1–26.

Guldin, W. O., Akbarian, S., & Grusser, O. J. (1992). Cortico-cortical connections and cytoarchitectonics of the primate vestibular cortex: A study in squirrel monkeys (Saimiri sciureus). *Journal of Comparative Neurology, 326(3),* 375–401.

Gulya, A. J. (1997). Anatomy and embryology of the ear. In G. B. Hughes & M. L. Pensak (Eds.), *Clinical otology* (2nd ed., pp. 3–34). New York, NY: Thieme.

Gulya, A. J. (2007). Anatomy and embryology of the ear. In G. B. Hughes & M. S. Pensak (Eds.), *Clinical otology* (3rd ed., pp. 3–34). New York, NY: Thieme.

Hain, T. C., & Helminski, J. O. (2007). Anatomy and physiology of the normal vestibular system. In S. J. Herdman (Ed.), *Vestibular rehabilitation* (3rd ed., pp. 2–18). Philadelphia, PA: F. A. Davis.

Hain, T. C., Zee, D. S., & Maria, B. L. (1988). Tilt suppression of vestibulo-ocular reflex in patients with cerebellar lesions. *Acta Otolaryngologica, 105(1–2),* 13–20.

Hallaran, W. S. (1810). *An enquiry into the causes producing the extraordinary addition to the number of insane together with extended observations on the cure of insanity: With hints as to the better management of public asylums for insane persons.* Cork, Ireland: Edwards & Savage, Cork, printer.

Hallaran, W. S. (1818). *Practical observations on the causes and cures of insanity* (2nd ed.). Cork, Ireland: Edwards & Savage, Cork, printer.

Hallpike, C. S., Hood, J. D., & Byford, G. H. (1952). The design, construction and performance of a new type of revolving chair; some experimental results and their application to the physical theory of cupular mechanism. *Acta Otolarnygologica, 42(6),* 511–538.

Halmagyi, G. M., & Curthoys, I. S. (2007). Otolith function tests. In S. J. Herdman (Ed.), *Vestibular rehabili-*

tation (3rd ed., pp. 144–161). Philadelphia, PA: F. A. Davis.

Harsch, V. (2006). Centrifuge "therapy" for psychiatric patients in Germany in the early 1800s. *Aviation, Space, and Environmental Medicine, 77*, 157–160.

Harsha, W. J., Phillips, J. O., & Backous, D. D. (2008). Clinical anatomy and physiology. In P. C. Weber (Ed.), *Vertigo and disequilibrium: A practical guide to diagnosis and management* (pp. 41–52). New York, NY: Thieme.

Hartmann, M., Grabherr, L., & Mast, F. (2012). Moving along the mental number line: Interactions between whole-body motion and numerical cognition. *Journal of Experimental Psychology: Human Perception and Performance, 38*(6), 1416–1427.

Hashiba, M. (2001). Control and modulation of canal driven vestibulo-ocular reflex. *Biological Sciences in Space, 15*(4), 382–386.

Hashiba, M., Watanabe, S., Watabe, H., Matsuoka, T., Baba, S., Wada, Y., . . . Sekiguchi, C. (1995). Imaginary gaze effects of eye movements induced by linear acceleration: Involvement of vestibular induced smooth pursuit eye movements. *Acta Otolarygologica Suppl, 520*, 372–376.

Henn, V. (1996). How does the brain detect and respond to head movement in three dimensions? In R. W. Baloh & G. M. Halmagyi (Eds.), *Disorders of the vestibular system* (pp. 62–72). New York, NY: Oxford University Press.

Highstein, S. (1996). How does the vestibular part of the inner ear work? In R. W. Baloh & G. M. Halmagyi (Eds.), *Disorders of the vestibular system,* (pp. 3–11). New York, NY: Oxford University Press.

Hirsch, B. E. (1986). Computed sinusoidal harmonic acceleration. *Ear and Hearing, 7*(3), 198–203.

Honrubia, V., Baloh, R. W., Yee, R. D., & Jenkins, R. A. (1980). Identification of the location of vestibular lesions on the basis of vestibulo-ocular reflex measurements. *American Journal of Otolaryngology, 1*(4), 291–301.

Honrubia, V., Jenkins, H. A., Baloh, R. W., Yee, R. D., & Lau, C. G. (1984). Vestibulo-ocular reflexes in peripheral labyrinthine lesions I: Unilateral dysfunction. *American Journal of Otolaryngology, 5*, 15–26.

Honrubia, V., Jenkins, H., Minser, K., Baloh, R., & Yee, R. (1984). Vestibulo-ocular reflexes in peripheral labyrinthine lesions. II. Caloric testing. *American Journal of Otolaryngology, 5*, 93–98.

Jacobson, G., McCaslin, D., Grantham, S., & Shepard, N. (2016). Within and between measure relationships between balance function tests—Illustrative cases. In G. P. Jacobson & N. T. Shepard (Eds.), *Bal-*ance function assessment and management, (pp. 833–855). San Diego, CA: Plural.

Jacobson, G., McCaslin, D., Patel, S., Barin, K., & Ramadan, N. (2004). Functional and anatomical correlates of impaired velocity storage. *Journal of the American Academy of Audiology, 15,* 324–333.

Jacobson, G. P., & Newman, C. W. (1990). The development of the Dizziness Handicap Inventory. *Archives of Otolaryngology Head and Neck Surgery, 116*(4), 424–427.

Jacobson, G., & Newman, C. (1997). Background and technique of caloric testing. In G. P. Jacobson, C. W. Newman, & J. M. Kartush (Eds.), *Handbook of balance function testing* (pp. 156–192). San Diego, CA: Singular.

Jacobson, G. P., Piker, E. G., Do, C., McCaslin, D. L., & Hood, L. (2012). Suppression of the vestibulo-ocular reflex using visual and nonvisual stimuli. *American Journal of Audiology, 21*(2), 226–231.

Jenkins, H., & Goldberg, J. (1988). Test-retest reliability of the rotatory test in normal subjects. *Advances in Otolaryngology, 41,* 190–195.

Johnson, G. D. (1998). Medical management of migraine-related dizziness and vertigo. *Laryngoscope, 108*(1, Pt. 2), 1–28.

Johnson, W. H. (1964). The importance of the otoliths in disorientation. *Aerospace Medicine, 35:* 874–877.

Jongkees, L. B. W., & Philipszoon, A. J. (1964). The rotational test. *Acta Otolaryngologica, 57*(Suppl. 189), 55–64.

Kanayama, R., Nakamura, T., Sano, R., Ohki, M., Okuyama, T., Kimura, Y., & Koike, Y. (1994). Effect of aging on smooth pursuit eye movement. *Acta Otolaryngologica, 114*(Suppl. 511), 131–134.

Kaplan, D. M., Marais, J., Ogawa, T., Kraus, M., Rutka, J. A., & Bance, M. L. (2001). Does high-frequency pseudo-random rotational chair testing increase the diagnostic yield of the ENG caloric test in detecting bilateral vestibular loss in the dizzy patient? *Laryngoscope, 111*(6), 959–963.

Kaufman, K. (2004). Objective assessment of posture and gait. In A. Bronstein, T. Brandt, M. Woollacott, & J. Nutt (Eds.), *Clinical disorders of balance, posture and gait* (2nd ed., pp. 130–145). London, UK: Arnold.

Kawano, K., Sasaki, M., & Yamashita, M. (1980). Vestibular input to visual tracking neurons in the posterior parietal association cortex of the monkey. *Neuroscience Letters, 17*(1–2), 55–60.

Kerber, K. A., Ishiyama, G. P., & Baloh, R. W. (2006). A longitudinal study of oculomotor function in normal older people. *Neurobiology of Aging, 27*(9), 1346–1353.

Kitahara, T., Fukushima, M., Takeda, N., Saika, T. & Kubo, T. (2000). Effects of pre-flocculectomy on fos expression and NMDA receptor-mediated neural circuits in the central vestibular system after unilateral labyrinthectomy. *Acta Otolaryngologica, 120*(7), 866–871.

Kitahara, T., Takeda, N., Uno, A., Kubo, T., Mishina, M., & Kiyama, H. (1998). Unilateral labyrinthectomy down-regulates glutamate receptor delta-2 expression in the rat vestibulocerebellum. *Brain Research. Molecular Brain Research, 61*(1– 2), 170–178.

Lackner, J. R. (1988). Some proprioceptive influences on the perceptual representation of body shape and orientation. *Brain, 111*, 281–297.

Lee, S. U., Choi, J. Y., Kim, H. J., Park, J. J., Zee, D. S., & Kim, J. S. (2016). Impaired tilt suppression of post-rotatory nystagmus and cross-coupled head-shaking nystagmus in cerebellar lesion: Image mapping study. *Cerebellum*. Advance online publication. doi:10.1007/s12311-016-0772-2

Leigh, R. J., & Zee, D. S. (2006). *The neurology of eye movements* (4th ed.). New York, NY: Oxford University Press.

Leigh, R. J., & Zee, D. S. (2015). *The neurology of eye movements* (5th ed.). New York, NY: Oxford University Press.

Leinonen, L., Hyvarinen, J., & Sovijarvi, A. R. (1980). Functional properties of neurons in the temporoparietal association cortex of awake monkey. *Experimental Brain Research, 39*(2), 203–215.

Lempert, T., Gianna, C. C., & Gresty, M. A. (1997). Effect of otolith dysfunction: Impairment of visual acuity during linear head motion in labyrinthine defective subjects. *Brain, 120*, 1005–1013.

Lim, D. J. (1984). The development and structure of the otoconia. In I. Friedmann & J. Ballantyne (Eds.), *Ultrastructural atlas of the inner ear* (pp. 249–269). London, UK: Buttersworth. In A. Sans, C. J. Dechesne & D. Demêmes. *The mammalian otolithic receptors: A complex morphological and biomechanical organization*. In P. Tran Ba Huy & M. Toupet (Eds.), *Otolith function and disorders* (pp. 1–14). New York, NY: Karger.

Lockette, W., Shepard, N. T., Lyos, A., Boismier, T., & Mers, A. (1991). Altered coriolis stress susceptibility in essential hypertension. *American Journal of Hypertension, 4*(8), 645–650.

Lorente de Nó, R. (1933). Vestibulo-ocular reflex arc. *Archives of Neurology and Psychiatry, 30*(2), 245–291.

Lysakowski, A., & Goldberg, J. M. (2004). Morphophysiology of the vestibular periphery. In S. M. Highstein, R. R. Fay, & A. N. Popper (Eds.), *The vestibular system* (pp. 57–152). New York, NY: Springer-Verlag.

Lysakowski, A., McCrea, R. A., & Tomlinson, R. D. (1998). Anatomy of vestibular end organs and neural pathways. In C. W. Cummings, J. M. Fredrickson, L. A. Harker, C. J. Krause, M. A. Richardson, & D. E. Schuller (Eds.), *Otolaryngology head and neck surgery* (3rd ed., pp. 2561–2583). St. Louis, MO: Mosby.

Mach, E. (1875). *Grundlinien der Lehre von den Bewegungsempfindungen*. Leipzig, Germany: Engelmann.

Maes, L., Dhooge, I., D'haenens, W., Bockstael, A., Keppler, H., Philips, B., . . . Vink, B. (2008). Normative data and test-retest reliability of the sinusoidal harmonic acceleration test, pseudorandom rotation test and velocity step test. *Journal of Vestibular Research, 18*, 197–208.

Markham, C. H. (1996). How does the brain generate horizontal nystagmus? In R. W. Baloh & G. M. Halmagyi (Eds.), *Disorders of the vestibular system* (pp. 48–61). New York, NY: Oxford University Press.

Mathog, R. H. (1972). Testing of the vestibular system by sinusoidal angular acceleration. *Acta Otolaryngologica, 74*(1), 96–103.

McCaslin, D. L. (2015). *Electronystagmography and videonystagmography: ENG/VNG*. San Diego, CA: Plural.

McCaslin, D. L., & Jacobson, G. P. (2016). Vestibular-evoked myogenic potentials (VEMPs). In G. P. Jacobson & N. T. Shepard (Eds.), *Balance function assessment and management*, (pp. 533–579). San Diego, CA: Plural.

McNally, W. J., & Stuart, E. A. (1967). *Physiology of the labyrinth*. Rochester, MN: American Academy of Ophthalmology and Otolaryngology.

Meng, H., Green, A. M., Dickman, J. D., & Angelaki, D. E. (2005). Pursuit-vestibular interactions in brainstem neurons during rotation and translation. *Journal of Neurophysiology, 93*, 3418–3433.

Merchant, S. N., & Nadol, J. B. (2010). *Schuknecht's pathology of the ear* (3rd ed.). Shelton, CT: People's Medical.

Miles, R. D., & Zapala, D. A. (2015). Vestibular function measurement devices. *Seminars in Hearing, 36*(1), 49–74.

Minor, L. B., & Goldberg, J. M. (1990). Influence of static head position on the horizontal nystagmus evoked by caloric, rotational and optokinetic stimulation in the squirrel monkey. *Experimental Brain Research, 82*(1), 1–13.

Moller, C., White, V., & Ödkvist, L. M. (1990). Plasticity of compensatory eye movments in rotary tests. II. The effect of voluntary, visual, imaginary, auditory and proprioceptive mechanisms. *Acta Otolaryngologica, 109*(3–4), 168–178.

Montandon, A., & Russbach, A. (1955). L'epreuve giratoire luminaire. *Practica Oto-Rhino-Laryngologica, 17*, 224–236.

Moon, I. S., Kim, J. S., Choi, K. D., Oh, S. Y., Lee, H., Lee, H. S., & Park, S. H. (2009). Isolated nodular infaction. *Stroke 40*(2), 487–491.

Moore, S. Clément, G., & Raphan, T. (2001). Ocular counterrolling induced by centrifugation during orbital space flight. *Experimental Brain Research, 137,* 323–335.

Mösges, R., & Klimek, L. (1993). Normal values of post-rotatory and per-rotatory ENG parameters. In I. K. Arenberg (Ed.), *Dizziness and balance disorders: An interdisciplinary approach to diagnosis, treatment and rehabilitation.* New York, NY: Kugler.

Nager, G. T. (1993). *Pathology of the ear and temporal bone.* Baltimore, MD: Williams & Wilkins.

Nashner, L. M. (1997). Practical biomechanics and physiology of balance. In G. P. Jacobson, C. W. Newman, & J. M. Kartush (Eds.), *Handbook of balance function testing* (pp. 261–279). San Diego, CA: Singular.

Nishiike, S., Guldin, W.O., & Baurle, J. (2000). Corticofugal connections between the cerebral cortex and the vestibular nuclei. *Journal of Comparative Neurology, 420*(3), 363–372.

Niven, J., Carroll Hixson, W., & Correia, M. J. (1965). *An experimental approach to the dynamics of the vestibular organs in the exploration of space.* U.S. Naval School of Aviation Medicine, Pensacola, FL: Washington, DC: National Aeronautics and Space Administration.

Nowé, V., Wuyts, F., Hoppenbouwers, M., Van de Heyning, P., De Schepper, A., & Parizel, P. (2003). The interutricular distance determined from external landmarks. *Journal of Vestibular Research, 13,* 17–23.

Nylen, C. O. (1965). *Historical vignette: Robert Bárány.* Retrieved February 17, 2016, from http://archotol.jamanetwork.com/

Ödkvist, L. (2001). Clinical and instrumental investigational otolith function. In P. Tran Ba Huy & M. Toupet (Eds.), *Otolith function and disorders* (pp. 68–76). New York, NY: Karger.

On acceleratory stimulation. (1955). *Acta Oto-Laryngologica, 45*(Suppl. 122), 22–44.

Paige, G. D. (1989). Nonlinearity and asymmetry in the human vestibulo-ocular reflex. *Acta Otolaryngologica, 108,* 1–8.

Peterka, R. (2002). Sensorimotor integration in human postural control. *Journal of Neurophysiology, 88*(3), 1097–1118.

Phillips, J., & Backous, D. (2002). Evaluation of vestibular function in young children. *Otolaryngologic Clinics of North America, 35,* 765–790.

Rabbitt, R. D., Damiano, E. R., & Grant, J. W. (2004). Biomechanics of the semicircular canals and otolith organs. In S. M. Highstein, R. R. Fay, & A. N. Popper (Eds.), *The vestibular system* (pp. 153–201). New York, NY: Springer-Verlag.

Raphan, T., & Cohen, B. (1996). How does the vestibulo-ocular reflex work? In R. W. Baloh & G. M. Halmagyi (Eds.), *Disorders of the vestibular system* (pp. 20–47). New York, NY: Oxford University Press.

Raphan, T., Matsuo, V., & Cohen, B. (1979). Velocity storage in the vestibulo-ocular reflex arc (VOR). *Experimental Brain Research, 35,* 229–248.

Raymond, J. & Demêmes, D. (1983). Efferent innervation of vestibular receptors in the cat: Radioautographic visualization. *Acta Otolarygologica, 96,* 413–419.

Reisine, H., & Raphan, T. (1992). Unit activity in the vestibular nuclei of monkeys during off-vertical axis rotation. *Annals of the New York Academy of Sciences, 656,* 954–956.

Robinson, D. A. (1971). Models of oculomotor neural organization. In P. Bach-y-Rita, C. C. Coffins, & J. Hyde (Eds.), *The control of eye movements* (pp. 519–538). New York, NY: Academic Press.

Robinson, D. A. (1976). Adaptive gain control of vestibuloocular reflex by the cerebellum. *Neurophysiology, 39*(5), 954–969.

Ross, H. E. (1989). Perceptual and motor skills of divers under water. *International Journal of Industrial Ergonomics, 2,* 155–181.

Ross, H. E., Crickmar, S. D., & Sills, N. V. (1969). Orientation to the vertical of free divers. *Aerospace Medicine, 40,* 728–732.

Ross W. D. (Ed.). (1927). *The works of Aristotle, volume 7.* Oxford, UK: Clarendon. In N. J. Wade, (2003). *Destined for distinguished oblivion: The scientific vision of William Charles Wells (1757–1817).* New York, NY: Springer.

Sans, A., Dechesne, C. J, & Demêmes, D. (2001). The mammalian otolithic receptors: A complex morphological and biomechanical organization. In P. Tran Ba Huy & M. Toupet, (Eds.), *Otolith Function and Disorders* (pp. 1–14). New York, NY: Karger.

Schönfeld, U., & Clarke, A. (2011). A clinical study of the subjective visual vertical during unilateral centrifugation and static tilt. *Acta Oto-Laryngologica, 131,* 1040–1050.

Schönfeld, U., Helling, K., & Clarke, A. (2010). Evidence of unilateral isolated utricular hypofunction. *Acta Oto-Laryngologica, 130,* 702–707.

Schubert, M., & Shepard, N. T. (2008). Practical anatomy and physiology of the vestibular system. In G. P Jacobson & N. T. Shepard (Eds.), *Balance function assessment and management* (pp. 1–12). San Diego, CA: Plural.

Schuknecht, H. F. (1993). *Pathology of the ear* (2nd ed.). Philadelphia, PA: Lea & Febiger.

Schwarz, D. W. F. & Tomlinson, R.D. (2005). Physiology of the vestibular system. In R. K. Jackler & D. E. Brackman (Eds.), *Neurotology* (2nd ed., pp. 91–121). Philadelphia, PA: Elsevier Mosby.

Shepard, N. T., Goulson, A. M., & McPherson, J. H. (2016). Clinical utility and interpretation of whole-body rotation. In G. P. Jacobson & N. T. Shepard, (Eds.), *Balance function assessment and management* (pp. 365–390). San Diego, CA: Plural.

Shepard, N. T., & Telian, S. A. (1996). *Practical management of the balanced disordered patient*. San Diego, CA: Singular.

Shoair, O. A., Nyandege, A. N., & Slattum, P. W. (2011). Medication-related dizziness in the older adult. *Otolaryngology Clinics of North America, 44*(2), 455–471.

Smith, S., Curthoys, I., & Moore, S. (1995). The human ocular torsion position response during yaw angular acceleration. *Vision Research, 35*(14), 2045–2055.

Söllner, C., & Nicolson, T. (2000). The zebrafish as a genetic model to study otolith formation. In E. Baeuerlein (Ed.), *Biomineralization: Progress in biology, molecular biology and application*. Weinheim, Germany: Wiley-VCH.

Stanfield, C. L. (2017). *Principles of human physiology* (6th ed.). London, UK: Pearson Education.

Stockwell, C. (2000, May). Incidence of ENG abnormalities. *Insights in practice, clinical topics in otoneurology*. Schaumburg, IL: ICS Medical.

Stockwell, C. W., & Bojrab, D. I. (1997a). Background and technique of rotational testing. In G. P. Jacobson, C. W. Newman, & J. M. Kartush (Eds.), *Handbook of balance function testing* (pp. 237–248). San Diego, CA: Singular.

Stockwell, C. W., & Bojrab, D. I. (1997b). Interpretation and usefulness of rotational testing. In G. P. Jacobson, C. W. Newman, & J. M. Kartush (Eds.), *Handbook of balance function testing* (pp. 249–258). San Diego, CA: Singular.

Swift, N. (2014). Centrifuging mental patients: A look back at twisting approaches to treating mental ailments. *Annals of Improbable Research, 20*(3). Retrieved from http://www.improbable.com/

Thalmann, R., Ignatova, E., Kachar, B., Ornitz, D. M., & Thalmann, I. (2001). Development and maintenance of otoconia: Biochemical considerations. *Annals of the New York Academy of Sciences, 942*, 162–178.

Timmann, D., & Diener, H. C. (2007). Coordination and ataxia. In C. G. Goetz *Textbook of clinical neurology* (3rd ed., 307–325). Philadelphia, PA: Saunders Elsevier.

Tran Ba Huy, P., & Toupet, M. (2001). Peripheral disorders in the otolith system. In P. Tran Ba Huy & M. Toupet (Eds.), *Otolith function and disorders* (pp. 110–127). New York, NY: Karger.

Tusa, R. J., Grant, M. P., Buettner, U. W., Herdman, S. J., & Zee, D. S. (1996). The contribution of the vertical semi-circular canals to high velocity horizontal vestibulo-ocular reflex (VOR) in normal subjects and patients with vestibular nerve section. *Acta Otolaryngologica, 116*(4), 507–512.

Valko, Y., Hegemann, S. C., Weber, K. P., Straumann, D., & Bockisch, C. J. (2011). Relative diagnostic value of ocular vestibular evoked potentials and the subjective visual vertical during tilt and eccentric rotation. *Clinical Neurophysiology, 122*, 398–404.

Van der Stappen, A., Wuyts, F. L., & Van de Heyning, P. (1999). Influence of head position on the vestibulo-ocular reflex during rotational testing. *Acta Otolaryngologica, 119*(8), 892–894.

Van Nechel, C., Toupet, M., & Bodson, I. (2001). The subjective visual vertical. In P. Tran Ba Huy & M. Toupet (Eds.), *Otolith function and disorders* (pp. 77–87). New York, NY: Karger.

Veits, C. (1929). Neue Untersuchungen über die kalorischen Vestibularisreaktionen [New investigations of caloric vestibular responses]. *Acto Otolaryngologica, 13*, 94–115.

Veits, C. (1931). Zur Drehprufung [On rotary testing]. *Hals-, Nas-, u. Ohrenheilk, 29*, 368.

Verpy, E., Leibovici, M., & Petit, C. (1999). Characterization of otoconin-95, the major protein of murine otoconia, provides insights into the formation of these inner ear biominerals. *Proceedings of the National Academy of Sciences of the United States of America, 96*(2), 529–534.

Vibert, D., Häusler, R., & Safran, A. B. (1999). Subjective visual vertical in peripheral unilateral vestibular diseases. *Journal of Vestibular Research, 9*(2), 145–152.

von Egmond, A. A. J., Van, Groenj, J., & Jongkees., B. W. (1948). The turning test with small regulable stimuli: The method of examination: Cupulometria. *Journal of Laryngology, 62*, 63.

Wade, N. J. (2003). *Destined for distinguished oblivion: The scientific vision of William Charles Wells (1757–1817)*. New York, NY: Springer.

Wade, N. J., Norrsell, U., & Presley, A. (2005). Cox's chair: "A moral and a medical mean in the treatment of maniacs." *History of Psychiatry, 16*(1), 73–88.

Waespe, W., Cohen, B., & Raphan, T. (1985). Dynamic modification of the vestibulo-ocular reflex by the nodulus and uvula. *Science, 228*, 199–202.

Wall, C. (1990). The sinusoidal harmonic acceleration rotary chair test. Theoretical and clinical basis. *Neurologic Clinics, 8*(2), 269–285.

Wall, C., III, Black, F. O., & Hunt, A. E. (1984). Effects of age, sex, and stimulus parameters upon vestibulo-ocular responses to sinusoidal rotation. *Acta Otolaryngologica, 98,* 270–278.

Wall, C., III, & Furman, J. M. R. (1989). Nystagmus responses in a group of normal humans during earth-horizontal axis rotation. *Acta Otolaryngologica, 108,* 327–335.

Wang, Y., Kowalski, P. E., Thalmann, I., Ornitz, D. M., Mager, D. L., & Thalmann, R. (1998). Otoconin-90, the mammalian otoconial matrix protein, contains two domains of homology to secretory phospholipase A_2. *Proceedings of the National Academy of Sciences of the United States of America, 95*(26), 15345–15350.

Wearne, S., Raphan, T., & Cohen, B. (1996). Nodulo-Uvular control of central vestibular dynamics determines spatial orientation of the angular vestibulo-ocular reflex. *Annals New York Academy of Sciences, 781,* 364–384.

Wearne, S., Raphan, T., Waespe, W., & Cohen, B. (1997). Control of the three-dimensional dynamic characteristics of the angular vestibulo-ocular reflex by the nodulus and uvula. *Progress in Brain Research, 114,* 321–334.

Wende, S., Nakayama, N., & Schwerdtfeger, P. (1975). The internal auditory artery (embryology, anatomy, angiography, pathology). *Journal of Neurology, 210,* 21.

Wetzig, J., Hofstetter-Degen, K., Maurer, J., & von Baumgarter, R. J. (1992). Clinical verification of a unilateral otolith test. *Acta Astronautica, 27,* 19–24.

Wetzig, J., Reiser, M., Martin, E., Bregenzer, N., & von Baumgarten, R. J. (1990). Unilateral centrifugation of the otoliths as a new method to determine bilateral asymmetries of the otolith apparatus in man. *Acta Astronautica, 21*(6/7), 519–525.

White, J. A. (2007). Laboratory tests of vestibular and balance function. In G. B. Hughes & M. L. Pensak (Eds.), *Clinical otology* (3rd ed., pp.132–149). New York, NY: Thieme.

White, W. J. (1964). *A history of the centrifuge in aerospace medicine.* Santa Monica, CA: Douglas Aircraft Company, Biotechnology Branch.

Wiest, G., Deecke, L., Trattnig, S., & Mueller, C. (1999). Abolished tilt suppression of the vestibulo-ocular reflex caused by selective uvulo-nodular lesion. *Neurology 52*(2), 417–419.

Wilmot, T. J. (1966). The application of modern vestibulometry to the problem of vertigo. *Journal of Laryngology, 80,* 1156–1172.

Wilson, V. J., & Jones, J. G. (1979). *Mammalian vestibular physiology.* New York, NY: Plenum Press.

Wong, A. M. F. (2008). *Eye movement disorders.* New York, NY: Oxford University Press.

Wuyts, F. L., Hoppenbrouwers, M., Pauwels, G., & Van de Heyning, P. H. (2003). Utricular sensitivity and preponderance assessed by the unilateral centrifugation test. *Journal of Vestibular Research, 13,* 227–234.

Yates, B. J., Aoki, M., & Burchill, P. (1999). Cardiovascular responses elicited by linear acceleration in humans. *Experimental Brain Research, 125,* 476–484.

Zalewski, C. K. (2015). Aging of the human vestibular system. *Seminars in Hearing, 36*(3), 175–196.

Zee, D. (2007). Vestibular adaptation. In S. J. Herdman, *Vestibular rehabilitation* (3rd ed., pp. 19–31). Philadelphia, PA: F. A. Davis.

Index

Note: Page numbers in **bold** reference non-text material.